W0036019

Comprehensive Review of

OTOLARYNGOLOGY

Comprehensive Review of
OTOLARYNGOLOGY

MICHAEL J. RUCKENSTEIN, MD, M.Sc, FACS, FRCSC
Associate Professor
Department of Otorhinolaryngology, Head and Neck Surgery
Hospital of the University of Pennsylvania
Philadelphia, Pennsylvania

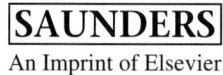

An Imprint of Elsevier

SAUNDERS

An Imprint of Elsevier

170 S Independence Mall W 300 E
Philadelphia, Pennsylvania 19106-3399

COMPREHENSIVE REVIEW OF OTOLARYNGOLOGY   ISBN 0-7216-9076-9
Copyright © 2004, Elsevier Inc. All rights reserved.

No part of this publication may be reproduced or transmitted in any form or by any means, electronic or mechanical, including photocopying, recording, or any information storage and retrieval system, without permission in writing from the publisher. Permissions may be sought directly from Elsevier's Health Sciences Rights Department in Philadelphia, PA, USA: phone: (+1) 215 238 7869, fax: (+1) 215 238 2239, e-mail: healthpermissions@elsevier.com. You may also complete your request on-line via the Elsevier Science homepage (http://www.elsevier.com), by selecting 'Customer Support' and then 'Obtaining Permissions'.

NOTICE

Otolaryngology is an ever-changing field. Standard safety procedures must be followed, but as new research and clinical experience broaden our knowledge, changes in treatment and drug therapy may become necessary or appropriate. Readers are advised to check the most current product information provided by the manufacturer of each drug to be administered to verify the recommended dose, the method and duration of administration, and contraindications. It is the responsibility of the licensed prescriber, relying on experience and knowledge of the patient, to determine dosages and the best treatment for each individual patient. Neither the publisher nor the editors assume any liability for any injury and/or damage to persons or property arising from this publication.

The Publisher

Library of Congress Cataloging-in-Publication Data
Ruckenstein, Michael J. (Michael Jay)
   Comprehensive review of otolaryngology / Michael J. Ruckenstein.– 1st ed.
      p.; cm.
   ISBN 0-7216-9076-9
      1. Otolaryngology. I. Title.
   [DNLM: 1. Otolaryngology–methods. 2. Otorhinolaryngologic Diseases. WV 100
R911c 2004]
RF46.R86 2004
617.5'1–dc22   2004040988

Developmental Editor: Suzanne Flint
Acquisitions Editor: Rebecca Schmidt Gaertner

Printed in the United States of America

Last digit is the print number: 9 8 7 6 5 4 3 2 1

To Debbie

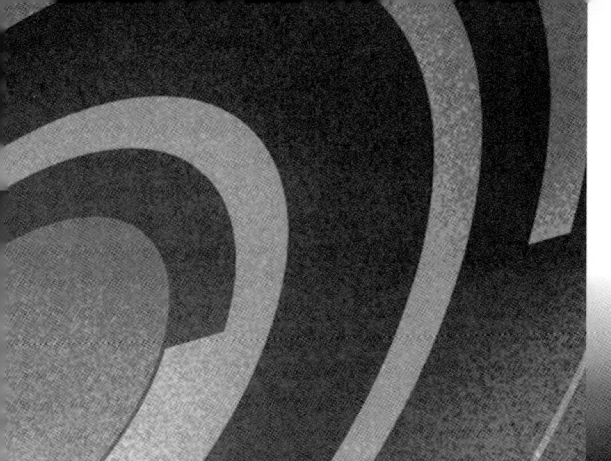

Contributors

 ASSOCIATE EDITORS

Natasha Mirza, MD, Associate Professor, Department of Otorhinolaryngology: Head and Neck Surgery, University of Pennsylvania, Philadelphia, Pennsylvania
Oral Cavity, Oropharynx, Larynx

Duane A. Sewell, MD, Assistant Professor, Department of Otorhinolaryngology: Head and Neck Surgery, University of Pennsylvania, Philadelphia, Pennsylvania
Disorders of the Head and Neck

Erica A. Thaler, MD, Associate Professor, Department of Otorhinolaryngology: Head and Neck Surgery, University of Pennsylvania, Philadelphia, Pennsylvania
Rhinology

 CONTRIBUTORS

All contributors listed below are current or former residents of
The Department of Otorhinolaryngology, Head and Neck Surgery
Hospital of the University of Pennsylvania
Philadelphia, PA

Soo H. Kim Abboud, MD

Timothy D. Anderson, MD
Lahey Clinic V&S Center

Anna Aronzon, MD

Eric Baum, MD

Michael Belmont, MD

Noam Cohen, MD, PhD

Orville H. Dyce, MD

Marc Eisen, MD, PhD

Kristin Gendron, MD

Neil Hockstein, MD

Masaru Ishii, MD, PhD

James Kallman, MD

Michael Kupferman, MD

Stephen Y. Lai, MD, PhD

David A. Litman, MD

Joel Perloff, MD

Robert Puchalski, MD

Adam T. Ross, MD

Daniel Sharya Samadi, MD

Ioana Schipor, MD

Jeffrey Shaari, MD

Anthony Sparano, MD

Ralph P. Tufano, MD

Stephen J. Wall, MD, PhD

Jeffrey Wise, MD

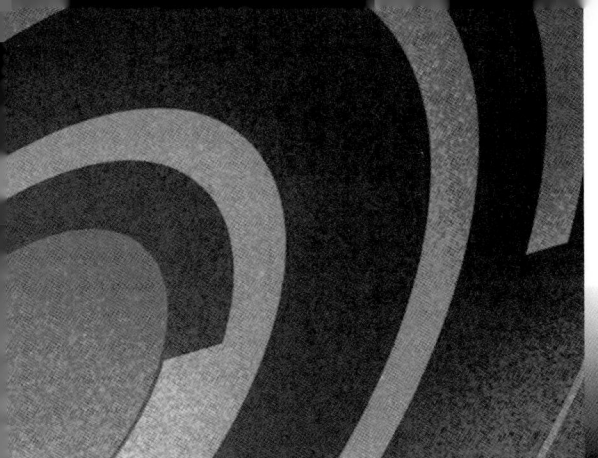

Preface

WHY THIS BOOK WAS WRITTEN

Otorhinolaryngology–Head and Neck Surgery, being a regional specialty, encompasses the medical and surgical treatment of diverse organ systems. The knowledge base pertaining to the management of otolaryngologic disease continues to expand, as manifested by the increasing size of the multi-volume general texts and the proliferation of specialty and subspecialty works. Amidst this deluge of information, how is the best resident or practicing clinician supposed to acquire and retain the factual knowledge base necessary to function as a competent otolaryngologist–head and neck surgeon? This book is an attempt to answer this question.

WHAT THIS BOOK IS

Comprehensive Review of Otolaryngology is an attempt to distill and render the factual basis of our specialty and to present it in a clear and organized fashion. It strives to be the *Dragnet* of otolaryngology texts (i.e., "Just the facts, Ma'am"). Chapters all maintain a standardized formatting designed to ensure that they are both inclusive and easy to read. This book contains no fluff; each line is written to provide the reader with a relevant fact. Sections are designed so that they can be reviewed rapidly, allowing the reader to review, refresh, and/or acquire the required knowledge base.

WHAT THIS BOOK ISN'T

This book is not designed for the novice. It assumes a general familiarity with the specialty that can be acquired by reading one of the general otolaryngology texts. However, it must be acknowledged that the chapters in these general tomes can be difficult to re-read, given the time constraints imposed by residency and clinical practice. Hence this book: a rendition of the core elements of our specialty.

This book will not provide a description of the nuances or controversies involving specific subjects. It is designed to provide an up-to-date summary of current standard of practice. Nor will you find historical treatises or references to personal/anecdotal experience.

It was decided that certain specific areas were best omitted from the text. Specifically, the areas of histopathology and imaging are not included. To properly address these areas, a vast library of images is required. These areas are better dealt with in currently available texts specifically dedicated to these subjects.

HOW THIS BOOK WAS WRITTEN

With the exception of the Otology/Neurotology section, for which I was completely responsible, the sections were written in the following fashion. Residents in the Department of Otorhinolaryngology–Head and Neck Surgery were given specific questions to answer. These answers were then reviewed, edited, and formatted, and then combined to create chapters. The chapters were then reviewed by the associate editors for accuracy and omissions. Instead of a standard bibliography, references to recent literature are provided to try to facilitate further reading.

WE NEED YOUR HELP!

We strove to make this book as accurate and complete as possible. However, this was a first effort and we acknowledge that there may be errors of omission and/or fact. To that end, we have set a dedicated e-mail site: *enttext@hotmail.com*. We would greatly appreciate any comments you have pertaining to general or specific ways this book can be improved. We will attempt to incorporate these changes in upcoming additions.

Thank you,

Michael J. Ruckenstein, MD, M.Sc, FACS, FRCSC
Philadelphia, Pennsylvania

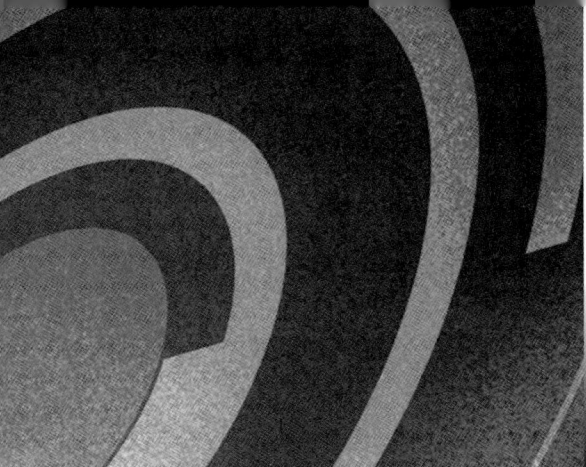

Contents

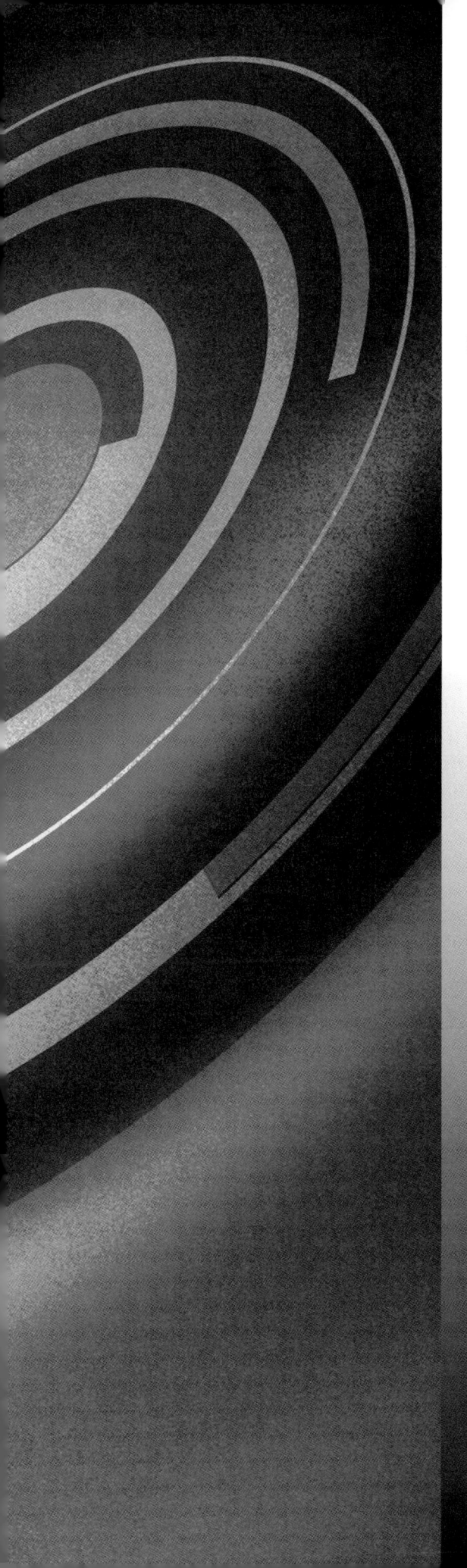

Otology/Neurotology

AUDITORY PHYSIOLOGY

Sound

- *Sound*, as we perceive it, represents a combination of waves that are generated by a vibrating sound source (or sources) and propagated through the air until they reach the ear.
- The most elementary sound wave is the *sinusoid*, or *sine wave*.
- The sine wave can be characterized by several properties, the most important of which are its *frequency* and *amplitude* (Fig. 1).
- The wave completes one cycle of vibration between points "A" and "B."
- *Frequency* (cycles/second or Hertz) is the time it takes for the wave to complete one cycle and corresponds to the pitch of the sound.
- The *amplitude* of the wave is the amount of displacement of the wave as it passes from its neutral position to its position of maximal displacement. It corresponds to the *intensity* of sound.
- A *Fourier transformation* is a mathematical process by which complex sounds can be analyzed and broken down into their composite sine waves. The ear itself performs just such an analysis when it is stimulated by sounds.

Sound Intensity

- A broad range of sound intensities can be detected by the ear, thus a measure of sound intensity is used that compresses the units of measurement into a practical range.
- This intensity scale uses the decibel (dB), which is defined as follows:

  # of dB = 10 Log_{10} Sound Intensity/Reference Intensity

  # of dB = 20 Log_{10} Sound Pressure/Reference Pressure

- Note the following characteristics of the decibel scale:
  - It is a relative scale; that is, it is based on a ratio that compares sound intensity or pressure to a standard reference level. The reference level used is the lowest sound pressure commonly detected by man and is equal to 2×10^{-5} Newtons/meter^2 (N/m^2). Thus the intensity level in dB sound pressure level (SPL) =

  20 Log_{10} Sound Pressure/2×10^{-5} N/m^2

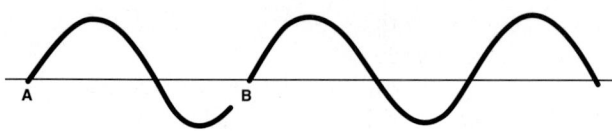

Fig. 1 Sine wave.

- It is logarithmic, not a linear scale. Thus, doubling the sound pressure results in a 6 dB increase in measured sound pressure, whereas a 10-fold change is reflected by a 20 dB change in measured sound pressure.
- The log of 1 is 0. Thus, 0 dB SPL does not correspond to the absence of sound but rather indicates that the sound pressure of the measured wave is equal to that of the reference sound pressure.
- When the reference sound pressure level just discussed is used, sound pressure is described in units of dB SPL.
- The ear's ability to detect sound waves differs for different frequencies, with the human ear being maximally sensitive from 1-5 kHz.
- The average, or *normal*, hearing thresholds for each hearing frequency serve as the reference values when determining auditory threshold in humans. When these reference values are used, thresholds are reported as *dB hearing level (dB HL)*, with a value of 0 dB HL indicating that, at the frequency being tested, the measured auditory threshold is equal to that of the average human hearing level.

The External and Middle Ears

- The external and middle ears form the conductive component of the auditory apparatus.
- They transmit sound waves from the external environment to the sensory organ of hearing (the inner ear), amplify sound, and modify its frequency spectrum.
- Amplification is required because of the differences in impedance between air (low impedance) and the liquid-filled inner ear (high impedance).
- Without the system of amplification, approximately 97% of the acoustic signal would be reflected back off the oval window and not enter the middle ear.

The External Ear

- The pinna, conchal bowl, and external ear canal each contribute to the amplification of the sound wave, maximally amplifying sound at frequencies from 2-5 kHz, with a maximal gain of 20 dB at 2.5 kHz.
- The external ear also plays a significant role in sound localization. Interaural differences in time and intensity, which are dependent on the angle of incidence of the sound wave on the head, are more pronounced for sound differences above 1 kHz and serve as important clues for sound localization.

The Middle Ear

- The middle ear confers the majority of sound amplification of the conductive system.
- Sound is transferred from the large surface area of the tympanic membrane (TM) and concentrated on the

small surface area of the oval window. The amplification conferred on the sound wave by the *area ratio* is 22:1.

- The long axis of the malleus is longer than that of the incus, creating a lever effect that further augments the amplitude of the wave. The *lever ratio* is 1.3:1.
- Although these are simple concepts to understand, several factors serve to modify their application.
  - The entire TM does not move in unison. Different parts of the TM move at different velocities in response to sound, thus decreasing the effective area of the TM and the efficiency of sound transfer. This "break up" of the TM increases with increasing frequency of sound.
  - The lever function of the ossicles becomes progressively less efficient at frequencies above 1 kHz. This results from laxity of the malleal-incudal joint system with consequent slippage of the joint and reduced efficiency of sound transfer.
  - The mastoid air cell system has a resonance that peaks at approximately 3 kHz, leading to a decrease in sound transmission of 5-6 dB at this frequency.
  - The impedance mismatch is not constant but in fact decreases with increasing frequency. That is, less amplification is required at higher frequencies to correct for the impedance of the cochlear contents.
- The middle ear pressure gain is relatively flat at frequencies below 1 kHz, averaging 23 dB and peaking at 26-27 dB at 0.9 kHz. At frequencies above 1 kHz, the gain decreases by 8-9 dB/octave, contributing little amplification above 7 kHz.

Eustachian Tube

- The functions of the eustachian tube are:
  - To equilibrate air pressure in the middle ear with that of the external environment.
  - To drain middle ear secretions into the nasopharynx.
  - To protect the middle ear from potentially infectious nasopharyngeal secretions.
- In its resting state the tube is closed, because of:
  - The elastic forces of the tube and its supporting structures.
  - The adhesive properties of the mucous blanket lining the tube.
- Contraction of the tensor veli palatini muscle, which can be elicited by swallowing or yawning, actively dilates the tube.
- The ability of the eustachian tube to perform its functions of ventilation, protection, and drainage can be influenced by variations in its own structure as well as by the conditions of the middle ear and the nasopharynx.

- An abnormally compliant eustachian tube would fail to protect the middle ear from reflux of nasopharyngeal secretions and would make it more prone to open in the face of changes in air pressure in the middle ear or nasopharynx.
- A partially or totally obstructed eustachian tube impedes passage of air or fluid. Either positive pressure within the ear or negative pressure in the nasopharynx promotes flow of air or secretions through the eustachian tube from the middle ear to the nasopharynx.
- Conversely, positive nasopharyngeal or negative middle ear pressure promotes air passage and/or reflux of nasopharyngeal secretion into the middle ear.

The Muscles of the Middle Ear

- Two small muscles are contained within the middle ear: the *tensor tympani* muscle that inserts on the malleus, and the *stapedius* muscle, which inserts on the stapes.
- Contraction of both muscles is activated primarily by acoustic stimulation.
- Other stimuli, such as tactile stimulation of the auricle and change in head posture can also activate contraction. Anticipation of speech production can also activate contraction.
- Sensory stimuli elicit contraction via an involuntary reflex mediated by the central nervous system at the level of the superior olivary complex.
- The superior olivary complex sends out crossed and uncrossed fibers, and thus, a unilateral sensory stimulus will elicit bilateral muscle contraction.
- Motor nerve fibers are carried to the tensor tympani via the Vth cranial nerve and to the stapedius via the VIIth nerve.
- Contraction of the middle ear muscles in the human is elicited by acoustic stimuli of 70-90 dB above threshold. Reflex contraction stiffens the ossicular chain, reducing sound transmission by 5-10 dB, primarily at frequencies below 1.2 kHz.
- The stapedius plays the dominant role in reducing sound transmission, with some arguing that the tensor tympani has little, if any, physiologic function.
- Although the nature of the acoustic middle ear muscle reflex has been well established, the physiologic role of the reflex has remained obscure.
- Proposed functions include:
  - Noise protection (unlikely given latency and minimal sound attenuation).
  - Alterations in the frequency spectrum of an acoustic stimulus.
  - Reduction in low-frequency harmonics and stabilization of the ossicular chain.
  - Reduction of the intensity of self vocalizations.

The Inner Ear

- The cochlea converts an acoustic waveform into an electrical stimulus that can be transmitted to the central nervous system (CNS).
- This *sensory transduction* process involves analyzing the sound stimulus in terms of its frequency, intensity, and temporal properties, and then transmitting this information to the CNS for further processing and interpretation.

The inner ear's microenvironment

- The cochlea consists of three fluid-filled ducts or *scalae*.
- These ducts are functionally divided into two spaces.
  - The *scala tympani* and *scala vestibuli* communicate with each other and are filled with *perilymph*. The *scala media* is isolated from the perilymphatic space and contains *endolymph*.
- Endolymph contains an electrolyte composition that is similar to that found in intracellular fluids; that is, it is high in K^+ and low in Na^+ and Ca^{2+}.
- The composition of perilymph resembles that of extracellular fluid and is high in Na^+ and low in K^+.
- For many years it was believed that the cochlear fluids were generated by filtration of blood or CSF, and then flowed longitudinally down the length of the cochlea to be absorbed through the endolymphatic sac.
- Current data suggest that substantial longitudinal flow of perilymph or endolymph does not occur. Instead, the maintenance of electrolyte concentrations within the scalae appears to be controlled locally via radial flow of the electrolytes.
- An anatomic barrier exists between perilymph and endolymph. It consists of Reissner's membrane, the stria vascularis, and the reticular lamina formed by tight junctions between the apices of hair cells and the adjacent supporting cells.
- The differences in electrolyte concentrations are maintained by the spiral ligament and stria vascularis.
- Pumping of K^+ into the endolymph occurs against a concentration gradient, and thus requires the expenditures of energy.
- Na, K-ATPase enzymes, located in the strial marginal cells and spiral ligament, use metabolic energy stores (ATP) to pump Na^+ and K^+ ions against their concentration gradients.
- A Na-Cl-K co-transporter located within the marginal cells also assists in electrolyte transport.
- Thus, the endolymph and perilymph electrolyte contents are regulated by local, radial flow of electrolytes, and not longitudinal flow of fluids along the length of the cochlea.
- Since electrolytes are charged particles (ions), differences in their concentrations also create electrical potentials between the perilymph and endolymph.
- The scala vestibuli has a potential of +5 mV with respect to the scala tympani, and the scala media has a relatively large positive potential of 80 mV.
- This positive 80 mV potential is known as the *endocochlear potential* and serves as the major driving force for signal transduction (see below).

The traveling wave and signal transduction

- A sound wave is transmitted to the middle ear, eliciting vibration of the ossicular chain.
- Vibration of the stapes transmits the sound wave, via the oval window, to the scala vestibuli, generating fluid waves within the perilymph.
- The displacement of the perilymph causes a wavelike displacement of the basilar membrane and organ of Corti, and ultimately distention of the round-window membrane.
- The frequency of basilar membrane motion is thus directly related to the frequency of the sound stimulus and represents the first stage of the transduction process.
- Studies performed on cadaveric specimens revealed that the amplitude of a sine wave traveling along the basilar membrane increased until it reach a maximum and then abruptly declined.
- The site at which the traveling wave reaches maximum amplitude is dependent on the specific frequency of the stimulus, with the high frequencies peaking toward the base of the cochlea and the lower frequencies more toward the apex.
- Thus, as frequency decreases, the distance from the base of the cochlea at which the amplitude of the wave reaches its maximum increases.
- Physical properties of the basilar membrane, related to changes in its stiffness and mass along its length, can account for these "passive" tuning properties.
- In an *in vivo* setting, there is not a gradual rise in amplitude of the wave as it travels to its point of maximal amplitude.
- The wave travels along the basilar membrane, causing minimal displacement until it reaches the site of the membrane that is maximally sensitive to a stimulus of that particular frequency—the *characteristic frequency* for that location on the basilar membrane.
- This fine-tuning mechanism depends on active (energy-dependent) processes and thus is not evident in cadaveric studies.
- The *outer hair cells (OHCs)* mediate the active processes that create the fine-tuning properties of the cochlea (see below).

Sensory Transduction and the Hair Cell

- The apical surface of the hair cells and their stereocilia lie within the endolymphatic space and are thus exposed to fluid with a potential of +80 mV.
- Intracellular recording reveals that hair cells have a resting potential of approximately −40 to −60 mV.
- Thus, the net potential difference across the hair cells apical membrane is 120-140 mV.
- According to Davis' battery theory of transduction, the stria vascularis contributes the metabolic energy necessary to maintain the positive endocochlear potential. The hair cell's apical surface functions as a *variable resistor*, whose impedance is altered by mechanical displacement of the stereocilia.
- Although the hair cell bodies move with the acoustically stimulated basilar membrane, the stereocilia are surrounded by the immobile endolymph and tectorial membrane.
- Thus, basilar membrane vibration will cause relative movement or shear of the hair cells with respect to the tectorial membrane and endolymph, causing a bending of the stereocilia.
- Bending toward the tallest row of stereocilia causes an opening of channels located within the stereocilia that provide a route for influx of K^+ ions into the cells, driven by the 120-140 mV potential gradient.
- The influx of positively charged K^+ ions causes a depolarization of the hair cell.
- Conversely, stereocilia bending in the opposite direction creates a hyperpolarization by closing those channels that are constantly open, even in the resting state, thus further obstructing K^+ flow down the electrical gradient.
- K^+ enters the cells via channels located within the stereocilia.
- Opening and closing of the channels is thought to be a mechanical process. Tip links, which join the middle of one stereocilia to the apex of an adjacent shorter stereocilia, serve as *gating springs* that stretch open the channels when bending occurs toward the tallest row of stereocilia.
- Stereociliar bending in the opposite direction relaxes the tension on the tip links, resulting in closure of channels.
- The functional outcome of depolarization differs in inner and OHCs.
  - Inner hair cells (IHCs) function primarily as *sensory receptors*.
  - Depolarization of the IHC results in the activation of voltage dependent ion channels located along the lateral cell membrane.
  - These channels allow for the efflux of K^+ from the cell and influx of Ca^{2+}.
  - Influx of Ca^{2+} activates neurotransmitter (likely *glutamate*) release from the base of the cell.
  - The amount of neurotransmitter release parallels the degree of depolarization and thus is proportional to the intensity of the stimulus.
  - The released neurotransmitter binds to the afferent nerve terminals that surround the base of the hair cell, resulting in an action potential being propagated down the afferent nerve fibers.
  - The vast majority of afferent nerve terminals (95%) synapse on the IHCs and serve to transmit the sensory signal.
- OHCs have minimal sensory function but possess energy-dependent motor properties responsible for the fine-tuning of the cochlea.
- OHCs perform this task by serving as *amplifiers* of the acoustic signal.
- This amplification process results from the unique motor properties of the OHC that allow it to change its length. As a result, voltage changes within the hair cell.
- Elongation and contraction of the OHC, resulting from acoustically driven depolarization and hyperpolarization of the cell, augments the displacement of the basilar membrane.
- The biological "motors" responsible for these length changes are felt to be proteins lodged within the lateral cell membrane. These proteins can change their shape (long and thin vs. short and fat) depending on voltage changes within the cell. Many protein motors are located within the lateral cell membrane and together act to elicit changes in cell length.
- OHCs exhibit the same frequency-specific response as seen in IHCs. The amplification they provide is, therefore, frequency specific.
- *Cochlear efferent fibers*, contained in the *olivocochlear bundles* and originating in the superior olivary complex of the brainstem, provide a route by which the CNS can influence cochlear function.
- The bundles are divided into *lateral* and *medial* groups, depending on their site of origin within the superior olivary complex.
- The medial groups of fibers are myelinated and synapse primarily on the *OHCs*.
- Stimulation of the medial efferent fibers decreases the amplification provided by the OHCs.

Cochlear Blood Flow

- The level of metabolic activity within the cochlea dictates the need for the maintenance of cochlear oxygenation, the provision of metabolic substrates (e.g., glucose), and the elimination of metabolic waste products.
- Various solutes can pass from blood to perilymph; however, a blood-perilymph barrier does exist that allows for selective transport between these two fluid

spaces. For example, glucose is preferentially taken up by the perilymph from blood. The perilymph serves as a reservoir for glucose, which can pass from it to the endolymphatic space for use by metabolically active cells.

- Regulation of cochlear blood flow is under both local (autoregulation) and systemic control. Systemic factors, such as blood pressure, heart rate, oxygenation, and hormones, can influence cochlear blood flow, just as they influence flow to any organ. Similarly, the autonomic nervous system, specifically sympathetic noradrenergic fibers, can control the state of vascular tone of the cochlear vessels. Local factors, such as hypoxia and acidosis, can also promote increases in circulation by causing vasodilation. Moderate sound stimulation leads to increased cochlear glucose use and blood flow.

Central Pathways

- The acoustic stimuli go through intense processing as they pass from the cochlea to the auditory cortex.
- Cochlear neuron cell bodies reside in the *spiral ganglion* of the cochlea. They are "bipolar" cells, giving rise to the afferent fibers that innervate the IHCs as well as the fibers that carry the signal to the cochlear nucleus.
- The *cochlear nucleus* of the brainstem is located near the cerebellopontine angle and is divided physiologically and anatomically into several divisions.
- From the cochlear nucleus, afferent fibers pass to the *ipsilateral and contralateral superior olivary complex*, consisting of the *medial superior olive* and the *lateral superior olive*.
- The *nucleus of the lateral lemniscus* receives input from the:
  - Contralateral cochlear nucleus.
  - Ipsilateral superior olivary complex.
  - Contralateral nucleus of the lateral lemniscus.
  - Inferior colliculus.
- The inferior colliculus receives input from the nuclei of the lateral lemniscus as well as the ipsilateral and contralateral superior olivary complexes. The inferior colliculus relays the processed stimuli to the ipsilateral and contralateral medial geniculate bodies.
- The medial geniculate bodies then relay the signal to the ipsilateral primary auditory cortex (Brodmann's areas 41 and 42) of the temporal lobe.

Vestibular Physiology

- The function of the vestibular system is to transduce forces, causing a head acceleration (including gravity) into a biologic signal.

- The brain uses this information to develop a subjective awareness of head position in relation to the environment and to produce motor reflexes to control equilibrium. In addition, the vestibular system functions to stabilize a visual image on the retina.
- The input from the vestibular system is coordinated with incoming information from other sensory systems (visual, proprioceptive) via higher centers and thus contributes to the subjective sensation of orientation.

Peripheral Vestibular System

- The peripheral vestibular system consists of five sensory organs, the three cristae of the semicircular canals (SCC), and the two maculae of the otolithic organs. The sensory cells within all these organs are the hair cells similar to those found in the organ of Corti, with the exception of the fact that kinocilia (KC) are present on the vestibular hair cells.
- *Type I hair cells* are chalice shaped and possess a single nerve terminal, whereas *Type II cells* are cylindrical and possess multiple nerve terminals.
- Afferent nerve fibers synapsing on these cells possess a baseline firing rate. A shearing force applied to the stereocilia that causes bending toward the KC results in depolarization of the cell and increased afferent nerve firing, whereas a force that bends stereocilia away from the KC results in hyperpolarization of the cells and a decrease in afferent firing rate.
- The function of the hair cells depends on the maintenance of the labyrinthine fluid compartments (see auditory section). These consist of perilymph, a filtrate of extracellular fluid from the vascular space and CSF (hi Na, low K), and an intracellular-like fluid, endolymph, which is produced by the dark cells of the vestibular labyrinth and the stria vascularis of the cochlea (hi K, low, Na). The maculae and cristae are bathed in endolymph. The differences in electrolyte concentrations are maintained by the dark cells, which function in a manner analogous to the stria vascularis of the cochlea.
- The labyrinthine artery is usually a branch of the anterior inferior cerebellar artery (AICA) but occasionally arises directly from the basilar artery.

The Otolith Organs

- These organs, which detect linear acceleration of the head, consist of the utricle and saccule. Each possesses a sensory organ called the *macule*. The utricular and saccular macules lie at right angles to each other (utricle = horizontal, saccule = vertical).
- The hair cell surfaces of the maculas are covered by an otolith membrane, which consists of a mesh of fibers

embedded in a mucopolysaccharide gel covered by a superficial otoconia (composed of calcium carbonate crystals). The stereocilia are embedded in the otolith membrane. Because the otoconia have a greater specific gravity than the surrounding endolymph, the otolithic macules respond to gravitational force.

- Each macule is divided into two areas by a curved *striola* with hair cells on each side of the striola lying in opposite directions. In the utricle, KC face the striola, whereas in the saccule they face away from the striola. Thus, displacement of the otolithic membrane has opposite physiologic effects on hair cells on either side of the striola.
- The curvature of the striola, as well as the fact that the utricle and saccule lie in perpendicular planes, ensures that the otoliths can respond to linear acceleration in any axis. The otoliths respond to linear acceleration forces, including those exerted by gravity. Thus, the net force acting on the otolithic macule is a result of two vector forces, one imposed by gravity and the other by linear head displacement.

The Semicircular Canals

- The superior, horizontal, and posterior canals are roughly perpendicular to each other so that they are aligned in the three planes of space (orthogonal arrangement). The horizontal canal makes a 30-degree angle with the horizontal plane, and the vertical canals make a 45-degree angle with the frontal plane.
- The anterior ends of the horizontal and superior canals widen to form the *ampullae*. The ampullated portion of the posterior canal lies at its inferior opening. The ampullae house the *cristae*, which are the sensory organs of the SCC. The sensory epithelium of the cristae is covered by a gelatinous mass (the *cupula*). The cupula extends from the hair cell surface to the roof of the ampulla, thus sealing the ampulla. The cupula has the same specific gravity as endolymph, thus the cristae do not respond to gravitational forces.
- Angular acceleration of the head causes endolymph movement relative to the canal wall. Head angular acceleration is paralleled by acceleration of the bony and membranous labyrinth. However, because of inertia and viscoelastic properties, endolymph movement lags behind the movement of the membranous labyrinth. This creates a relative flow of endolymph in a direction *opposite* to that of head acceleration. The cupula moves with the endolymph, resulting in bending of the stereocilia.
- Hair cells within the cristae are oriented with their KC in the same direction. In the horizontal canal, the KC are directed toward the utricular side of the ampulla, whereas in the superior and posterior canals, the KC are oriented toward the canal side of the ampulla.

Therefore, ampullopetal (utricular) endolymphatic flow within the horizontal canal results in hair cell depolarization and increased afferent firing, whereas ampullofugal (away from the ampulla) flow causes excitation of afferents coming from the posterior and superior canals.

- The SCCs are functional pairs, with the two members of each pair being in parallel planes. The three functional pairs are:
  1. The two horizontal canals.
  2. The superior canal and the contralateral posterior canal.
  3. The posterior canal and the contralateral superior canal.

Central Vestibular Physiology

- The *vestibular nuclei* lie on the floor of the fourth ventricle, bounded rostrally by the brachium conjunctivum, medially by the pontine reticular formation, laterally by the restiform body, and ventrally by the nucleus and spinal tract of the trigeminal nerve.
- They receive input from the vestibular afferents, vestibular cerebellum (flocculus, nodulus, fastigial nucleus), reticular formation, and commissural fibers from the contralateral nuclei. They send fibers to the cerebellum, reticular formation, contralateral vestibular nuclei, oculomotor nuclei, and vestibulospinal tracts.
- There are four groups of neurons that comprise the nuclei (superior, medial, lateral, and descending). The superior nucleus is mainly involved in the vestibuloocular reflex (VOR). The lateral vestibular nucleus mainly functions in the vestibulospinal reflexes. The medial vestibular nucleus functions in the VOR and vestibulospinal reflexes, coordinating the head, neck, and eye movements. The descending nucleus functions to integrate signals from bilateral vestibular afferents, cerebellum, and reticular formation.

The Vestibuloocular Reflex

- The function of the VOR is to stabilize a visual image on the retina during head movement. Ideally, the proper function of the VOR ensures that an angular head acceleration results in an equal and opposite angular eye movement (i.e., gain = 1).
- At a simple level, it represents a three-neuron arc, with the vestibular afferent from a SCC synapsing on an interneuron in the vestibular nucleus, which in turn synapses with a neuron in an oculomotor nucleus.
- Activation of a canal produces eye movement in the plane of movement of that canal. This pattern of eye

movement is affected by excitatory and inhibitory pathways (Fig. 2). This would be the situation involved, for example, in head rotation to the right.

- Stimulation of the ipsilateral horizontal canal (e.g., right) results in eye deviation to the contralateral side (e.g., left) by stimulation of the ipsilateral medial rectus (IIIrd nerve) and the contralateral lateral rectus (VIth nerve), as well as by relaxation of the ipsilateral lateral rectus.
- Because of symmetry of the canals, an angular head acceleration that stimulates one of the horizontal canal results in decreased output from the contralateral canal. This results in a relaxation of the left medial rectus and right lateral rectus and disinhibition of the left lateral rectus. The relationship between the SCCs and the ocular muscles is detailed in Table 1.
- The function of the VOR is much more complex than a three-neuron arc, because it involves multisynaptic pathways from the cerebellum and reticular formation. These pathways are important in the integration of visual and proprioceptive stimuli with those from the vestibular end organs (see following text).

Peripheral Vestibular Nystagmus

- If the magnitude of the stimulation of the SCC is greater than what can be compensated for by eye movement, the slow compensating eye movement is interrupted by a fast *saccadic* movement in the opposite direction.
- This rhythmic slow/fast movement is known as *nystagmus*. Nystagmus is always defined by the direction of the fast saccade. The fast saccadic movements are generated by neurons in the parapontine reticular formation and vestibular cerebellum, which monitor vestibular activity and periodically discharge. The principles of the VOR and corrective saccades can be illustrated as follows.

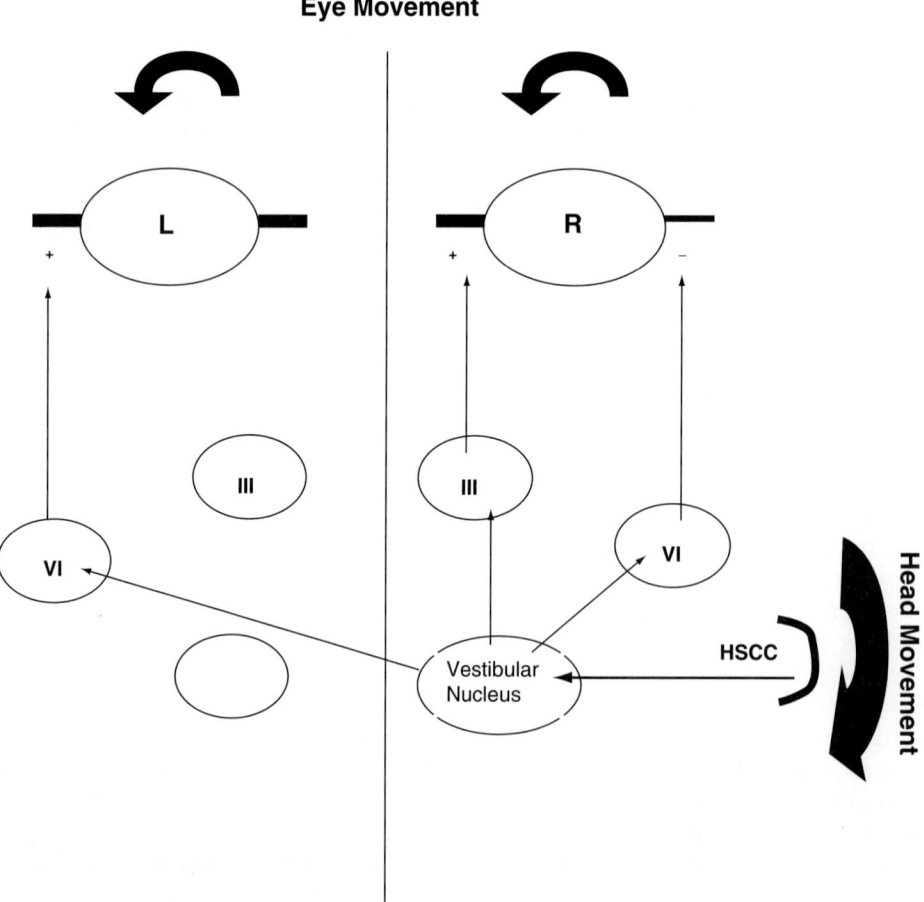

Fig. 2 Pathway for stimulation of right horizontal canal.

TABLE 1. Relationship Between Semicircular Canals and Ocular Muscles

	Excitation	Inhibition
Horizontal	Ipsilateral: Medial rectus Contralateral: Lateral rectus	Ipsilateral: Lateral rectus Contralateral: Medial rectus
Posterior	Ipsilateral: Superior oblique Contralateral: Inferior rectus	Ipsilateral: Inferior oblique Contralateral: Superior rectus
Superior	Ipsilateral: Superior rectus Contralateral: Inferior oblique	Ipsilateral: Inferior rectus Contralateral: Superior oblique

▫ If a person undergoes an *angular acceleration* to the right, the VOR will produce a corrective eye movement to the left. When the eye reaches a maximal displacement to the left, a saccade will be produced to the right to reset the eye position. As long as the acceleration continues, the VOR-generated slow leftward eye movement, and the fast resetting rightward saccades will continue, creating a *right-beating jerk nystagmus*. Once head acceleration is stopped and the head moves at a constant velocity, the perception of movement and nystagmus will gradually resolve over 25-30 seconds. Similarly, if after obtaining a constant angular velocity, the rotation is suddenly stopped, the perception of movement and nystagmus will continue for approximately 25-30 seconds. Cupular mechanics *(cupula time constant)* can only account for a portion of the observed perpetuation of the nystagmus. The prolongation of the nystagmus beyond what is expected based on cupular mechanics is due to neural firing rate asymmetry that persists within the vestibular nuclei *(canal-ocular time constant)*. This neural firing within the vestibular nuclei is known as the *velocity storage integrator,* which is controlled by the vestibular cerebellum (nodulus).

Interaction of the VOR with other systems
Cervical ocular reflex (COR)

▪ Nerve endings in ligaments and capsules of upper cervical joints project to vestibular nuclei (descending and medial). Although the COR is not believed to play a major role in humans, the COR and VOR generally act synergistically to maintain eye position.

Visual vestibular interaction

▪ Relationship between head and object may change as follows:
  ▫ Head moves in relation to object.
  ▫ Object moves in relation to head.
  ▫ Both head and object move.
▪ Visual and vestibular signals usually interact synergistically to stabilize gaze. Occasionally, visual and vestibular signals conflict, in which case the visual system overrides the vestibular input. Three visually controlled systems interact to stabilize gaze by producing versional eye movements.
  1. Saccadic: Responds to an error in the direction of gaze with respect to a position of an object of interest by initiating a rapid eye movement (saccade) to correct the retinal positional error. It is generated by neurons in the paramedian pontine reticular formation.
  2. Smooth Pursuit: Maintains foveal visual field on a moving target. Compares eye and target velocities to produce a match between eye and target velocities. It functions optimally (i.e., gain = 1) at lower target velocities (peak 30 degrees/sec), whereas the VOR acts optimally (gain = 1) at higher velocities (100 degrees/sec). To remember this, just contrast your ability to maintain focus on your finger by moving your finger back and forth at increasing speed versus your ability to maintain your focus on your stationary finger when oscillating your head back and forth at increasing speed.
  3. Optokinetic System: Phylogenetically older system. Primitive form of smooth pursuit involving whole retina rather than fovea. Eye motion is periodically interrupted by saccades to relocate gaze on new targets coming into visual field.

Interaction of visual and vestibular systems

▪ Information coming from visual and vestibular receptors must be integrated to allow for accurate maintenance of gaze and a consistent sense of orientation. Thus, this sensory information is processed by a common integrator center. Both visual and vestibular receptors send input to and receive output from the cerebellum (flocculus, nodulus, posterior vermis) and the parapontine reticular formation. These centers are responsible for the integration and coordination of this sensory information and allow the visual system to override the VOR. It also explains why damage to these centers results in symptoms of vertigo and imbalance.

Compensation to an acute vestibular lesion

▪ A lesion of the labyrinth or VIIIth nerve nucleus will result in an imbalance of peripheral vestibular activity, both at rest *(static state)* and during head movement *(dynamic state)*.

- With regard to the *static state,* a pathologic spontaneous nystagmus that beats away from the side of the lesion develops.
- This nystagmus will increase in amplitude when eye position is directed away from the lesion (i.e., toward the direction of the nystagmus [Alexander's law]).
- The nystagmus results from asymmetries between the tonic discharge rates in the right and left vestibular afferents.
- Compensation to these static asymmetries occurs over a course of 24-72 hours and is manifested by a resolution of symptoms of vertigo and nausea and an elimination of the spontaneous nystagmus.
- Even once static compensation occurs, movement will still provoke symptoms of imbalance.
- The ability to compensate to pathology evoked in the dynamic state is variable, in terms of both its completeness and the duration of recovery.
- Dynamic compensation is highly dependent on an intact contralateral peripheral vestibular system. For dynamic compensation to occur, the CNS must undergo a process of *adaptive plasticity.* This ability of the CNS to adapt to changes in its sensory environment is triggered by "error messages" sent to the CNS during head movement. These error messages result from asymmetric vestibular inputs being sent to the CNS by the left and right peripheral vestibular systems. The conflicting information must be resolved by the CNS, and the CNS's ability to adapt to these asymmetric inputs is facilitated by repeated exposure to these sensory stimuli.
- An unusual form of adaptation is required in situations of bilateral vestibular loss (Dandy's syndrome). In this situation, the VOR becomes nonfunctional. These patients become highly dependent on visual and proprioceptive inputs to maintain balance and postural control. Thus the smooth pursuit system will become important to these patients. However, recall that the smooth pursuit system functions optimally with low-frequency stimulation. Thus these patients develop *oscillopsia,* an ability to maintain gaze stability during more rapid head movements, such as those occurring when walking.
- Compensation to a bilateral vestibular loss is difficult and often incomplete. Compensation mechanisms include:
  - Incorporation of the cervical ocular reflex (seen in animals, but not prominent in humans).
  - Substitution of other oculomotor control systems, such as the saccadic system that is capable of functioning at higher frequencies.
  - Cognitive strategies, which prevent gaze overshoot by incorporating preplanned volitional eye

movements that accompany anticipated head movement.

Vestibulospinal Reflexes

Lateral vestibulospinal tract
- Originates in the lateral vestibular nucleus.
- Largely an uncrossed pathway.
- Function: Ipsilateral monosynaptic excitation of extensors contralateral inhibition of flexors (disynaptic).

Medial vestibulospinal tract
- Originates in the medial vestibular nucleus.
- Uncrossed and crossed pathway running in descending medial longitudinal fasciculus (MLF). Most of the fibers terminate at level of cervical cord.
- Function: Important in interaction of neck-vestibular-ocular reflexes. Polysynaptic excitation and inhibition of neck flexors and extensors can be elicited by fibers in this pathway.

Reticulospinal tract
- Originates in neurons from the bulbar reticular formation, which are neurons that receive input from the vestibular fibers (mainly from vestibular nuclei).
- It is a crossed and uncrossed pathway, the excitation of which results in inhibition of flexors and extensors at all levels of the cord.
- Function: The lateral ventral spinothalamic tract and the reticulospinal tract are heavily influenced by input from the vestibular cerebellum. The cerebellum, in turn, receives input from the vestibular nuclei, spinal cord, and pontomedullary reticular formation. This results in a system that integrates and coordinates multiple sensory inputs to maintain normal equilibrium and locomotion.

AUDIOLOGY

Pure Tone Audiogram

- **X axis:** stimulus frequency (Hertz [Hz]). Frequencies tested are at octave intervals between 250 and 8000 Hz.
- **Y axis:** threshold of sound intensity that can be heard by the patient 50% of the time. Measured in dB hearing level units (see section of Auditory Physiology)
- Air conduction tested by an earphone placed in ear. Thresholds for right ear are marked by an *"O,"* and thresholds for the left ear are marked by an *"X."*
- *The Pure Tone Average* = Mean of air conduction thresholds obtained at 500, 1000, and 2000 Hz.

- Bone conduction thresholds are obtained by a stimulation provided by a bone oscillator placed just behind the tested ear. Thresholds for right ear are marked by a "<," and thresholds for the left ear are marked by ">."
- In bone conduction testing, if a patient responds to feeling the vibration of the oscillator rather that actually hearing the stimulus, this is noted by initials *"VT"* (for vibrotactile) on the audiogram.
- An air-bone gap is considered significant if air conduction thresholds exceed bone conduction thresholds by 10 dB or more. It is indicative of a conductive hearing loss.
- A reliability measure is provided by the audiologist based on the replicability of thresholds at one or more frequencies. Replicability within 5 dB is considered good, replicability within 10 dB is considered fair, and a difference of greater than 10 dB in repeated threshold measures is considered poor.
- Because the dB is a log scale, the numbers derived from the test cannot be used to calculate a percentage of hearing loss, much to the confusion of most patients. Thus, hearing loss is typically classified in terms of the categories listed in Table 2.

Masking

- Masking noise is used to prevent the nontest ear from hearing the stimulus provided to the test ear.
- The *interaural attenuation* of sound is 40 dB for air conduction and 0 dB for bone conduction. Therefore, in *air-conduction testing,* the better hearing ear must be masked if the asymmetry in air conduction thresholds is *40 dB or greater. Bone stimuli* must be masked with *any* asymmetries in air conduction thresholds.
- A *masking dilemma* occurs when the masking sound crosses over to the test ear and is perceived by the test ear. This typically occurs when testing a patient with a maximal bilateral conductive hearing loss. The masking sound will crossover to the test ear, affecting the test ear's ability to hear the stimulus. Thus the intensity of the test stimulus is increased to try to

determine the threshold. The increase in the test frequency intensity requires an increase in the masking intensity, thus making the derivation of threshold in the test ear impossible. The use of insert earphones, as opposed to circumaural headphones, increases the interaural attenuation and therefore decreases the likelihood of encountering a masking dilemma.

Speech Testing

Speech reception threshold (SRT)

- Measures the ability to correctly repeat 50% of common, bisyllabic words that are delivered at with equal emphasis on both syllables.
- SRT should correspond to the pure tone average (PTA). If the SRT is better than the PTA, the patient may be malingering (see pseudohypacusis)

Word recognition (speech discrimination)

- Percentage of phonetically balanced monosyllabic words (25 or 50) repeated correctly by a patient.
- Words are presented at an intensity of 40 dB above SRT or at a comfortable level for the patient.
- Words may be spoken by the audiologist or may be provided by a tape recording.
- A retrocochlear hearing loss may be suspected if the word recognition is disproportionately poorer than the pure tone testing.
- A retrocochlear hearing loss may be suspected if word recognition testing becomes worse as intensity is increased *(rollover).*

Immittance testing

- Performed by ear insert tube connected to an impedance bridge capable of providing a sound stimulus.
- Measuring the amount of sound reflected back while varying the pressure within a sealed ear canal.
- The device may provide a measure of sound *impedance* (the amount of sound reflected back) or the reciprocal sound *admittance* (the amount of sound transferred through the middle ear).

Tympanometry

- A *tympanogram* is a graph presenting *ear canal pressure* on the X axis and *sound admittance* on the Y axis.
- The amount of sound transmitted to the middle ear is maximal when the TM is free to vibrate (i.e., when air pressures on the external and middle ear sides are equal).
- In a normal ear, the middle ear pressure = atmospheric pressure = 0. Therefore the maximal sound admittance will occur when the external ear pressure is 0 *(Type A).*

TABLE 2. Categories of Hearing Loss	
Hearing Loss Range (dB)	**Category**
−10-25	Normal
26-40	Mild loss
41-55	Moderate loss
56-70	Moderately severe loss
71-90	Severe loss
91+	Profound loss

- In a middle ear with restricted movement of the TM (e.g., when the ossicles are fixed because of otosclerosis), the pressure at which the middle ear maximally conducts sound will also be 0. However, the degree of variation in sound transmission will be restricted because of the stiffness of the TM *(Type As)*.
- Conversely, if a TM is flaccid because of, for example, ossicular discontinuity, there is a high peak in admittance *(Type Ad),* which is also centered at the 0 pressure point.
- An ear filled with fluid will not provide much sound admittance, regardless of the pressure, and therefore will have a relatively flat tympanogram *(Type B)*.
- A *negative middle ear pressure* will allow good admittance only if the pressure in the ear canal is set at the same pressure on the middle ear. In this form of tympanogram, the peak admittance will be recorded at a negative pressure *(Type C)*.

Acoustic reflexes

- An ipsilateral sound stimulus carried to the brainstem via the VIIIth nerve will elicit contraction of the ipsilateral (IL) and contralateral (CL) stapedius muscle (via the VIIth nerves).
- The ipsilateral reflex is referred to as the *uncrossed reflex.*
- The contralateral reflex is referred to as the *crossed reflex.*
- If the pressure is set at a constant within the external ear so that sound admittance is maximal, a contraction of the stapedius muscle will elicit a change in admittance that can be recorded.
- The crossed and uncrossed reflexes are tested at 70-100 dB HL.
- A reflex decay test is performed by presenting a 500- or 1000-Hz signal to the ear for 10 seconds at 10 dB higher than reflex threshold. If the amplitude of the *crossed reflex* declines more than 50% during the 10-second stimulus, the test is abnormal and considered to be consistent with the presence of a retrocochlear lesion.
- A conductive loss of 30 dB or more should eliminate the reflex whether the affected or unaffected side is stimulated. If the acoustic reflex *is present* with this degree of hearing loss, one may consider a diagnosis of *cochlear conductive hearing loss.* This phenomenon has been associated with the presence of a "third" labyrinthine membranous window, such as seen in superior canal dehiscence syndrome. These patients will demonstrate clinical and audiometric findings of conductive hearing loss, except for the present reflexes, in the absence of external or middle ear pathology.

Otoacoustic Emissions (OAEs) and Evoked Potential Audiometry

OAEs

- See section on physiology.
- OAEs are acoustic signals emitted by the OHCs of the cochlea and transmitted down the basilar membrane, to the oval window, then to the ossicles, the TM, and finally to the external ear canal.
- They are recorded using a probe microphone placed near the TM.
- OAEs cannot be recorded in patients with middle ear pathology, despite the presence of a normal inner ear.
- They are classified as follows:
  - *Spontaneous OAEs* can be recorded in approximately 50%-60% of people. The presence, or absence, of these OAEs is not indicative of any inner ear pathology.
  - *Transient-evoked OAEs (TOAEs)* are recorded after the ear is stimulated by a transient "click" sound stimulus. The stimulus is broad spectrum and so is the response. Little can be said about TOAEs, other than whether they are present or absent. A 30-dB sensorineural hearing loss (SNHL) will generally eliminate TOAEs, as will a conductive hearing loss.
  - *Distortion product OAEs (DPOAEs).* If two different pure tones (F1 and F2) are used to simultaneously stimulate the cochlea, an acoustic signal will be generated by the cochlea. The acoustic signal has a different frequency than the two stimulating frequencies and is known as the *distortion product.* The most commonly recorded DPOAE is the acoustic signal with a frequency = $2F1 - F2$, where $F2 = 1.2 \times F1$. By varying F1 and F2, DPOAEs with different frequencies can be recorded. Although DPOAEs do provide frequency-specific information pertaining to cochlear function, they cannot be correlated with audiometric thresholds.

Indications for OAEs

- Neonatal hearing screening.
- Evaluation of pseudohypacusis (malingering or somatization).
- Individual ear information on pediatric patients tested in sound field.
- Ototoxic drug monitoring.
- Evaluation of auditory neuropathy: a disorder in which the cochlea is intact but central pathology results in hearing loss. In these cases, the auditory brainstem response (ABR) is normal, with normal OAEs.

Evoked potential audiometry
Electrocochleography (ECOG)
- Records electrical potentials generated by the cochlea and the VIIIth nerve afferent fibers.
- Stimulus may be a rapid, broad-spectrum click or frequency-specific tone-pips or tone bursts.
- The recording electrode may be placed on the TM (peritympanic) or through the TM placed on the promontory (transtympanic). Transtympanic recordings provide more accurate and reproducible waveforms but require a physician to place the electrode. A variety of peritympanic electrodes have been developed, but they tend to provide less consistent results.
- The components of the ECOG are:
  - The cochlear microphonic (CM). The CM is an AC potential that parallels the properties of the acoustic signal. It is generated by the OHCs. It is rarely recorded in the clinical setting. The stimulus required to record the CM is a pure tone (sine wave).
  - The compound action potential (CAP). The CAP (or AP) is generated by the synchronous firing of multiple cochlear nerve fiber afferents. Thus, it is the sum of the all the action potentials generated by the afferent fibers. It represents the same neural activity that generates Wave 1 of the ABR. The stimuli required to generate the CAP are either a rapid, broad spectrum click or a more frequency-specific tone-pip or tone-burst.
  - The summating potential (SP). When stimulated by a pure tone (sine wave), hair cells undergo recurrent depolarization and repolarization (see section on auditory physiology). During these cycles, the level of repolarization never quite reaches the cell's resting potential. Thus, when compared to its resting state, the stimulated hair cell is always slightly depolarized. This persistent depolarization is a DC potential and is referred to as the *summating potential*.

Indications for ECOG
  - The CAP can be used to monitor hearing during resection of acoustic neuromas and other similar procedures. Because it is recorded by an electrode placed near the cochlea, the CAPs are of larger amplitude and can be recorded with fewer stimuli than an ABR.
  - Meniere's disease. An elevation in the SP/AP ratio has been noted to be a relatively consistent finding in patients with well-established Meniere's disease. The clinical value of this recording is of questionable significance (see section on Meniere's disease).

The Auditory Brainstem Response
- The ABR represents the recording of electrical potentials generated by the simultaneous firing of auditory pathway neurons of the lower CNS.
- Like the CAP, it requires a rapid "on-off" stimulus such as a click or tone-pip.
- An active recording is placed on the vertex of the skull, a neutral electrode is placed on the ipsilateral mastoid, and a ground electrode may be placed on a variety of sites, such as the contralateral mastoid.
- The ABR consists of seven positive waves (I-VII):
  - Waves I and II are generated by the proximal and distal portions of the VIIIth nerve.
  - Wave III is generated primarily by the cochlear nucleus.
  - Wave IV is generated by the superior olivary complex as well as the cochlear nucleus and the nucleus of the lateral lemniscus.
  - Wave V is primarily generated by the lateral lemniscus.
  - Waves VI and VII are primarily generated by the inferior colliculus.

Measures used in the ABR
- Typically only waves I, III, and V are used clinically.
- Latencies.
  - Waves I-III: Normal = 2 ms.
  - Waves III -V: Normal = 2 ms.
  - Waves I-V: Normal = 4 ms.
- The ILD V (IT_5) = Difference between absolute latencies of wave V recorded from the two ears. Normal = < 0.2-0.3 ms.
- Morphology: the presence or absence of the waveform, or abnormal waveform morphology, is typically recorded by the audiologist.

Indications for ABR
- *Threshold estimation:* Thresholds of ABR waveforms can be determined that approximate thresholds of behavioral testing. Thus ABR can be used to estimate behavioral thresholds in difficult-to-test patients (e.g., comatose, pediatric, pseudohypacusis).
- *Intraoperative monitoring:* ABR is typically used to monitor hearing during resections of acoustic neuromas and other similar operations.
- ABR may be used to assess the comatose patient to help establish *brain death status*.
- *Neonatal screening:* ABR is the major tool used for neonatal screening.
- Evaluation for *retrocochlear lesions:* For many years, ABR was the test of choice to screen for retrocochlear lesions in the presence of an asymmetric hearing loss. Prolongation in latencies and absent or abnormal waveforms were considered consistent with a retrocochlear lesion (e.g., an acoustic neuroma).

Because of its lack of sensitivity and specificity when compared with MRI, it is generally no longer used for retrocochlear lesion screening in the United States.

Pediatric Audiology

Hearing screening

- The National Institutes of Health currently recommends neonatal hearing screening be performed on all newborns.
- Currently, a screening ABR, where the ABR response is recorded to one (or two) stimulus intensity(ies) is the most frequently used neonatal screening test.
- OAEs may also be used as a screening tool.
- If neonates fail these tests, they are referred back for a repeat screen at 2-4 weeks of age.
- If they fail this evaluation, a formal ABR evaluation for threshold is performed along with an otolaryngology examination to rule out any medical causes of the hearing loss (e.g., middle ear effusion).

Behavioral observation audiometry (BOA)

- Used in neonates to 5 months of age.
- Observe a startle response to an intense sound stimulus (90-100 dB).

Visual reinforcement audiometry (VRA)

- Used in children 6-24 months.
- Uses sound field stimuli, therefore only provides estimate of hearing in the better-hearing ear.
- Stimuli are warble tones, speech, or narrow band noise.
- Sounds are presented at moderately intense levels through speakers placed at 45-degree angles to the child.
- If the child turns towards the sound stimulus, his/her behavior is rewarded by a light turning on or movement of an animated toy.
- Once the child is conditioned, thresholds can be determined for the better-hearing ear.

Visually reinforced operant conditioning audiometry (VROCA)

- 18 months to 3 years.
- Same as VRA, except instead of turning to the sound, the child is conditioned to push a button when a sound is heard. When correct, pushing the button will cause the toy to activate.

Tangibly reinforced operant conditioning audiometry (TROCA)

- 18 months to 3 years.
- Same as VROCA, except the child is conditioned with a reward of food.

Play audiometry

- Age 2-5 years.
- Child is conditioned to respond to a sound stimulus with a play activity (e.g., dropping a toy in a bucket).
- Is usually performed with headphones and allows determination of hearing in individual ears.

OAEs and ABR

- Note that OAEs and ABR can be used at any age during pediatric assessment.

Pseudohypacusis (functional or nonorganic hearing loss)

- Seen in patients who are malingering (e.g., disability claimants) or in patients with a psychiatric disorder (e.g., somatization disorder).
- Clues that hearing loss may not be organic.
  - Poor *reliability* on pure tone testing.
  - SRT > 10 dB *better* than PTA.
  - Speech discrimination scores significantly *better* than pure tone testing.
  - Patient conversing at *normal* volumes of speech and claiming significant pure tone hearing loss.
  - Bone-conduction thresholds *worse* than air-conduction thresholds.

Tests for pseudohypacusis

- OAEs provide an excellent initial screening.
- ABR can be used to derive thresholds.
- Behavioral tests are less commonly used, given the advent of the above-mentioned tests, but include:
  - Stenger test:
    - For unilateral hearing loss.
    - Principle: if patient presented with binaural stimuli of unequal intensities, only the louder stimulus will be "heard."
    - The patient is presented with a stimulus 10 dB above threshold in the better ear and 10 dB below threshold in the "poorer"-hearing ear.
    - If the patient doesn't respond, it means he/she is hearing the stimulus in the "poorer"-hearing ear.
    - By decreasing the intensity of the stimulus in the "poorer"-hearing ear, the true threshold can be derived.
  - Other behavioral tests are of historic significance.

Balance Function Testing

- Laboratory tests used to evaluate the balance system include electronystagmography (ENG).
- Rotational chair.
- Dynamic posturography.
  - Although these data are valuable, the reader must recognize important limitations of vestibular

testing that distinguish it from other laboratory tests.

- ❑ The diagnosis of vestibular disorders primarily rests on the acquisition of an accurate patient history.
- ❑ The accuracy of individual balance function tests must be considered when interpreting the significance of the results.
  - Balance function testing incorporates a spectrum of individual tests, with each individual test possessing a specific false-positive and false-negative rate. Thus abnormalities on testing must be considered in light of the results of the entire testing protocol and the clinical presentation.
- ❑ The diagnosis of specific vestibular disorders *cannot* be made based on the results of vestibular testing alone.
- ❑ The degree of patient disability from a vestibular disorder *cannot* be directly correlated with the degree of pathology detected on vestibular function tests.
- ❑ Given these limitations, balance function testing can provide a considerable amount of useful information pertaining to vestibular dysfunction. Such information includes:
  - Site of lesion: Vestibular function tests (specifically ENG) can provide important information confirming the side involved in a peripheral vestibular lesion.
  - Extent of lesion: Balance function tests can provide a quantitative measure of the extent of a vestibular lesion.
  - Information pertaining to functional integration of sensory inputs: Balance function tests that evaluate postural control can provide the clinician with a measure of the patient's ability to integrate sensory information pertaining to balance and effect a postural response. Such information correlates strongly with the patient's subjective perception of his/her disability.
  - Indications for vestibular rehabilitation.

Electronystagmography

- Consists of a battery of tests designed to record eye movements in response to visual or vestibular stimuli.
- Eye movements have traditionally been recorded with electrodes that record changes in the polarity of the corneal-retinal potential.
- Recordings can also be made using infrared video cameras mounted on goggles, which enhance the ability of evaluating the torsional components of eye movements.

OCULOMOTOR EVALUATION

Saccades

- Saccades (see physiology section) are rapid eye movements designed to focus objects in the periphery of the visual field onto the fovea.
- Most systems today use a computer-generated paradigm for testing saccades in which patients are asked to focus on target dots.
- The resulting saccades are characterized in terms of their velocity, accuracy, and latency.
- Abnormalities in saccade generation and control result from pathology within the central nervous system.
  - ❑ Saccades may *undershoot* (hypometria) or *overshoot* (hypermetria) their targets, typically implicating pathology in the cerebellum (or less commonly, the brainstem or basal ganglia).
  - ❑ *Slow saccades* can result from a variety of etiologies including medications, or pathology within the brainstem, cerebellum, or basal ganglia.
  - ❑ *Rapid saccades* may be observed in myasthenia gravis and mechanical syndromes restricting eye movement.
  - ❑ *Long latencies* in the initiation of saccades can result from a variety of neurodegenerative conditions (e.g., Alzheimer's disease, Parkinson's disease, Huntington's chorea).

Pursuit Testing

Two forms of ocular pursuit testing are used during ENG evaluation.

1. *Smooth pursuit testing.* Currently performed using computerized regimens, smooth pursuit testing involves tracking a target that is focused on the fovea as it moves back and forth in a horizontal plane at varying frequencies and intensities. Inability to smoothly track the target, resulting in frequent corrective saccades, can result from pathology throughout the CNS, most commonly localized to the cerebellum or brainstem. As the ability to maintain smooth pursuit declines with age, it is important that results be compared with appropriate normative data.

2. *Optokinetic nystagmus.* Optokinetic testing involves the stimulation of virtually the entire retina (as opposed to just the fovea) with continuously moving repetitive stimuli. Rotating stripes are traditionally used. The eye targets the stripe and then makes a quick saccade to catch the next stripe entering the visual field. The resulting pattern of eye movement is called *optokinetic nystagmus (OKN)*. In general, abnormalities in the slow phase of the OKN mimic abnormalities in the

smooth pursuit mechanism, whereas abnormalities in the rapid phase parallel abnormalities in saccade testing.

SPONTANEOUS AND GAZE-EVOKED NYSTAGMUS

Eyes are evaluated for nystagmus in the:
- Primary position (looking straight forward) with and without visual fixation.
- Gaze: testing is performed by having the patient fixate on a target 30 degrees to the right, left, above center, and below center.
- Currently, most centers consider the presence of spontaneous nystagmus to be abnormal if its peak slow component velocity exceeds 5 to 6 degrees/second. Spontaneous nystagmus that is peripheral in origin typically displays the following characteristics:
  - It has combined torsional and horizontal components.
  - It is inhibited by visual fixation.
  - It follows Alexander's law (its amplitude increases when gaze is directed toward the direction of the nystagmus).
- Spontaneous nystagmus of central origin may be purely horizontal, vertical, or torsional. It does not suppress with fixation, and it may change direction with gaze.
- Congenital nystagmus.
  - Is usually purely horizontal with a pendular or sawtooth waveform.
  - Is present with fixation and typically disappears when the patient is not fixating.
  - May present when one eye is covered and the contralateral eye beats in the direction of the covered eye.
- Nystagmus that appears only when looking away from the primary position may be physiologic (end point nystagmus) or pathologic.
- Symmetric gaze-evoked nystagmus (equal amplitude to the left and right) commonly results from drug ingestion (e.g., phenobarbital, alcohol, diazepam, phenytoin) or from a variety of CNS lesions.
- Asymmetric gaze-evoked nystagmus most commonly results from structural lesions in the brainstem or cerebellum.

POSITIONAL TESTING

- *Static positional testing* is designed to detect nystagmus evoked when the head is maintained in different positions.
- *Paroxysmal positioning testing* (the Dix-Hallpike maneuver) is designed to detect nystagmus provoked by a rapid change in head position.

- In static positional testing, eye movements are recorded while the patient is placed in the following positions:
  1. Supine.
  2. Supine with head turned to left.
  3. Supine with head turned to right.
  4. Lying in left lateral position.
  5. Lying in right lateral position.
- Nystagmus resulting from static positional testing can be classified based on whether it is:
  - Direction changing vs. direction fixed.
  - Intermittent vs. persistent.
  - Geotropic vs. ageotropic
- The interpretation of static positional testing is complicated by the determination of what truly represents clinically significant positional nystagmus, and whether the pattern of nystagmus is most consistent with central or peripheral disease. Positional nystagmus is a fairly common finding in the normal population, and the different patterns of positional nystagmus can be seen in either central or peripheral disease. Although various centers have established criteria as to what they consider to be significant degrees and patterns of nystagmus, the results of positional testing must be correlated with the results of other balance testing and the clinical presentation of the patient.
- In general, if oculomotor testing is normal (i.e., smooth pursuit), most findings of positional nystagmus are felt to be peripheral in origin
- A positive Dix-Hallpike maneuver (indicative of benign positional vertigo) will display nystagmus with a latency of 10 seconds and fatigue within 1-2 minutes.
- The pattern of nystagmus will indicate the canal affected:
  - Posterior SCC = torsional and upbeating.
  - Superior canal = torsional and downbeating.
  - Horizontal canal = pure horizontal nystagmus.

CALORIC TESTING

- In *alternate bithermal caloric* testing, each ear is stimulated with either water or air equally above (warm: 44° C) and below (cool: 30° C) body temperature. In cases of poor response to stimulation, ice water may be substituted for cool water.
- Testing is done in both ears with and without fixation.
- Caloric stimulation creates a temperature gradient between the two sides (ampullary vs. utricular) of the horizontal SCC. This creates a difference between the specific gravities of the endolymph in these two sections of the canal. The differences in specific gravities make the endolymph potentially sensitive to gravitational forces. To take advantage of this, the

head is positioned 30 degrees up so that the horizontal canal is essentially vertical.

- The direction of the nystagmus elicited by caloric stimulation follows the COWS mnemonic: Cold: *opposite*; *warm*: *same*. That is, cold water stimulation to the right ear will elicit left-beating nystagmus.
- Stimulation of the horizontal SCCs results in nystagmus that can be quantified and used to calculate a *unilateral peripheral weakness* or a *bilateral vestibular loss*. In both situations, testing centers must establish criteria as to what values represent a true loss of function. In general, a unilateral weakness of 20%-25% is considered significant.
- The *unilateral weakness (UW) index* is calculated as follows:

$$\frac{(RW + RC) - (LW + LC)}{RW + RC + LW + LC} \times 100 = UW$$

where RW = right warm, RC = right cold, LW = left warm, and LC = left cold.

- Cases of suspected bilateral vestibular loss should undergo rotational chair testing to confirm and quantify the finding (see below).
- Caloric testing may also reveal that one side responds more strongly to bithermal stimuli than does the other ear. This finding of *directional preponderance* is most often associated with the presence of spontaneous nystagmus or a unilateral weakness. When it occurs as an isolated finding, it is nonlocalizing and must be correlated with the results of the remainder of the testing.
- *Directional preponderance (DP)* is calculated as follows:

$$\frac{(RW + LC) - (LW + RC)}{RW + RC + LW + LC} \times 100 = DP$$

- In general a DP of 20%-30% is considered significant.

Rotational Chair

- The SCCs of the inner ear are designed to detect angular accelerations. Thus caloric irrigations represent a nonphysiologic stimulus to the horizontal canal. In fact, standard caloric irrigations are equivalent to a low-frequency rotation of 0.002-0.004 Hz. Rotational chair testing offers the opportunity to test the response to a range of rotational stimuli, using a quantifiable physiologic stimulus (rotation).
- Rotational chair testing is performed in the dark, with eye movements recorded with an infrared camera or scleral coil. The chair is rotated at frequencies of 0.01-1.28 Hz, with the velocity of the slow phase of the nystagmus being the outcome measured.

- Comparing head velocity to eye velocity at the various tested frequencies allows the derivation of *phase* measurements. Given that the sinusoidal rotations are repetitive, eye movements actually anticipate head movements and occur slightly before, or *lead*, the head movement. This phase lead is known as the *phase angle* and is measured in degrees.
- *Increases* in the phase angle are associated with peripheral vestibular pathology or, less commonly, with isolated lesions in the brainstem vestibular nuclei. The significance of decreases in the phase angle is less clear but may be associated with cerebellar lesions focused in the nodulus.
- *Gain* measurements are derived by comparing head and eye velocities for specific frequencies of rotation. Significant reductions in gain are consistent with a bilateral peripheral vestibular weakness and are thus useful in confirming and quantifying results obtained from caloric testing.
- The velocities of rightward and leftward eye movements can be compared to derive a measure of *asymmetry*, analogous to the measurement of directional preponderance obtained in ENG testing. Like the directional preponderance measurement, asymmetries may be noted in both central and peripheral disease and must be correlated with the results of other testing.

Dynamic Posturography

- Tests such as ENG and rotatory chair measure the function of specific components of the balance system but do not provide information pertaining to the functional ability of the patient to maintain balance.
- *Dynamic posturography* is designed to provide quantitative information pertaining to the patient's functional ability to maintain balance.
- With dynamic posturography the patient stands on force plates. As the patient's weight distribution over his/her feet changes, the plates measure these changes in vertical and horizontal forces placed on the surface of the plate. These force measurements can be used to calculate the patient's center of mass.
- The *sensory organization test* measures the ability of the patient to maintain the position of his/her center of mass when visual and somatosensory inputs are altered. Six conditions are tested. In the first three the platform is fixed, providing stable somatosensory (proprioceptive) inputs.
  - Condition 1: the patient maintains stable position with eyes open.
  - Condition 2: stance is maintained with eyes closed.
  - Condition 3: the visual surround moves in a pattern designed to match the postural sway of the patient. This creates a sensory conflict in which

proprioceptive and vestibular inputs indicate that the patient is swaying, whereas the visual input is consistent with a stationary position.

- Conditions 4, 5, and 6 replicate 1, 2, and 3 with one exception: instead of being fixed, the platform is allowed to move in a pattern dictated by the sway pattern of the patient. This limits the contribution of proprioceptive sensory inputs in maintaining a stable stance.

- Each paradigm is repeated three times because the normal improvement in performance that takes place as the tasks are repeated improves the validity of the test.

- The patterns of performance may indicate an inability to use certain information (e.g., vestibular, visual) to maintain balance, a preferential reliance on particular cues to maintain balance, or inconsistent results not attributable to physical pathology.

- It is important to emphasize that the sensory organization test provides *no information* pertaining to the site of lesion. Instead, it provides information about the type of stimuli (visual, vestibular, proprioceptive) that the patient can or cannot use to maintain balance.

- In the motor control test, the patient is subjected to abrupt changes in his/her center of gravity through horizontal translations and rotations in the floor plate. The floor plate measures the muscle responses to these perturbations, with outcome measures being the latency of the muscle response, the weight distribution onto the right or left leg, and a relative measure of the strength of the response.

- Abnormalities in latency implicate potential pathology anywhere along the long loop pathways that extend from the afferent proprioceptors to the CNS and back to the efferent nerves controlling the motor response.

- Results pertaining to weight distribution and strength of response may identify maladaptive balance strategies that can be addressed through rehabilitation.

Otitis Externa

Definition
An inflammatory (typically infectious) disorder of the external ear canal.

Incidence and epidemiology
- Acute otitis externa affects approximately 4 in 1000 children and adults per year.
- Eighty percent of the cases occur in the summer.
- Predisposing factors:
  - Warm, humid environments.
  - Anatomic obstructions of the ear canals (stenosis, exostoses, impacted cerumen).
  - Hearing aid or ear plug use.
  - Self-induced trauma (e.g., by cotton swabs).
  - Swimming.

Pathogenesis
1. Abrogation of the hydrophobic ceruminous coating of the external canal (e.g., trauma, water).
2. Exposure of the underlying epithelium to water and other contaminants.
3. Edema and excoriation of the epithelial layer.
4. Bacterial infection.
   - *Fungal* infections of the external canal are generally considered to be opportunistic, occurring subsequent to treatment of bacterial infection.
   - *Chronic otitis externa* may result from an allergic reaction to a topical agent (e.g., neomycin), a contact dermatitis (e.g., hairsprays, shampoos), an extension of psoriasis or other systemic dermatitides (e.g., seborrhea), or a chronic granular bacterial/fungal infection.

Microbiology
See Table 3.

Symptoms
- Pain.
- Itching.
- Aural fullness.
- Decreased hearing.
- Otorrhea.

Clinical findings
- An erythematous canal with scant discharge in cases of early bacterial otitis externa.
- An edematous canal filled with purulent-squamous debris in cases of well-established bacterial otitis externa.
- An accumulation of white debris sprouting hyphae best seen with the otologic microscopic, typical of candidal otitis externa.

TABLE 3. Microbiology of Otitis Externa	
Microbes	**Frequency**
Pseudomonas aeruginosa	40%
Staphylococcus epidermidis	9%
Staphylococcus aureus	8%
Staph species: other	8%
Coryneform (diphtheroids)	9%
Other gram-negative rods (e.g., *Enterobacter, Klebsiella, Proteus, Escherichia coli*)	9%
Streptococcus, Enterococcus	4%
Aspergillus/Candida	2%

- An accumulation of a moist white plug dotted with black debris ("wet newspaper") typical of *Aspergillus niger*.
- A maculopapular eruption on conchal bowl and in the ear canal consistent with an allergic reaction to a topical agent (e.g., neomycin).
- A thickened, erythematous canal associated with an allergic or contact dermatitis.
- Granulation tissue in the canal and on the TM caused by chronic infection.

Investigations

Cultures for bacteria and fungus are indicated in cases of persistent or refractory infection, particularly to identify cases of fungal infection. Sensitivities of bacteria to particular antibiotics as provided by microbiology laboratories should generally be disregarded. They are determined based on typical serum concentrations obtained by systemic administration of the antibiotic and are not based on the many-fold higher antibiotic concentrations obtained with topical use.

Treatment

- Debridement.
- Insertion of a wick (e.g., Merocel) to facilitate drug transport.
- Acidification of the ear canal is toxic to many bacterial (including pseudomonas) and fungal species.
- Antibiotic drops continue to be the mainstay of treatment for otitis externa. Examples of available topical medications include:
  - A combination solution or suspension of polymyxin, neomycin, and hydrocortisone (e.g., Cortisporin). Polymyxin provides coverage against *Pseudomonas,* whereas both the polymyxin and neomycin are effective against *Staphylococcus aureus* and other gram-negative organisms. A contact dermatitis resulting from neomycin exposure can occur. Hydrocortisone may remain as a precipitate in the canal, thus obscuring visualization, creating an impression of persistent infection, and even causing a conductive hearing loss if a caste of the precipitate adheres to the TM. Neomycin is potentially ototoxic, which is an issue if prolonged use is required in the presence of a perforated TM.
  - Other aminoglycoside antibiotics are available in ophthalmic solutions and can be used for the treatment of otitis externa. Both gentamicin and tobramycin are available in solutions with and without topical steroids.
  - Quinolone antibiotics are available in both otic and ophthalmic solutions. They offer single-agent coverage for pathogenic bacteria, with virtually no risk of contact dermatitis or ototoxicity. Floxin (ofloxacin) is available for treatment of both external and middle ear disease. It has been shown to be as effective as PMH for the treatment of bacterial otitis externa. Its main disadvantages are a relatively neutral pH (6.2-6.8), the absence of a steroid, and expense. Ciprofloxacin is available as an otic preparation combined with hydrocortisone and a newer formulation combined with dexamethasone (Cipro-HC, Ciprodex). These solutions are acidic and contain a steroid. The hydrocortisone in Cipro-HC may leave a precipitate in the canal, and both solutions are expensive.
  - Oral antibiotics should be reserved for complications of otitis externa (see below).
- Fungal otitis externa can be treated with meticulous debridement and acidification of the ear. Antifungal solutions or creams (e.g., clotrimazole, nystatin) may prove effective in candidal infections but do not offer coverage against aspergillus. Aspergillus infections may prove difficult to treat. Many infections will resolve with frequent debridement and administration of an acidic drop (e.g., VoSol, Domeboro). An alternative popular treatment is painting the canal and TM with dyes that possess antifungal properties (e.g., gentian violet, "triple blue"). Persistent aspergillus infections associated with considerable canal edema may require the administration of oral itraconazole.
- Contact or allergic dermatitis should be treated by elimination of the offending agent, debridement, and administration of a topical corticosteroid solution/lotion.
- Chronic granular otitis externa can be a difficult entity to treat.
  - This is seen most frequently in people who are dependent on their hearing aids.
  - Minimizing or alternating hearing aid use should be advised.
  - Culture of the ear for bacteria and fungus may provide evidence of the causative organisms.
  - Repeated debridement, cauterization of the granulations, and filling the canal with topical antibiotic or antifungal creams can be effective.
  - Topical gentian violet may also be effective at drying the ear canal and eliminating the chronic infection.
  - Surgical therapy may be required, involving resection of the affected skin and placement of split skin grafts.

Complications

- *Cellulitis, perichondritis,* or even *chondritis* may result from otitis externa.
  - In adults, treat with a quinolone antibiotic.
  - In children, in the case of a cellulitis, an oral antistaphylococcal drug may be initiated; however,

if pseudomonas is detected on ear culture, parenteral administration of antipseudomonal antibiotics is required. For specific treatment of perichondritis and chondritis, see below.

- **Medial canal fibrosis**
  - ▫ Chronic otitis externa may result in the formation of a thick fibrous scar that obstructs the medial aspect of the canal.
  - ▫ Physical examination will reveal what appears to be a lateralized TM as well as an absence of typical landmarks.
  - ▫ Surgical treatment of this disorder can be challenging. The affected portion of the canal lining is resected, a bony canaloplasty is performed, and the canal is relined with split skin grafts. Recurrence after surgical treatment is common.
- Aspergillus infection may result in *TM perforation*. Elimination of the offending fungus allows for a high rate of spontaneous healing of these perforations.
- *Malignant otitis externa (see below).*

Malignant Otitis Externa

Definition
An aggressive and potentially fatal infection originating in the external canal, with progressive spread along the soft tissues and bone of the skull base, ultimately involving intracranial structures. It is also known as *necrotizing otitis externa.*

Incidence and epidemiology
- A rare disorder occurring in *immunocompromised patients.*
- Most common population involved is the elderly with *diabetes mellitus.*
- Myeloid malignancies.
- Iatrogenic immunosuppression caused by pharmacologic treatment of malignancies and organ transplant recipients and in patients with HIV/AIDS.
- Reported in *immunocompetent* patients.

Microbiology
- The vast majority of cases are caused by *Pseudomonas aeruginosa.*
- Other bacteria (e.g., *S. aureus* and *Staphylococcus epidermidis*) are rarely implicated.
- Aspergillus species are the most common fungal pathogens to cause this disorder.

Clinical manifestations
- Otalgia that can be severe.
- Otorrhea.
- Granulation tissue protruding through the floor of the ear canal at the bony-cartilaginous junction.

- Initial stages of the infection involve the skin and soft tissues of the ear canal.
- With progression, the infection will lead to involvement of the bony structures of the temporal bone along the skull base.
- In the most advanced stages, it will extend beyond the temporal bone along the skull base and/or intracranially.
- The *facial nerve* is the most common cranial nerve involved (at the stylomastoid foramen).
- Further progression will lead to involvement of the *lower cranial nerves* at the jugular foramen.
- *Intracranial spread* will result in headaches, fever, neck stiffness, and altered levels of consciousness.

Investigations
- Traditionally, malignant otitis externa was diagnosed with a *Technetium-99m* bone scan and a *Gallium-67* scan. The Gallium-67 scan was also used to follow the progression of the infection and its response to treatment.
- In most centers, the Gallium-67 scan has been supplanted by an *Indium-111-labelled leukocyte* scan.
- *High-resolution computed tomography (CT) scans* have been shown to be fairly accurate in diagnosing and following the course of infection and can be used as the sole method of radiographic evaluation.
- A greater degree of diagnostic accuracy seems to be afforded by the use of simultaneous acquisition of *single photon emission tomographs (SPECT)* using two radionuclide tracers (Indium-111-labelled leukocytes and Technetium-99m).
- Bacterial and fungal *cultures* of the otorrhea should be obtained at the time of initiation of treatment.

Treatment
- Administration of antipseudomonal antibiotics remains the cornerstone of treatment. Early infections may be treated solely with oral ciprofloxacin.
- In more advanced stages, parenteral antibiotics may be indicated initially, with discharge of the patients on oral ciprofloxacin. Resistance of bacteria to quinolones may occur.
- Total duration of treatment is typically 6 weeks, or as indicated by the results of radiologic studies.
- Hyperbaric oxygen therapy has been shown to be a useful adjuvant in more advanced cases.
- The role of surgical treatment for this disorder is unclear. Mastoid debridement may play a role in certain resistant infections.

Herpes Zoster Oticus

Definition
A recrudescent herpes zoster infection involving the external ear.

Incidence and epidemiology

- It is a relatively uncommon infection that more frequently affects immunosuppressed patients.
- Other stimuli for viral reactivation involve a variety of physical and psychological stressors.
- Often, no precipitating event will be identified.

Pathogenesis

- Virus is harbored in a latent state in sensory ganglia and will reactivate with infection spreading along dermatomes.
- When the ear is involved, virus is most commonly believed to be harbored in the geniculate ganglion and spread along the sensory fibers of the facial nerve.
- Other sensory ganglia have also been implicated, including those in the Vth and VIIIth cranial nerves.

Clinical manifestations

- A prodrome of otalgia, which may be very severe.
- A vesicular eruption will be seen in the canal and concha. Ultimately, these vesicles will rupture and form crusts.
- A subgroup of patients will manifest *Ramsay Hunt syndrome,* defined as a facial paralysis in the presence of herpes zoster oticus.
- VIIIth nerve involvement results in SNHL and/or vertigo.

Treatment

- Treatment is somewhat empiric and not based on many scientific studies.
- Local ear care.
- Topical antibiotic/steroid drops (e.g., TobraDex).
- Antiherpetic agent at the onset of the syndrome (e.g., valacyclovir 1000 mg tid × 7 days).
- High-dose steroids (e.g., prednisone 1 mg/kg/day) should be added in the presence of facial paralysis and/or SNHL.
- Particular attention should be directed toward eye care, and an ophthalmologic consult should be obtained with any evidence of a herpetic keratitis.
- Postherpetic neuralgia can be a significant problem.

Bullous Myringitis

Definition

Bullous myringitis is an inflammatory/infectious condition involving the lateral surface of the TM and the medial portion of the canal wall.

Incidence and epidemiology

Bullous myringitis is typically associated with upper respiratory infections and is more common in winter. The etiology is believed to be primarily viral; however, mycoplasma has been identified in some cases.

Clinical manifestations

- Acute, severe otalgia.
- Serosanguineous otorrhea.
- Hearing loss (in the majority of cases).
- Physical examination reveals bulla(e) on the TM that is (are) filled with serous or serosanguineous fluid.
- Spontaneous rupture of the bullae leads to the observed discharge.
- Primary care practitioners frequently mistake the disorder for an acute otitis media (AOM). A serous otitis media is a frequently associated finding in 30%-40% of cases.
- Between 60% and 65% of patients will manifest a sensorineural or mixed hearing loss, with the sensorineural component recovering completely in approximately 60% of these patients.

Treatment

- Analgesics, topical antibiotic/steroid drops to prevent bacterial superinfection, and lancing of the bullae, which may result in some pain relief.
- Because mycoplasma can be associated at times with this infection, the administration of a macrolide or quinolone antibiotic may be indicated.
- The role of systemic steroids has never been established.

Cellulitis

Cellulitis of the ear typically results from a spreading otitis externa or a penetrating injury. It is distinguished from perichondritis by the lack of induration. It will present as an erythematous ear. Treatment is with systemic, antistaphylococcal antibiotics.

Erysipelas

Erysipelas is a dermal infection that may involve the skin of the head and face, including the ear, caused by β-hemolytic streptococcus. The involved tissue is erythematous, indurated, and tender. The hallmark of the infection is that it spreads along a well-demarcated border. The treatment is with oral systemic antibiotics (e.g., penicillin)

Perichondritis and Chondritis

- Perichondritis and chondritis represent infections of the auricular perichondrium or cartilage.
- They result from blunt or penetrating trauma to the ear, or via direct extension from an otitis externa.
  - In the case of a blunt trauma, a hematoma on the lateral surface of the pinna is usually the initiating event. The pinna then becomes infected.

- ❑ Penetrating trauma may result from a variety of injuries, including ear piercing, assaults, bites, and iatrogenic injuries.
- *Pseudomonas* is the most frequent causative organism.
- Physical exam reveals a tender, erythematous, indurated pinna.
- Fluctuance indicates the presence of an abscess and possible chondritis.
- Treatment of perichondritis consists of elimination of any foreign bodies and the administration of an oral quinolone antibiotic.
- An abscess must be drained and any necrotic cartilage resected.
- The wound can be packed with antibiotic impregnated ribbon gauze or, when cartilage is resected, a through-and-through Penrose drain may be placed.
- A permanent deformity of the cartilage ("cauliflower ear") may result.
- Recurrent or bilateral auricular swelling should prompt a rheumatologic work-up for *relapsing polychondritis*.

Furunculosis

A furuncle (abscess or boil) is a walled-off collection of pus that presents as a painful, firm, or fluctuant mass. It arises from the hair follicles of the lateral ear canal. The causative organism is typically *S. aureus*. Clinical manifestations include localized pain, particularly to touch. Early manifestations include a nodular swelling that proceeds to fluctuance. Treatment includes the application of warm compresses and topical antibiotic ointment. Antistaphylococcal oral antibiotics should be administered. A fluctuant lesion should be incised and drained under local anesthetic.

Selected References from the Recent Literature

1. Bellini C, Antonini P, Ermanni S *et al*. Malignant otitis externa due to *Aspergillus niger*. [Review] [21 refs]. *Scandinavian Journal of Infectious Diseases* 2003;35(4):284-288.
2. Dohar JE. Evolution of management approaches for otitis externa. [Review] [49 refs]. *Pediatric Infectious Disease Journal* 2003;22(4):299-305.
3. Schrader N, Isaacson G. Fungal otitis externa—its association with fluoroquinolone eardrops. [Review] [6 refs]. *Pediatrics* 2003;111(5 Pt 1):1123.
4. Sudhoff H, Linthicum FH, Jr. Malignant external otitis: temporal bone histopathology case of the month. *Otology & Neurotology* 2003;24(2):346-347.
5. Finer G, Greenberg D, Leibovitz E *et al*. Conservative treatment of malignant (invasive) external otitis caused by *Aspergillus flavus* with oral itraconazole solution in a neutropenic patient. *Scandinavian Journal of Infectious Diseases* 2002;34(3):227-229.
6. Hopsu E, Pitkaranta A. Idiopathic inflammatory medial meatal fibrotizing otitis. *Archives of Otolaryngology—Head & Neck Surgery* 2002;128(11):1313-1316.
7. Pond F, McCarty D, O'Leary S. Randomized trial on the treatment of oedematous acute otitis externa using ear wicks or ribbon gauze: clinical outcome and cost. *Journal of Laryngology & Otology* 2002;116(6):415-419.
8. Berenholz L, Katzenell U, Harell M. Evolving resistant pseudomonas to ciprofloxacin in malignant otitis externa. *Laryngoscope* 2002;112(9):1619-1622.
9. Roland PS, Stroman DW. Microbiology of acute otitis externa. *Laryngoscope* 2002;112(7 Pt 1):1166-1177.
10. Tsikoudas A, Jasser P, England RJ. Are topical antibiotics necessary in the management of otitis externa? *Clinical Otolaryngology & Allied Sciences* 2002;27(4):260-262.
11. Hurst WB. Outcome of 22 cases of perforated tympanic membrane caused by otomycosis. *Journal of Laryngology & Otology* 2001;115(11):879-880.

ACUTE OTITIS MEDIA AND ITS COMPLICATIONS

Definition
Bacterial infection of the middle ear of less than 3 weeks in duration.

Incidence
- Occurs in 65% of children by age 2.
- Highest incidence at 6-24 months of age.
- Slight increase at 5-6 years of age.

Epidemiology
- Male > female.
- Native Americans, Hispanic > Whites, Asians > African Americans.
- High-density populations.
- Familial.
- Season: winter and spring.
- Breast-feeding decreases incidence.

Bacteriology
- *Streptococcus pneumoniae:* 35%.
- *Haemophilus influenzae:* 23%.
- *Moraxella catarrhalis:* 14%
- Other gram-positive: 7%.
- No growth: 16%.

Pathology
- Acute inflammatory infiltrate.

Pathogenesis
- Mechanical suboptimal eustachian tube function.
- Local and systemic immune factors.
- Bacterial source:
  - Nasopharynx.

Clinical stages
1. Hyperemia
   - Otalgia.
   - Fullness.
   - Fever.
   - Injection of the TM along manubrium and periphery.
2. Exudation
   - Between 12 and 24 hours.
   - Inflammatory exudate (serum, polymorphonuclear neutrophils).
   - Otalgia, fever, decreased hearing.
   - Red, thickened, bulging TM.
     - Loss of landmarks.
   - Clouding of middle ear and mastoid cells.
     - May be pain/erythema over mastoid.
3. Suppuration
   - Spontaneous perforation and drainage.
   - Decreased pain.
   - Mucopurulent discharge.
   - Hearing loss.
4. Coalescence and surgical mastoiditis
   - Two weeks after onset.
   - Mucopurulent discharge.
   - Mastoid tenderness and thickening of periosteum.
   - Sagging of posterosuperior wall.
   - Protrusion of TM because of granulations.
   - Caused by chronic suppuration and osteoclastic resorption of bone.
   - Treated with cortical mastoidectomy.
5. Complications (see below)
   - Intratemporal.
   - Extratemporal, extradural.
   - Extratemporal, intradural.

Complications, intratemporal
- Chronic otitis media: Otitis media with effusion (OME) vs. chronic suppurative otitis media (CSOM)
- Tympanosclerosis: Scarring of the TM and/or middle ear space with hyalinized collagen. If the tympanosclerosis is extensive, with involvement of the ossicles, it can result in a maximal conductive hearing loss.
- Petrositis
- Gradenigo's syndrome: Severe unilateral retro-orbital pain (Vth nerve), VIth nerve paralysis, and otorrhea. Treatment is with mastoidectomy, which may allow drainage of the petrous apex. Occasionally, decompression of the petrous apex by exenteration of the perilabyrinthine cell tracts may be required.
- Facial paralysis: Acute facial paralysis is treated by myringotomy with or without ventilation tube and systemic antibiotics. The use of corticosteroids is empiric but generally advocated.
- Labyrinthitis: Suppurative labyrinthitis is treated by myringotomy with or without a tube, parenteral antibiotics, corticosteroids, and vestibular suppressants. Even with aggressive treatment, the prognosis for salvaging hearing is poor. Vestibular rehabilitation physical therapy may be required.

Complications, extratemporal, extradural
- Abscess
  - Subperiosteal.
  - Zygomatic.
  - Mastoid tip (Bezold's).
Treatment of these complications is by incision and drainage and cortical mastoidectomy.

Complications, extratemporal, intradural

- *Meningitis:* Treatment is by myringotomy and tube and appropriate parenteral antibiotics.
- *Extradural abscess:* Treatment is by decompression via a mastoidectomy.
- *Intracranial abscess*
  - Temporal: cerebellar = 2:1.
  - Spread of infection via direct extension or thrombophlebitis.
  - Four stages:
    1. Encephalitis.
    2. Latent.
    3. Expansion
       - Fever, headache, nausea, and vomiting.
       - Altered mental status.
       - Papilledema.
       - Cerebellar
         - Ataxia, intention tremor.
       - Temporal
         - Seizures, aphasia.
       - Treatment: neurosurgical drainage, myringotomy and tube, mastoidectiomy with coalescence.
    4. Rupture
- Sigmoid (lateral) sinus thrombophlebitis
  - Bone erosion over sinus can lead to localized phlebitis that progresses to a mural thrombus.
  - Griesinger's sign
    - Postauricular edema.
  - Fever (had "picket fence" pattern prior to antibiotics).
  - Otorrhea.
  - Tender mastoid/neck.
  - Unreliable signs
    - Papilledema.
    - Queckenstedt's test (occlusion of the internal jugular vein on the affected side using manual pressure fails to lead to increased intracranial pressure).
  - Diagnosis
    - CT with contrast.
    - MRV.
    - Angiography.
  - Treatment
    - Administer parenteral antibiotics.
    - Mastoidectomy, expose needle sinus to determine if flow is present.
    - If thrombus present and localized, open and remove.
    - Perform internal jugular vein ligation if septic emboli are occurring.
    - Anticoagulants are not recommended unless the thrombosis is propagating throughout the intracranial venous system.

Otitic Hydrocephalus

- Uncommon complication.
- Presents with signs of increased intracranial pressure in the *presence* of chronic ear infection and in the *absence* of intracranial infection.
- Treatment is cortical mastoidectomy and possible neurosurgical intervention for shunt.

CHRONIC OTITIS MEDIA

Otitis Media with Effusion

Definition
- Acute: 3 weeks (e.g., AOM).
- Subacute: 3 weeks – 3 months.
- Chronic: >3 months.

Incidence
- 10% have effusion persistent for 3 months after AOM.

Etiology
- Infection
  - Eustachian tube dysfunction.
  - Persistence of bacterial products and inflammatory mediators.
  - Allergy.
  - Recent attention has focused on the role of biofilms in the generation of OME. Biofilms are a complex organization of bacteria anchored to a surface (in this situation, the mucosa of the middle ear). The biofilm largely consists of an exopolysaccharide matrix secreted by the bacteria. This matrix protects the bacteria from host immune cells and inflammatory mediators. The reduced metabolic rate of the bacteria residing within the biofilm contributes to their being impervious to antibiotics and recalcitrant to culture. Alterations in bacterial metabolism within the biofilm allow for recrudescence of infection.
  - Barotrauma.
  - Tumors obstructing the eustachian tube.

Pathology
- Serous fluid
  - Yellow; short-term disease; minimal mucosal changes.
- Mucoid (glue ear)
  - Secretory, hypertrophy of lining with increased goblet cells.

Diagnosis
- Otoscopy.
- Tuning forks (adult).
- Tympanometry.
- Audiometry.

Treatment

- Child:
  - Prophylactic antibiotics or bilateral myringotomy tubes (BMTs) if persists longer than 3 months.
  - Adenoidectomy.
- Adult:
  - Trial of steroids plus antibiotics.
  - BMTs.
  - Rule out malignancy.

Complications

- Atrophy and atelectasis of the TM
- Ossicular erosion
- Tympanosclerosis
- Cholesterol granuloma
- Cholesteatoma
- Sensorineural hearing loss (SNHL) (?)

Chronic Suppurative Otitis Media

Definition

- History of chronic suppurative infection of the middle ear.
- Must have (or have had) TM perforation.
- Can be:
  - Active.
  - Intermittent.
  - Quiescent (dry perforation).
  - Resolved (healed perforation).

Pathology

- Thickened mucosa.
- Submucosal inflammatory infiltrate.
- Submucosal fibrosis.
- Mucosal edema leading to polyps.
- Resorption of ossicles.
- Deposits of hyalinized collagen (tympanosclerosis).
- Decreased aeration of mastoid.

Bacteriology

- Typically gram-negative infection.
  - High incidence of pseudomonas (67%).
- S. aureus.

Symptoms

- Chronic drainage (or history thereof).
- Hearing loss:
  - TM perforation and atelectasis.
  - Ossicular erosion or fixation.
  - Tympanosclerosis.
  - SNHL (?).
- Complications (as described in the previous section)
  - Particularly with cholesteatoma.

Investigations

- Audiogram.

- Culture and sensitivity (C & S) if otorrhea persistent.
- CT if cholesteatoma is present on clinical examination.

Treatment

- Topical drops are the cornerstone of management. Efforts should be made to limit the duration of exposure to aminoglycoside antibiotic drops because of the potential for ototoxicity.
- Oral antibiotics are rarely required. Oral quinolones may help in resolving infections in adults.
- Systemic antibiotics (children) may be required in recalcitrant cases.
- Tympanoplasty.
- Ossiculoplasty.
- Mastoidectomy, in the presence of coalescence or in the case of infection that has failed maximal medical treatment.

Complications of OME and CSOM

- Same as those for OME.

Selected References from the Recent Literature

1. Kotikoski MJ, Palmu AA, Puhakka HJ. The symptoms and clinical course of acute bullous myringitis in children less than two years of age. *International Journal of Pediatric Otorhinolaryngology* 2003;67(2):165-172.
2. Jose J, Coatesworth AP, Anthony R *et al.* Life threatening complications after partially treated mastoiditis. *BMJ* 2003;327(7405):41-42.
3. Veenhoven R, Bogaert D, Uiterwaal C *et al.* Effect of conjugate pneumococcal vaccine followed by polysaccharide pneumococcal vaccine on recurrent acute otitis media: a randomised study [comment]. *Lancet* 2003;361(9376): 2189-2195.
4. Grewal DS, Hathiram BT, Dwivedi A *et al.* Labyrinthine fistula: a complication of chronic suppurative otitis media. *Journal of Laryngology & Otology* 2003;117(5):353-357.
5. Weber SM, Grundfast KM. Modern management of acute otitis media. [Review] [54 refs]. *Pediatric Clinics of North America* 2003;50(2):399-411.
6. Daly KA, Hunter LL, Lindgren BR et al. Chronic otitis media with effusion sequelae in children treated with tubes. *Archives of Otolaryngology—Head & Neck Surgery* 2003;129(5):517-522.
7. Paradise JL, Feldman HM, Campbell TF *et al.* Early versus delayed insertion of tympanostomy tubes for persistent otitis media: developmental outcomes at the age of three years in relation to prerandomization illness patterns and hearing levels. *Pediatric Infectious Disease Journal* 2003;22(4):309-314.
8. Heikkinen T, Chonmaitree T. Importance of respiratory viruses in acute otitis media. [Review] [141 refs]. *Clinical Microbiology Reviews* 2003;16(2):230-241.
9. Poe DS, Metson RB, Kujawski O. Laser eustachian tuboplasty: a preliminary report. *Laryngoscope* 2003;113(4): 583-591.
10. Papp Z, Rezes S, Jokay I et al. Sensorineural hearing loss in chronic otitis media. *Otology & Neurotology* 2003;24(2): 141-144.

11. Dawes PJ. Myringostapediopexy: surgical expectation. *Journal of Laryngology & Otology* 2003;117(3):182-185.

12. Khan I, Shahzad F. Mastoiditis in children. *Journal of Laryngology & Otology* 2003;117(3):177-181.

13. Arnold W, Bredberg G, Gstottner W et al. Meningitis following cochlear implantation: pathomechanisms, clinical symptoms, conservative and surgical treatments. [Review] [33 refs]. *ORL Journal of Otorhinolaryngology & Its Related Specialties* 2002;64(6):382-389.

14. Bluestone CD. Prevention of meningitis: cochlear implants and inner ear abnormalities. *Archives of Otolaryngology—Head & Neck Surgery* 2003;129(3):279-281.

15. Klein JO. Changes in management of otitis media: 2003 and beyond. [Review] [10 refs]. *Pediatric Annals* 2002;31(12):824-826.

16. DeRosa J, Grundfast KM. Surgical management of otitis media. [Review] [29 refs]. *Pediatric Annals* 2002;31(12):814-820.

17. Pelton SI. Vaccination for the prevention of acute otitis media: proof of concept and current challenges. [Review] [28 refs]. *Pediatric Annals* 2002;31(12):804-809.

18. Barnett ED. Antibiotic resistance and choice of antimicrobial agents for acute otitis media. [Review] [27 refs]. *Pediatric Annals* 2002;31(12):794-799.

19. Carbonell R, Ruiz-Garcia V. Ventilation tubes after surgery for otitis media with effusion or acute otitis media and swimming. Systematic review and meta-analysis. [Review] [24 refs]. *International Journal of Pediatric Otorhinolaryngology* 2002;66(3):281-289.

20. Ford-Jones EL, Friedberg J, McGeer A et al. Microbiologic findings and risk factors for antimicrobial resistance at myringotomy for tympanostomy tube placement—a prospective study of 601 children in Toronto. *International Journal of Pediatric Otorhinolaryngology* 2002;66(3):227-242.

21. Tarantino V, D'Agostino R, Taborelli G et al. Acute mastoiditis: a 10 year retrospective study. *International Journal of Pediatric Otorhinolaryngology* 2002;66(2):143-148.

22. Redaelli de Zinis LO, Gamba P, Balzanelli C. Acute otitis media and facial nerve paralysis in adults. *Otology & Neurotology* 2003;24(1):113-117.

23. Agarwal A, Lowry P, Isaacson G. Natural history of sigmoid sinus thrombosis. *Annals of Otology, Rhinology & Laryngology* 2003;112(2):191-194.

CHOLESTEATOMA

Definition

- Accumulation of keratinizing debris arising from a squamous epithelial lining (matrix) within the middle ear or other pneumatized areas of the temporal bone.
- Congenital, primary acquired, or secondary acquired.

Congenital cholesteatoma

- Epidermoid cyst behind an intact TM.
- No retraction pockets.
- No otorrhea or perforation.
- No previous ear surgery.
- No external canal atresia.
- Prior bouts of OM not grounds for exclusion.

Presentation

- Presents as a white mass behind an intact TM, usually in anterosuperior quadrant.
  - Incidental, noted on otoscopy (two thirds) with no other findings.
  - Persistent OME.
  - Hearing loss.
  - Other complications more uncommon .

Epidemiology

- Male:female ratio: 3:1.
- Mean age: 4.5 years.

Etiology

- Epidermoid rest (Michael's body) at distal end of eustachian tube normally involutes during development.

Treatment

- Wide tympanotomy: may need to remove TM from malleus to access anterosuperior quadrant.
- Mastoidectomy if large.

Acquired cholesteatoma

- Primary acquired
  - Retraction pocket may form in posterosuperior quadrant or directly superior into attic. Retraction pocket typically initially forms in Prussak's space, a space formed between the pars flaccida laterally and the neck of the malleus medially.
- Secondary acquired
  - Epithelial migration through perforation or implantation post-trauma or post-surgery.

Cholesteatoma growth

- Local expansion via accumulation of desquamated keratin.
- Growth promoted by infection and inflammation.

- Erosion of bone as growth progresses through secretion of lytic enzymes, inflammatory mediators, pressure necrosis.

Complications

- CHL secondary to bone erosion.
- Facial paralysis: treated with mastoidectomy, facial nerve decompression.
- Perilabyrinthine fistula: typically forms because of erosion of cholesteatoma into lateral canal. Presents with vertigo and/or SNHL. Treated with canal wall–down mastoidectomy with preservation of matrix over fistula or canal wall–up mastoidectomy with removal of matrix and patching of fistula with fascia.
- SNHL.
- Invasion of posterior or middle cranial fossa.
  - Complications as per AOM.

Treatment (see later section)

- Tympanomastoidectomy.
  - Canal wall up.
  - Canal wall down.
    - Types II-V.
- Radical mastoidectomy.

SURGERY FOR CHRONIC EAR DISEASE

Bilateral Myringotomy and Tubes

Indications

- Persistent otitis media with effusion (lasting greater than 3 months in a child)
- Chronic retraction and atelectasis
- Prophylaxis for barotraumas (e.g., hyperbaric oxygen treatment)
- Complications of otitis media (see above)

Contraindications

- Intratympanic fluid secondary to CSF leak.
- High jugular bulb or dehiscent carotid artery.
- Some authorities believe that OME secondary to radiation of the nasopharynx should not be treated with a tube because there is a high propensity for these ears to drain chronically.

Technique

- In adults, local anesthesia is used (phenol, EMLA cream, lidocaine injection). In children, general anesthesia is used.
- The myringotomy can be placed anterosuperiorly, anteroinferiorly, or posteroinferiorly. Few data exist that suggest that the position of the myringotomy makes a difference in terms of the longevity of the tube.
- A variety of tubes are available, and the choice of the tube is up to the surgeon. In general, long-shank

tubes are less prone to water contamination but are also more prone to becoming plugged by thicker secretions. Classic "T tubes" have long flanges that tend to erode the TM, leaving a large perforation. When long-term ventilation is required, a *subannular tube* may be preferential. In this procedure, a short, inferior tympanomeatal flap is raised; a groove is drilled or curetted in the posteroinferior aspect of the ear canal; and a long-shank tube is placed in the ear, with the flange in the middle ear and the shaft passing under the ear canal skin, exiting in the ear canal.

Complications

- *Hemorrhage:* usually minor and controlled by an epinephrine-soaked pledget. Any major hemorrhage would implicate a dehiscent carotid artery or high-rising jugular bulb. If the jugular bulb is violated, a tympanomeatal flap is elevated and the bleeding packed off with Gelfoam. If the carotid is cut, it is packed off with gauze packing and an emergency interventional radiology consult is obtained for angiogram. Angiogram will determine if the carotid is indeed violated and if the bleeding persists. Tolerance for occlusion of the carotid can also be determined. If the bleeding persists, a direct vascular repair may be required after the intratemporal carotid is drilled out.
- *Otorrhea:* minimal postoperative otorrhea is a common complication. In general, otorrhea should be treated with topical, nonototoxic drops. The value of "water precautions" to prevent infection has been questioned. Persistent otorrhea may require removal of the tube.
- *Persistent perforation:* approximately 1% of children having tubes will have a residual perforation requiring surgical repair.
- *Retained tube:* most tubes will fall out within 6-18 months. A tube that has been present for over 2 years in a patient whose contralateral ear has no recurrence of OME likely should removed and a myringoplasty performed.

Myringoplasty

Definition

- Repair of the TM without entering the middle ear space.

Indications

- Small perforation.

Contraindications

- None.

Technique

- The perforation is rimmed with trichloroacetic acid (TCA) or an otologic pick. A piece of cigarette paper or Steri-Strip is used to cover the perforation and serve as a template for an epithelial closure to take place.

Complications

- Failure.

Tympanoplasty

Definition

- Repair of the TM and/or the ossicular chain.

Indications

- Chronic perforation or retraction of the TM and/or the disruption of the ossicular chain secondary to infection, trauma, or neoplasm.

Contraindications

- There are no absolute contraindications. However, some ears defy repair, and thus multiple attempts at repair should be discouraged.

Technique

- Multiple techniques exist with no one technique demonstrating superiority. They can be divided as follows
  - **Approach**
    - *Transcanal* surgery involves incisions restricted to the ear canal and all the surgery performed through the ear canal. It offers the lowest morbidity but offers the most restricted access.
    - A *postauricular* approach involves an incision 5 mm off the postauricular crease as well as access to the ear canal and TM via an incision in the posterior ear canal.
    - *Endaural* incisions are less popular in North America. The incision is made from the ear canal through the cartilaginous incisura, between the tragus and the helix, and extended superiorly in a vertical line close to the helix.
  - **Graft material**
    - *Temporalis fascia* is the most common material used.
    - *Superficial areolar tissue,* lying lateral to the temporalis fascia, is a good alternative.
    - Other materials used include *perichondrium, cartilage,* or *pericranium.*
  - **Graft position**.
    - The position of the graft may be placed medial or lateral to the TM remnant.

○ In the *medial graft technique,* the perforation is rimmed, a tympanomeatal flap is elevated, the middle ear space is filled with Gelfoam, the graft is laid medial to TM remnant, and the tympanomeatal flap is returned to position.

○ In the *lateral graft technique,* a "vascular strip" of canal skin, located between the tympanomastoid and tympanosquamous suture lines, is back-elevated. The remaining skin of the medial ear canal is excised, and the anterior canal overhang is drilled away. The layer of squamous epithelium of the TM is elevated off the fibrous layer of the TM. The TM is then resurfaced by placing fascia on (lateral to) the fibrous TM, and the canal skin is then repositioned.

- The techniques just described are performed in isolation when the ossicular chain is intact. With the classic Wullstein definitions of tympanoplasty, these techniques would be referred to as a *Type 1* tympanoplasty. In a *Type 2* tympanoplasty, the graft is laid on the incus. The graft is laid on the stapes superstructure in a *Type 3* tympanoplasty and is placed into the oval window in a *Type 4* tympanoplasty. In a *Type 5a* tympanoplasty, which is currently not performed, the graft is laid over a lateral canal fenestration. In a *Type 5b* tympanoplasty, the graft is placed on a stapedectomy prosthesis. In general, Types 1, 3, and 4 tympanoplasties are currently performed procedures, with Types 3 and 4 tympanoplasties typically performed along with a mastoidectomy.

- *Ossicular reconstruction* can be performed with a variety of materials while replacing any or all of the ossicles. Currently, most prostheses are constructed of hydroxyapatite, hybrids of hydroxyapatite and Teflon, or titanium. Partial ossicular reconstruction prostheses (PORPs) may connect the TM and stapes superstructure, the malleus to the stapes superstructure, or a partially eroded incus to the stapes. A total ossicular reconstruction prosthesis (TORP) connects the TM to the oval window. When a prosthesis is run to the TM, a thin piece of cartilage is typically interfaced between the TM and the prosthesis head. Autogenous bone may also be fashioned into a prosthesis. Currently, this is most commonly performed when the incus is removed, reshaped, and interposed between the malleus and stapes superstructure *(incus interposition).*

Complications

- Failure of graft to close the perforation. Primary Type 1 tympanoplasties are generally successful in 90%-95% of cases. Success rates are reduced by 10% in revision cases. Active drainage at the time of tympanoplasty does not affect success rates.
- Failure to resolve the conductive hearing loss. *Tympanosclerosis* within the middle ear, resulting in fixation of the ossicles, is a common and typically irreversible cause of conductive hearing loss. Fibrous scarring of the ossicles and the failure to recognize an ossicular discontinuity are other causes of persistent conductive hearing loss. Lateral graft technique is prone to *"blunting,"* a process in which a thick scar is formed at the junction of the anterior TM and the ear canal, obliterating the anterior tympanic angle and restricting TM motion. Results of PORPs and TORPs vary widely. In general, PORPs achieve a superior hearing result compared with TORPs. A PORP can achieve a near-perfect closure of the air-bone gap, whereas a TORP will not achieve better than a 20-dB closure.
- Infection.
- Hemorrhage.
- Alteration in taste caused by damage to the chorda tympani.
- Facial paralysis (rare).
- SNHL.
- Vertigo/imbalance.
- Secondary acquired cholesteatoma caused by retained squamous epithelium medial to the graft; more common in lateral graft techniques.

Mastoidectomy (Cortical Mastoidectomy)

Definition

- Exenteration of the mastoid air cells, leaving the external canal wall intact.

Indications

- Acute coalescent mastoiditis.
- Chronic otitis media with chronic mastoiditis manifested by purulent otorrhea refractory to medical treatment.
- As an initial step for more aggressive mastoidectomy and skull base approaches.

Contraindications

- There are no absolute contraindications; however, care must be taken prior to this procedure in an ear that is congenitally malformed or in a mastoid that manifests a significant degree of osteoneogenesis secondary to chronic infection.

Technique

- Typically performed via a postauricular approach.
  □ The mastoid cortex is removed.

- □ Koerner's septum (junction between squamous and mastoid portions of the temporal bone) is opened.
- □ The antrum is opened, revealing the lateral SCC and the incus.
- □ The tegmen is skeletonized and the epitympanum is opened, exposing the malleal-incudal joint.
- □ The sigmoid sinus is identified.
- □ The sinodural (Citelli's) angle is opened.
- □ The digastric ridge is identified.
- □ The remaining air cells inferior to the labyrinth and posterior to the facial nerve are opened.

Complications

- ▪ Infection.
- ▪ Hemorrhage: if from the sigmoid sinus, control with bone wax or Gelfoam covered by a cottonoid.
- ▪ Hearing loss (conductive or sensorineural).
- ▪ Vertigo/imbalance (if lateral canal is entered).
- ▪ Facial paralysis: wait for several hours to ensure that it is not due to injection of lidocaine. If it does not resolve, decompression and repair (reanastomosis or graft with greater auricular nerve) is indicated.
- ▪ Altered taste.

Facial Recess Approach (Posterior Tympanotomy)

- ▪ The facial recess is a triangular space bound anteriorly and inferiorly by the chorda tympani, superiorly by the incus bridge, and posteriorly by the facial nerve.

Indications

- ▪ The facial recess is opened:
  - □ During canal wall–up surgery for removal of cholesteatoma.
  - □ For cochlear implant insertion.
  - □ For removal of certain middle ear tumors (e.g., glomus tumors).

Contraindications

- ▪ If the disease process has already violated the external canal wall, there is no indication for a facial recess approach.

Technique

1. The facial nerve and the chorda tympani are identified using a high-speed drill along their vertical components in the mastoid.
2. Running from superior to inferior, the facial nerve is anteroinferior to the lateral canal, 2 mm anterior to the posterior canal, and anterior to the retrofacial air cells. It exits via the stylomastoid foramen. The stylomastoid foramen is identified in the mastoid by finding the digastric ridge and sweeping anteriorly along it.

3. The triangle is opened, beginning superiorly, using a small cutting burr.
4. Once opened, the incus, pyramidal eminence and stapedius tendon, stapes, oval window, promontory, and round window should be visible through the recess.

Complications

- ▪ Same as for canal wall–up mastoidectomy.

Modified Radical Mastoidectomy

- ▪ A modified radical mastoidectomy (MRM) creates a cavity that includes the mastoid and middle ear contents. A tympanoplasty is performed.

Indications

- ▪ Cholesteatoma.
- ▪ For certain tumors of the middle ear and mastoid.

Contraindications

- ▪ Tympanoplasty should not be undertaken if residual cholesteatoma is present.

Technique

- ▪ As per cortical mastoidectomy.
- ▪ Locate the descending portion of the facial nerve.
- ▪ Remove the posterior and superior portions of the ear canal to the level of the facial nerve.
- ▪ Reconstruct the middle ear with tympanoplasty with and without ossiculoplasty.
- ▪ Perform a meatoplasty to allow for adequate cleaning of the cavity.

Complications

- ▪ As per cortical mastoidectomy.

Radical Mastoidectomy

Indications

- ▪ Residual cholesteatoma that cannot be cleared from cavity (e.g., oval window penetration).
- ▪ As part of tumor surgery.

Technique

- ▪ As modified MRM, except that a tympanoplasty is not performed. The mucosa is stripped and the eustachian tube is plugged (mucosa, muscle, fascia).

Complications

- ▪ Same as for cortical mastoidectomy.

A note on canal wall–up vs. canal wall–down surgery for cholesteatoma: A prevalent misconception is that canal wall–up surgery offers a consistently better hearing result.

However, even the individual who developed canal wall–up surgery concedes that this is not the case. Hearing results depend on the degree of destruction caused by the cholesteatoma, not on whether the canal wall is taken down. The main differences between the techniques relate to recurrence rate (approximately 30% for canal wall up vs. < 5% for canal wall down) and the need for routine cavity maintenance and cleaning (not required for canal wall up) and activities such as swimming (more easily undertaken with canal wall up).

Otosclerosis

Definition
- Bony dysplasia of the temporal bone characterized by an initial resorptive phase (spongiosis) followed by a deposition phase (sclerosis).

Incidence
- Clinical
  - White: 1%.
  - African American: 0.1%.
  - Native Americans, Asians: approximately 0%.
- Pathologic
  - White: 10%.
  - African American: 1%.
- Female:male ratio
  - Clinical: 2:1.
  - Pathology: 1:1.
- Bilateral
  - >90%.
- Age
  - Onset between puberty and 40 years.

Etiology
- Genetic
  - Autosomal dominant with incomplete penetrance.
    - Penetrance = 20%-40%.
  - Genetic mutation linked to the *COL1A1* gene associated with the mild form of osteoneogenesis imperfecta.
- Measles virus
  - Viral material found in bone.
  - (?) Double hit: viral infection in the face of a genetic predisposition.

Pathology
- Disease of endochondral bone unique to the otic capsule.
- Three stages:
  - Stage 1 (spongiotic phase): osteoclast-mediated bone resorption with vascular basophilic connective tissue.
  - Stage 2: decreased vascularity with deposition of collagen and osteoid.
  - Stage 3 (sclerosis): bone deposition (acidophilic).

- Location
  - Fissula ante fenestram (70%-90%)
    - Anterior to oval window.
  - Spreads
    - Posteriorly across annular ligament to fix stapes.
    - Anteriorly to promontory.
    - Medially (vestibule): ? significance.
- Cochlear involvement
  - Degeneration of spiral ligament and stria vascularis in region of endosteal involvement.
  - OHC degeneration.
- Vestibular otosclerosis
  - Degeneration of vestibular nerve fibers
    - Not related to endosteal involvement of vestibular end organs.

Clinical presentation
- Otosclerosis is a disease in which the "patient hears nothing and physician sees nothing."
- History
  - Progressive hearing loss in young adult.
  - Usually begins in one ear.
  - Family history.
  - Vestibular complaints (20%).
- Physical examination
  - Schwartze's sign: red blush on promontory seen through the TM during the spongiotic phase.
  - Tuning forks: some debate exists as to whether a 256-Hz or a 512-Hz fork should be used. In general, the 512 Hz is more accurate because patients tend to respond to the vibrotactile components of the 256-Hz fork.
- Audiogram
  - Tympanogram = normal or As.
  - Acoustic reflex = absent. It is important to check reflexes in these patients. The presence of reflexes in the face of a significant conductive hearing loss is seen in fractures of the stapes distal to the insertion of the stapedius muscle and, importantly, in superior SCC dehiscence.
  - Pure conductive or mixed loss.
    - Carhart's notch is a "sensorineural" loss found predominantly at 2 kHz in patients with otosclerosis. It does not represent a true sensorineural loss but rather an artifact induced by footplate fixation. Stapedectomy will result in a resolution of the "sensorineural" loss, a phenomenon referred to as **overclosure.**

Differential diagnosis
- Congenital malleal fixation.
- Congenital stapes fixation.
  - Syndromal (bilateral, sex linked; DFN3; stapes fixation with gusher).
  - Sporadic.

- Tympanosclerosis (COM).
- Ossicular discontinuity (trauma).
- Superior SCC dehiscence.
- Rare: osteogenesis imperfecta (OI), Paget's disease.

Treatment

- Observation.
- Hearing amplification.
- Sodium fluoride: generally reserved for patients with significant progressive sensorineural component. Most commonly used formulation is Florical 1 tablet tid × 1 year.
- Surgery.
  - Stapedectomy vs. stapedotomy. A full stapedectomy was the originally described procedure. It is associated with a higher complication rate than a small fenestra stapedotomy. Options for fenestration include removing the posterior half of the footplate or creating a small hole in the footplate using a hand drill, low-speed electric drill, or laser (CO_2, argon, KTP).

Intraoperative complications

- Hemorrhage: pack with pledget soaked with 1:1000 epinephrine.
- Dislocated incus: options for treatment include aborting the procedure, completing the stapedectomy in hopes that the joint will re-adhere, or running the prosthesis from the malleus to the fenestra.
- Flap too short or TM perforated: graft with fascia or perichondrium.
- Floating footplate: abort procedure or use laser to fenestrate.
- Perilymph (CSF) gusher: pack oval window with perichondrium or fascia and elevate bed; a lumbar drain is rarely necessary. Most physicians would abort the procedure in the face of a gusher.
- Facial nerve dehiscence: most authorities would abort the procedure in the face of a dehiscence. Some have advocated transposing the nerve.

Postoperative complications

- Persistent vertigo (>3 days)
  - Benign positional vertigo (BPV): treat with Epley maneuver.
  - Prosthesis too long (saccule): change the prosthesis.
  - Prosthesis too short (fistula): revise the procedure with a longer prosthesis and patch.
- Dysgeusia
- Sudden SNHL (1%).
- Otitis media.
- Facial paralysis: may be secondary to thermal injury from laser, direct trauma, or lidocaine injection.

Reexploration is indicated only if direct trauma to the nerve is considered likely.

- Reparative granuloma: seen 7-10 days postsurgery; was more common when full stapedectomies were routinely performed, particularly when Gelfoam was used as a patch. It is an inflammation resulting in granuloma formation on the footplate, and it manifests with vertigo and hearing loss. Treatment includes the administration of corticosteroids and reexploration of the ear with removal of the granuloma.
- Tinnitus.
- TM perforation.
- Long-term failure rate is 5%-10%, usually because of a displaced prosthesis. Incus necrosis is the second most common cause. Other causes include closure of the fenestra in the absence of dislocation of the prosthesis and scar formation around the prosthesis.

Selected References from the Recent Literature

1. Battaglia AS, Sabri AN, Jackson CG. Management of chronic otitis media in the only hearing ear. *Laryngoscope* 2002;112(4):681-685.
2. Chen W, Campbell CA, Green GE *et al*. Linkage of otosclerosis to a third locus (OTSC3) on human chromosome 6p21.3-22.3. *Journal of Medical Genetics* 2002;39(7): 473-477.
3. Chole RA, Faddis BT. Evidence for microbial biofilms in cholesteatomas. *Archives of Otolaryngology—Head & Neck Surgery* 2002;128(10):1129-1133.
4. Chole RA, McKenna M. Pathophysiology of otosclerosis. [Review] [90 refs]. *Otology & Neurotology* 2001;22(2):249-257.
5. Copeland BJ, Buchman CA. Management of labyrinthine fistulae in chronic ear surgery. [Review] [38 refs]. *American Journal of Otolaryngology* 2003;24(1):51-60.
6. Cruz OL, Kasse CA, Leonhart FD. Efficacy of surgical treatment of chronic otitis media. *Otolaryngology—Head & Neck Surgery* 2003;128(2):263-266.
7. Daniels RL, Krieger LW, Lippy WH. The other ear: findings and results in 1,800 bilateral stapedectomies. *Otology & Neurotology* 2001;22(5):603-607.
8. De La CA, Fayad JN. Revision stapedectomy. *Otolaryngology—Head & Neck Surgery* 2000;123(6):728-732.
9. Elluru RG, Dhanda R, Neely JG *et al*. Anterior subannular T-tube for prolonged middle ear ventilation during tympanoplasty: evaluation of efficacy and complications. *Otology & Neurotology* 2001;22(6):761-765.
10. House HP, Hansen MR, Al Dakhail AA *et al*. Stapedectomy versus stapedotomy: comparison of results with long-term follow-up. *Laryngoscope* 2002;112(11):2046-2050.
11. Koltai PJ, Nelson M, Castellon RJ *et al*. The natural history of congenital cholesteatoma. *Archives of Otolaryngology—Head & Neck Surgery* 2002;128(7):804-809.
12. Liang J, Michaels L, Wright A. Immunohistochemical characterization of the epidermoid formation in the middle ear. *Laryngoscope* 2003;113(6):1007-1014.

13. Lippy WH, Berenholz LP, Burkey JM. Otosclerosis in the 1960s, 1970s, 1980s, and 1990s. *Laryngoscope* 1999;109(8):1307-1309.

14. Mallet Y, Nouwen J, Lecomte-Houcke M *et al*. Aggressiveness and quantification of epithelial proliferation of middle ear cholesteatoma by MIB1. *Laryngoscope* 2003;113(2):328-331.

15. McKenna MJ, Kristiansen AG, Tropitzsch AS. Similar COL1A1 expression in fibroblasts from some patients with clinical otosclerosis and those with type I osteogenesis imperfecta. *Annals of Otology, Rhinology & Laryngology* 2002;111(2):184-189.

16. Nadol JB, Jr. Histopathology of residual and recurrent conductive hearing loss after stapedectomy. *Otology & Neurotology* 2001;22(2):162-169.

17. Nelson M, Roger G, Koltai PJ *et al*. Congenital cholesteatoma: classification, management, and outcome. *Archives of Otolaryngology—Head & Neck Surgery* 2002;128(7):810-814.

18. Niedermeyer HP, Arnold W. Etiopathogenesis of otosclerosis. [Review] [50 refs]. *ORL; Journal of Otorhinolaryngology & Its Related Specialties* 2002;64(2):114-119.

19. O'Leary S, Veldman JE. Revision surgery for chronic otitis media: recurrent-residual disease and hearing. *Journal of Laryngology & Otology* 2002;116(12):996-1000.

20. Potsic WP, Samadi DS, Marsh RR *et al*. A staging system for congenital cholesteatoma. *Archives of Otolaryngology—Head & Neck Surgery* 2002;128(9):1009-1012.

21. Potsic WP, Korman SB, Samadi DS *et al*. Congenital cholesteatoma: 20 years' experience at The Children's Hospital of Philadelphia. *Otolaryngology—Head & Neck Surgery* 2002;126(4):409-414.

22. Ruckenstein MJ, Rafter KO, Montes M *et al*. Management of far advanced otosclerosis in the era of cochlear implantation. *Otology & Neurotology* 2001;22(4):471-474.

23. Sakagami M, Sone M, Tsuji K *et al*. Rate of recovery of taste function after preservation of chorda tympani nerve in middle ear surgery with special reference to type of disease. *Annals of Otology, Rhinology & Laryngology* 2003;112(1):52-56.

24. Shohet JA, de Jong AL. The management of pediatric cholesteatoma. [Review] [45 refs]. *Otolaryngologic Clinics of North America* 2002;35(4):841-851.

25. Stimmer H, Arnold W, Schwaiger M *et al*. Magnetic resonance imaging and high-resolution computed tomography in the otospongiotic phase of otosclerosis. *ORL; Journal of Otorhinolaryngology & Its Related Specialties* 2002;64(6):451-453.

26. Tokuriki M, Noda I, Saito T *et al*. Gene expression analysis of human middle ear cholesteatoma using complementary DNA arrays. *Laryngoscope* 2003;113(5):808-814.

27. Van Den BK, Govaerts PJ, De Leenheer EM *et al*. Otosclerosis: a genetically heterogeneous disease involving at least three different genes. *Bone* 2002; 30(4):624-630.

28. Van Den BK, Govaerts PJ, Schatteman I *et al*. A second gene for otosclerosis, OTSC2, maps to chromosome 7q34-36. *American Journal of Human Genetics* 2001;68(2):495-500.

29. Wang PC, Merchant SN, McKenna MJ *et al*. Does otosclerosis occur only in the temporal bone? *American Journal of Otology* 1999;20(2):162-165.

30. Yetiser S, Tosun F, Kazkayasi M. Facial nerve paralysis due to chronic otitis media. *Otology & Neurotology* 2002;23(4):580-588.

TEMPORAL BONE TRAUMA

Incidence
- Temporal bone fractures comprise 20% of all skull fractures.
- Inner ear is the sensory organ most frequently affected by severe head trauma.

Etiology
- Motor vehicle accidents (MVAs): 40%.
- Falls: 20%.
- Syncopal episodes, altercations, athletic injuries: approximately 10% each.

Pathology
- Traditional classification divides temporal bone fractures into longitudinal and transverse fractures.
  - *Longitudinal* (classically 70%-90%)
    - Result from blow to the temporoparietal region.
    - Run parallel to petrous ridge, through roof of external and middle ears.
    - Pass anterior to labyrinth.
    - Terminate in foramen lacerum or foramen spinosum.
  - *Transverse* (classically 10%-30%)
    - Generated by powerful blow to parietoccipital region or, less commonly, the frontal region.
    - Run perpendicular to the petrous ridge.
    - Begin in foramen magnum or jugular bulb.
    - Pass through the labyrinth or IAC.
    - Terminate in foramen lacerum or foramen spinosum.
- Although useful in explaining the clinical manifestations of temporal bone fractures, high-resolution CT scans of the temporal bone have revealed the majority of temporal bone fractures to be *mixed* or *oblique*.

Clinical manifestations and treatment
External ear
- Seen in longitudinal fractures.
- Lacerations of the external canal.
- Step deformities caused by bony displacement.
- No treatment is advocated for these pathologies at acute presentation, because probing may result in more extensive damage to surrounding structures (e.g., brain, middle ear).
- May be complicated by external canal stenosis.
  - This is generally treated with a meatoplasty with or without canaloplasty once the stenosis is stable. If severe disruption to the anterior ear canal (posterior TMJ) occurs, a canal wall–down mastoidectomy may be required to open the ear and prevent a cholesteatoma forming behind the stenosis.

Tympanic membrane
- Seen in longitudinal fractures.
- Most heal by 3 weeks.
- Persistent perforation may require tympanoplasty.

Middle ear
- Hemotympanum.
- Ossicular chain.
- Incus is the most vulnerable (fracture or dislocation), causing separation of the incudostapedial joint.
- Fracture of the stapes superstructure is the second most common pathology.
- The malleus is rarely affected.
- Transverse fractures may involve the stapes footplate, resulting in a perilymphatic fistula.
- Ossicular chain abnormalities are managed by ossiculoplasty performed once the patient and fracture have stabilized.
- If a disruption of the oval window is suspected based on CT scan results, an immediate exploration and patching of the oval window is advisable, if the patient is stable.

CSF leak
- Occurs in approximately 15% of temporal bone fractures.
- Results from a fracture in the tegmen and a laceration of the middle fossa dura.
- Will drain through the eustachian tube into the nose or into the external ear via a laceration in the TM.
- Treatment includes head rest, avoidance of straining, and a lumbar drain.
- Prophylactic antibiotics *are* indicated.
- Most resolve within 3 weeks.
- If CSF leaks fail to resolve, closure can be effected as follows:
  - Via a craniotomy and dural repair if the hearing is intact.
  - Via a mastoid obliteration and closure of the ear canal and eustachian tube if there is no residual hearing.
  - Some advocate a combined approach, with a dural repair, a repair of middle fossa floor with fascia and bone (harvested from the mastoid cortex) or cartilage (from the concha), and obliteration of the mastoid with fat. This approach can preserve hearing.

Inner ear
Auditory function
- A transverse fracture may cross the inner ear of IAC, resulting in profound hearing loss.
- A temporary, primarily high-frequency SNHL may seen as a result of concussive trauma.

Vestibular function

- Acute vertigo may result from an acute vestibular loss secondary to a labyrinthine fracture. This may not be obvious because these patients frequently suffer from altered levels of consciousness in the immediate post-traumatic period.
- Once patients have recovered their mental status, symptoms of a noncompensated vestibular loss (positional imbalance) may be present subsequent to an acute vestibular loss. Treatment is via vestibular rehabilitation physical therapy.
- Benign positional vertigo is a common sequela of head trauma.
- A perilymph fistula may occur, as noted previously.

Facial nerve

- Management of the facial nerve is the most controversial aspect of treatment of temporal bone fractures.
- Facial nerve paralysis occurs in 10%-30% of longitudinal fractures (perigeniculate region) and in a greater proportion of transverse fractures (perigeniculate, often just proximal to the geniculate ganglion in the intralabyrinthine segment).

Investigations

- Topognostic tests (lacrimation, stapedius reflex, taste, salivary flow) are unreliable and have been discarded as a method of determining site of lesion.

Electrical tests

- Electrical tests are performed by applying an electrical stimulus in the region of the stylomastoid foramen and observing or recording the resulting muscle contractions.
- The nerve excitability test (NET) is performed by determining the smallest current required to elicit any muscle contraction. It has largely been abandoned.
- The maximal stimulation test (MST) is performed by applying a supramaximal electrical stimulus and visually observing and comparing the muscle contractions elicited from the normal and affected sides. The contraction on the affected side is classified as 0%, 25%, 50%, 75%, or 100% of the control side.
- Electroneurography (ENOG) is essentially an electrically evoked electromyogram (EMG). The stimulus is the same as that used in MST, with the resulting compound action potential (CAP) recorded using a bipolar electrode placed in the nasolabial fold. The amplitude and latency of the CAPs recorded from the normal and affected sides can be quantified and compared.
- EMG is a useful tool. Any detectable motor units firing in response to volitional stimulation indicate

that the nerve is intact. Fibrillation potentials, present at 10-14 days postinjury, indicate neural degeneration. Polyphasic reinnervation potentials that appear 4-6 weeks after injury indicate neural recovery and may precede visible muscle contractions.

The following is a protocol for managing facial nerve paralysis resulting from blunt trauma to the temporal bone. This analysis is based on a critical review of the current literature.

- Any incomplete paralysis has an excellent prognosis and will not benefit from surgical exploration.
- Any delayed-onset complete paralysis has an excellent prognosis and will not benefit from surgical exploration.
- Any complete paralysis with retained ENOG activity (CAP of affected side >5%-10% of control) has a good prognosis for recovery and will not benefit from surgical exploration.
- Any complete paralysis with retained volitional EMG activity has an excellent prognosis, regardless of ENOG results, and will not benefit from surgical exploration.
- An immediate-onset, complete paralysis without ENOG or volitional EMG activity has a poor prognosis for recovery (best outcome = House-Brackmann 3-4/6), and *may* benefit from surgical exploration.
  - The decision to explore the patient must be based on the patient's overall medical condition and the results of the CT scan.
  - The CT scan may reveal the specific site of lesion, which then can be approached, decompressed, and grafted (greater auricular nerve) if necessary.
  - If there is no residual hearing, a translabyrinthine exploration is the safest and most direct method of exploration.
  - If hearing is intact, a combined transmastoid and middle fossa exploration is indicated, with particular attention to the intralabyrinthine segment.

Selected References from the Recent Literature

1. Lin TF, Huang YC, Wang PC. Isolated transverse transcochlear temporal bone fracture. *Otology & Neurotology* 2002;23(4):615-616.
2. Jager L, Reiser M. CT and MR imaging of the normal and pathologic conditions of the facial nerve. [Review] [33 refs]. *European Journal of Radiology* 2001;40(2):133-146.
3. Swartz JD. Temporal bone trauma. [Review] [8 refs]. *Seminars in Ultrasound, CT & MR* 2001;22(3):219-228.
4. Okizaki A, Shuke N, Aburano T *et al.* Detection of cerebrospinal fluid leak by dual-isotope spect with In-111 DTPA and Tc-99m HMDP. *Clinical Nuclear Medicine* 2001;26(7): 628-629.

5. Vrabec JT. Otic capsule fracture with preservation of hearing and delayed-onset facial paralysis. *International Journal of Pediatric Otorhinolaryngology* 2001;58(2):173-177.

6. Harrison SE, Anand VK. Pediatric temporal bone fractures. *Annals of Otology, Rhinology & Laryngology* 2000;109(10 Pt 1):988-990.

7. Li ST, Baxter AB. Traumatic ossicular disruption. *AJR American Journal of Roentgenology* 2000;174(5):1296.

8. Jones RM, Rothman MI, Gray WC *et al.* Temporal lobe injury in temporal bone fractures.[comment]. *Archives of Otolaryngology—Head & Neck Surgery* 2000;126(2):131-135.

NOISE-INDUCED HEARING LOSS (NIHL)

Definition
- NIHL: auditory deficit induced by chronic noise exposure.
- Acoustic trauma: auditory deficit sustained secondary to exposure to an acute, explosive noise trauma.

Incidence and epidemiology
- NIHL affects approximately 2% of the population.
- Male > female.
- Offending chronic noise exposure may be:
  - Industrial.
  - Recreational
    - Firearms.
    - Lawn care.
    - Hobbies (e.g., woodworking).
- Examples of acoustic trauma include:
  - Gunshot.
  - Bomb explosion.
  - Note: There is little to no evidence that personal stereos/CD players cause NIHL.
- OSHA standards for permissible chronic noise exposures are listed in Table 4.
- Acoustic trauma generally occurs at intensities > 110-120 dB.
- Individuals possess different sensitivities to noise trauma. This may be due in part to underlying disease states that *may* predispose to sensitivity to acoustic trauma. Such disease states include:
  - Diabetes mellitus.
  - Hyperlipidemia.
- Concurrent administration of ototoxins may predispose to increased sensitivity to acoustic trauma.

TABLE 4. OSHA Standards for Permissible Chronic Noise Exposures

Duration (hr)	Intensity (dBA)*
16	85
8	90
6	92
4	95
3	97
2	100
1.5	102
1	105
0.5	110
0.25	115

*High-frequency sounds are more damaging to the ear than lower-frequency sounds. Sound pressure level meters that measure environmental noise are equipped with a filter that decreases the importance of the lower frequencies of sound, resulting in the dBA sound intensity scale.

- People with darker skin pigmentation may experience less NIHL than people with lighter pigmentation.

Pathophysiology
Temporary threshold shift (TTS)
- A TTS is a reversible SNHL that resolves 24-72 hours after noise exposure.
- There are no morphologic correlates to the TTS.
- TTS appears to result from a temporary loss of hair cell stereociliar stiffness.
  - Maintenance of normal stereociliar stiffness is an energy-dependent process. Noise exposure resulting in TTS results in a temporary exhaustion of energy supplies (ATP) that can be reversed once the individual is extricated from the noise exposure.
- Other evidence suggests that a TTS may result from an uncoupling of the stereocilia from tectorial membrane

Permanent threshold shift (PTS)
- PTS presumably results from an irreversible exhaustion of hair cell metabolic processes.
- Stereocilia of OHCs are more sensitive than those of IHCs, with loss of stereocilia being followed by cell death. A secondary deafferentation and Wallerian degeneration of the VIIIth nerve afferents occurs.
- Some evidence exists that noise may also be primarily toxic to the afferent fibers.
- After hair cell death, supporting cells produce a cellular "scar" in the region of the hair cells.
- Avian and lower animal species have shown the ability to regenerate their hair cells after noise exposure. This has not been demonstrated in mammalian cells.

Acoustic trauma
- An acoustic trauma may result in physical disruption of the cochlea, including the organ of Corti, the tectorial membrane, and Reissner's membrane.

Clinical manifestations
- Tinnitus will often be the patient's first complaint.
- Hearing loss may be an initial manifestation or may only become clinically apparent after the onset of presbycusis.
- Audiometric findings reveal a SNHL that is maximal at 4 kHz (the 4-kHz notch). The hearing loss will spread to the higher and then lower frequencies as the noise exposure continues.
- The hearing loss should be symmetric in most situations. However, patients with asymmetric noise exposure (e.g., gun shooters, truck drivers) may show an asymmetric hearing loss.

- Hearing loss from noise exposure rarely exceeds 75 dB in the high frequencies and 40 dB in the low frequencies.
  - After cessation of noise exposure, the hearing loss should not progress.
  - An acoustic trauma may result in a profound hearing loss.

Investigations

- Audiometric assessment is typically the only test required in the patient suffering from NIHL.
- An MRI with paramagnetic enhancement is indicated in patients with asymmetric SNHL.

Treatment

- Hearing conservation program at work.
- Earplugs or earmuffs for any noise exposure.
- Hearing aid assessment.

Selected References from the Recent Literature

1. Niu X, Canlon B. Activation of tyrosine hydroxylase in the lateral efferent terminals by sound conditioning. *Hearing Research* 2002;174(1-2):124-132.
2. Ohinata Y, Miller JM, Schacht J. Protection from noise-induced lipid peroxidation and hair cell loss in the cochlea. *Brain Research* 2003;966(2):265-273.
3. Hamernik RP, Qiu W, Davis B. Cochlear toughening, protection, and potentiation of noise-induced trauma by non-Gaussian noise. *Journal of the Acoustical Society of America* 2003;113(2):969-976.
4. Chen GD. Effect of hypoxia on noise-induced auditory impairment. *Hearing Research* 2002;172(1-2):186-195.
5. Wang J, Ding D, Salvi RJ. Functional reorganization in chinchilla inferior colliculus associated with chronic and acute cochlear damage. [Review] [69 refs]. *Hearing Research* 2002;168(1-2):238-249.
6. Wang Y, Hirose K, Liberman MC. Dynamics of noise-induced cellular injury and repair in the mouse cochlea. *Journal of the Association for Research in Otolaryngology: JARO* 2002;3(3):248-268.
7. Kopke RD, Coleman JK, Liu J et al. Candidate's thesis: enhancing intrinsic cochlear stress defenses to reduce noise-induced hearing loss. *Laryngoscope* 2002;112(9): 1515-1532.
8. Wang Y, Hirose K, Liberman MC. Dynamics of noise-induced cellular injury and repair in the mouse cochlea. *Journal of the Association for Research in Otolaryngology: JARO* 2002;3(3):248-268.
9. Hsu CJ, Chen YS, Shau WY et al. Impact of activities of Na(+)-K(+)-ATPase and Ca2(+)-ATPase in the cochlear lateral wall on recovery from noise-induced temporary threshold shift. *Annals of Otology, Rhinology & Laryngology* 2002;111(9):842-849.
10. Lefebvre PP, Malgrange B, Lallemend F et al. Mechanisms of cell death in the injured auditory system: otoprotective strategies. *Audiology & Neuro-Otology* 2002;7(3):165-170.
11. Toppila E, Pyykko I, Starck J. Age and noise-induced hearing loss. *Scandinavian Audiology* 2001;30(4):236-244.
12. Hamernik RP, Qiu W. Energy-independent factors influencing noise-induced hearing loss in the chinchilla model. *Journal of the Acoustical Society of America* 2001;110(6): 3163-3168.
13. Kaygusuz I, Ozturk A, Ustundag B et al. Role of free oxygen radicals in noise-related hearing impairment. *Hearing Research* 2001;162(1-2):43-47.
14. Bartels S, Ito S, Trune DR et al. Noise-induced hearing loss: the effect of melanin in the stria vascularis. *Hearing Research* 2001;154(1-2):116-123.
15. Davis RR, Newlander JK, Ling X et al. Genetic basis for susceptibility to noise-induced hearing loss in mice. *Hearing Research* 2001;155(1-2):82-90.

OTOTOXICITY

Aminoglycosides

Clinical Manifestations

All aminoglycosides have the potential for both cochlear and vestibular toxicity.

- Cochleotoxicity > vestibulotoxity:
  - Amikacin.
  - Kanamycin.
  - Dihydrostreptomycin.
- Vestibulotoxicity > cochleotoxicity:
  - Gentamicin.
  - Streptomycin.
- Vestibulotoxicity = cochleotoxicity:
  - Tobramycin.

Note: Netilmicin may be the least ototoxic of all the aminoglycosides.

- Patients with cochleotoxicity will typically present with high-frequency hearing loss and tinnitus.
- Patients with vestibulotoxicity will typically present with imbalance. Symptoms of a bilateral vestibular loss (Dandy's syndrome), including oscillopsia and imbalance. are particularly devastating.
- Individuals vary in their sensitivity to aminoglycoside ototoxicity:
  - Carriers of a specific mitochondrial gene mutation are particularly prone to aminoglycoside ototoxicity.
  - Other factors that predispose to aminoglycoside (AG) toxicity include:
    - Age extremes.
    - Prolonged use.
    - Coadministration of other ototoxins: loop diuretics, vancomycin.
    - Elevation of peak/trough levels.
    - Febrile state.
    - Renal failure.
    - Liver failure.

Pathology

- AGs result in hair cell death.
- In the cochlea:
  - OHC > IHC.
  - Base > apex.

Pathophysiology

- Ototoxic effects are mediated by free radicals.
- AGs generation of free radicals appears to depend on the chelation of the aminoglycoside to Fe. When AGs are administered systemically, this chelation is performed by the liver.

Chemoprotection

- In animal models, chemoprotection against AG ototoxicity is afforded by:
  - Fe-chelators-deferoxamine, salicylic acid.
  - Free-radical scavengers or inhibitors of free-radical formation:
    - Growth factors, neurotrophins.
    - D-methionine.
    - Caspase inhibitors.

Vancomycin

- Vancomycin mainly serves to potentiate the ototoxicity of other ototoxic agents (e.g., coadministration of vancomycin and an aminoglycoside).
- Given alone at therapeutic levels, vancomycin does not seem to pose a risk of ototoxicity.

Erythromycin

- Cochleotoxicity is associated with high-dose intravenous administration (>4 g/day) and is generally reversible with the discontinuation of the drug.
- The site of lesion is unknown. The stria vascularis and the central auditory pathways have been implicated.

Loop diuretics (furosemide, bumetanide, ethacrynic acid)

- May cause tinnitus and hearing in loss at high doses.
- Site of lesion: the stria vascularis (edema and degeneration).
- More dangerous as a potentiator of ototoxic effects of other drugs (e.g., aminoglycosides)
- May produce irreversible ototoxicity in the neonatal population.

Cisplatin

Clinical presentation

- Primarily cochleotoxic.
- Patients present with tinnitus and high-frequency hearing loss.
- Profound hearing loss possible.
- Increased ototoxicity seen in patients with:
  - High individual dose.
  - High cumulative dose.
  - Age extremes.
  - Dehydration.
  - Renal failure.
  - Concurrent or past cranial radiation.
  - Coadministration of other ototoxic agents.

Pathology

- Sites of lesion are the stria vascularis and sensory hair cells.
- Hair cells:
  - Base > apex.
  - OHC > IHC.

Pathophysiology

- Cisplatin results in free radical formation within the cochlea, which appears to cause the ototoxicity.

Chemoprevention

- Clinical human and animal experimental studies have demonstrated that a variety of agents can exert chemoprotective effects, largely by preventing free radical formation.
- Such agents include:
  - Thiosulfate.
  - Diethyldithiocarbamate.
  - Glutathione.
  - D-methionine.
  - Ebselen.

Carboplatin

- Less nephrotoxic and cochleotoxic than cisplatin.
- May cause cochleotoxicity at high doses.
- Appears to preferentially affect IHCs rather than OHCs.

Salicylates

- Although any of the NSAIDs can cause ototoxicity, the salicylates are much more prone than any other of these compounds to result in inner ear pathology.
- Salicylates are primarily cochleotoxic.
- Patients will present with tinnitus and, rarely, a flat SNHL.
- The cochleotoxic effects are generally reversible.
- Cochleotoxicity is directly related to unbound salicylate serum levels.
- There are no observable morphologic changes attributable to salicylate cochleotoxicity.
- The pathophysiologic affects of salicylates may be attributable to a reduction in stiffness of the lateral portion of the cell membrane of OHCs.

Quinine

- Quinine may cause reversible tinnitus, hearing loss, and vertigo.
- The site of lesion is not known.
- Treatment is by discontinuation of the drug.

Selected References from the Recent Literature

1. McFadden SL, Ding D, Jiang H *et al*. Chinchilla models of selective cochlear hair cell loss. *Hearing Research* 2002; 174(1-2):230-238.
2. Bodmer D, Brors D, Pak K *et al*. Gentamicin-induced hair cell death is not dependent on the apoptosis receptor Fas. *Laryngoscope* 2003;113(3):452-455.
3. Hilton M, Chen J, Kakigi A *et al*. Middle ear instillation of gentamicin and streptomycin in chinchillas: electrophysiological appraisal of selective ototoxicity. *Clinical Otolaryngology & Allied Sciences* 2002;27(6):529-535.
4. Plontke SK, Wood AW, Salt AN. Analysis of gentamicin kinetics in fluids of the inner ear with round window administration. *Otology & Neurotology* 2002;23(6):967-974.
5. Hellier WP, Wagstaff SA, O'Leary SJ *et al*. Functional and morphological response of the stria vascularis following a sensorineural hearing loss. *Hearing Research* 2002;172 (1-2):127-136.
6. Kalkandelen S, Selimoglu E, Erdogan F *et al*. Comparative cochlear toxicities of streptomycin, gentamicin, amikacin and netilmicin in guinea-pigs. *Journal of International Medical Research* 2002;30(4):406-412.
7. Becvarovski Z, Bojrab DI, Michaelides EM *et al*. Round window gentamicin absorption: an in vivo human model. *Laryngoscope* 2002;112(9):1610-1613.
8. Cunningham LL, Cheng AG, Rubel EW. Caspase activation in hair cells of the mouse utricle exposed to neomycin. *Journal of Neuroscience* 2002;22(19):8532-8540.
9. Wu WJ, Sha SH, Schacht J. Recent advances in understanding aminoglycoside ototoxicity and its prevention. *Audiology & Neuro-Otology* 2002;7(3):171-174.
10. Matsui JI, Ogilvie JM, Warchol ME. Inhibition of caspases prevents ototoxic and ongoing hair cell death. *Journal of Neuroscience* 2002;22(4):1218-1227.

CONGENITAL AND GENETIC SENSORINEURAL HEARING LOSS

Etiology
- Congenital
  - 50% Genetic.
  - 50% Acquired.
- Childhood
  - 50% Genetic.
  - 20%-25% Acquired.
  - 25%-30% Unknown.

Genetic
- 75% Nonsyndromal.
- 25% Syndromal.
- 75% Autosomal recessive.
- 20%-25% Autosomal dominant.
- 1%-2% X-linked.
- Rare: Mitochondrial.

Autosomal recessive
- "Horizontal pattern."
- Monogenic, 25% risk to offspring.
- Severe to profound SNHL, prelingual onset.
- **Nonsyndromal**
  - DFNB, with number designating the phenotype (e.g., DFNB1).
- **Syndromal**
- **Usher syndrome**
  - Retinitis pigmentosa (RP): early diagnosis with electroculogram.
  - Retinal degeneration with pigment deposition on retinal examination.
  - Night blindness > field cut > central blindness.
  - SNHL.
- **Four types**
  - **Type I**
    - Profound SNHL with no vestibular function.
    - Onset of RP early in childhood.
    - Results from production of an *atypical myosin (myosin 7A)* that interferes with mechanoelectrical transduction within labyrinthine hair cells.
  - **Type II**
    - Congenital sloping SNHL.
    - Normal vestibular function.
    - RP onset in teens.
  - **Type III**
    - Progressive SNHL and vestibular dysfunction.
    - Vestibulocerebellar ataxia.
  - **Type IV**
    - Mental retardation and hypotonia.
- **Pendred**
  - May be responsible for up to 10% of hereditary hearing loss.
  - Nontoxic goiter that may appear at birth, in childhood, or after puberty.
  - Typically euthyroid.
  - Congenital profound SNHL.
  - Associated with Mondini malformations and enlarged vestibular aqueduct syndrome.
  - Can be diagnosed using the perchlorate challenge test.
  - Gene mutation affects the production of pendrin, a molecule that has a role in the regulation of Cl-I transport.
- **Jervell and Lange Nielsen syndrome**
  - Congenital profound SNHL.
  - Prolonged QT interval and syncope.
  - Gene mutation = KVKQT1 = abnormal K + channel involved in repolarization.

Autosomal dominant
- "Vertical pattern."
- Offspring risk: 50%.
- Variable penetrance and expressivity.
- More commonly presents with postlingual hearing loss. The hearing loss may be moderate to profound and is generally progressive.
- **Nonsyndromal**
  - DFNA, with number designating phenotype (e.g., DFNA1).
- **Syndromal**
  - **Waardenburg's syndrome**
    - Autosomal dominant with variable expressivity.
    - **Type 1**
      - Dystopia canthorum.
      - Synophrys.
      - Broad prominent nasal root.
      - Heterochromia of the iris.
      - White forlock.
      - Vitiligo.
      - Pigmentary changes of the fundus.
      - Associated with mutations in the PAX3 gene (2q35) that are important in embryonic neural development
    - **Type 2**
      - 20% of Waardenburg's.
      - Similar to Type I but does not manifest with dystopia canthorum.
      - Hearing loss: more common but less severe in Type II.
      - Not associated with PA3 mutations, but rather with MITF mutation.
    - **Type 3 (severe variant)**
      - Unilateral ptosis and multiple skeletal abnormalities.
      - Also associated with PAX3 mutations.
    - **Type 4**
      - Similar to Type 2+ Hirschsprung's disease (aganglionic megacolon).

- **Treacher Collins syndrome**
  - Mandibulofacial dysostosis.
  - Hypoplasia of mandible and facial bones.
  - Downsloping palpebral fissures.
  - Atretic external and middle ear.
  - Mixed hearing loss.
  - Cleft palate (35%).
  - Gene mutation located on chromosome 5q; mutant gene *TCOF1* codes for a transport protein that shuttles between the nucleolus and cytoplasm.
- **Alport's syndrome**
  - Autosomal dominant or X-linked.
  - Progressive glomerulonephritis and SNHL.
  - Some ocular pathology.
  - Six types.
  - Autosomal dominant form accounts for 20% of cases of Alport's syndrome (see below).
- **Stickler's syndrome**
  - Tall, thin body habitus.
  - Severe myopia (retinal detachment).
  - Flat midface.
  - Hypermobile joints.
  - Progressive SNHL: 80%.
- **Neurofibromatosis Type 2 (NF2)**
  - Defined by the presence of:
    - Bilateral acoustic neuromas, or
    - A first-degree relative with NF2 and a unilateral acoustic neuroma, or
    - A first-degree relative with NF2 and two of the following:
      - Neurofibroma.
      - Meningioma.
      - Glioma.
      - Schwannoma.
      - Juvenile posterior subcapsular lenticular opacity
  - Gene mutation is located at 22q12 and represents a mutation in a tumor suppressor gene.
- **Branchio-oto-renal syndrome**
  - Branchial cleft cysts.
  - Preauricular pits.
  - Renal pathology: mild hypoplasia to bilateral aplasia.
  - Hearing loss.
    - Penetrance: 80%
    - Mixed: 50%.
    - Pure conductive: 30%.
    - Pure SNHL: 20%.

X-linked
- Only males affected; females are carriers.
- **Nonsyndromal**
  - DFN, with number designating the phenotype (e.g., DFN1).

- **Syndromal**
  - **Alport's syndrome**
    - 80% X-linked.
    - Hearing loss and glomerulonephritis.
    - Results from gene mutations in specific collagens, leading to abnormal basement membrane formation.
    - Associated with mutation in the collagen gene COL4A5.
  - **Otopalatal-digital**
    - May present with prelingual or postlingual deafness
  - **DFN3** = Mixed hearing loss with stapes fixation and stapes "gusher" during stapedectomy.

Mitochondrial
- Carried by oocyte, therefore follows maternal line.
- Affected females produce affected males and females.
- Affected males produce normal progeny.
- Generally presents with postlingual hearing loss, associated with systemic metabolic disorders such as myopathies, aminoglycoside sensitivity.
- Examples of mitochondrial syndromes that include hearing loss are:
  - MELAS: Mitochondrial encephalopathy, lactic acidosis, and strokelike syndrome.
  - MIDD: Maternally inherited diabetes and deafness.

Acquired
Prenatal
- **Infection**
- Congenital cytomegalovirus (CMV)
  - 1%-2% of live births.
  - 90% asymptomatic (10% hearing loss).
  - Cytomegalovirus inclusion disease (CID) (50% hearing loss).
- Rubella
  - First- or second-trimester infection.
  - Cataracts, heart, hearing loss.
- Toxoplasmosis
- Syphilis
  - Menigoneurlabyritnhitis (profound SNHL).
- *Herpes simplex* encephalitis.

Teratogens
- Alcohol.
- Thalidomide.
- Radiation.
- Aminoglycosides.

Perinatal
- Severe perinatal disease
  - NICU admission.
  - Hypoxia.
  - Kernicterus.

❑ Persistent fetal circulation.

❑ Hypoxia.

Postnatal

- Meningitis
  ❑ Results in a suppurative labyrinthitis.
  ❑ Causes 25% of severe to profound cases of hearing loss in children.
  ❑ Results in progressive ossification of the labyrinth that may impair cochlear implant placement.
  ❑ Bacteria: *S. pneumoniae, H. influenzae, Neisseria meningitidis, Escherichia coli* (neonatal).
  ❑ Decrease incidence and severity of hearing loss with concomitant administration of systemic corticosteroids.
- Viral infection.
- Ototoxin: most commonly seen as a complication of chemotherapy.
- Trauma (acoustic, blunt, penetrating).
- Perilymph fistula (PLF).
- Neoplasm.
  ❑ Medulloblastoma, acoustic neuroma, fibrous dysplasia, histiocytosis.
- Autoimmune (rare in children).

Congenital anomalies of the labyrinth

- Congenital anomalies may involve the:
  ❑ Membranous labyrinth.
  ❑ Osseous and membranous labyrinth.
- Etiology is either genetic or teratogenic.

Membranous

- *Complete dysplasia of labyrinth*
  ❑ Rare.
  ❑ Also known as Bing Siebenmann.
  ❑ Associated with the following syndromes: Jervell and Lange-Nielsen, Usher
- *Cochleosaccular (Schiebe)*
  ❑ Most common inner ear anomaly.
- *Basal turn anomaly (Alexander)*
  ❑ High-frequency hearing loss.

Membranous and osseous

- *Complete Aplasia (Michel)*
  ❑ Rare, associated with thalidomide exposure.
  ❑ Must be differentiated from acquired labyrinthitis ossificans.
- *Hypoplasia (small bud of cochlea).*
- *Incomplete partition (Mondini)*
  ❑ Most common cochlear anomaly.
  ❑ Fewer turns, interscalar septum incomplete.
- *Common cavity.*

Labyrinthine

- *Superior SCC or lateral SCC dysplasia.*

❑ Frequently associated with cochlear dysplasia.

- *SCC aplasia (rare).*

Aqueduct and IAC

- *Enlarged vestibular aqueduct*
  ❑ Most common anomaly identified on CT.
  ❑ Defined by a diameter of the aqueduct >2 mm at midpoint.
  ❑ Associated with progressive cochleovestibular loss.
  ❑ No treatment available to abort progressive loss.
- *IAC*
  ❑ Widened canal significant if associated with stapes fixation.
  ❑ Narrow, absent VIIIth nerve.

Selected References from the Recent Literature

1. Smith RJ, Hone S. Genetic screening for deafness. [Review] [70 refs]. *Pediatric Clinics of North America* 2003;50(2): 315-329.
2. Petersen MB. Non-syndromic autosomal-dominant deafness. [Review] [127 refs]. *Clinical Genetics* 2002;62(1): 1-13.
3. Li XC, Friedman RA. Nonsyndromic hereditary hearing loss. [Review] [49 refs]. *Otolaryngologic Clinics of North America* 2002;35(2):275-285.
4. Libby RT, Steel KP. The roles of unconventional myosins in hearing and deafness. [Review] [28 refs]. *Essays in Biochemistry* 2000;35:159-174.
5. Kenneson A, Van Naarden BK, Boyle C. GJB2 (connexin 26) variants and nonsyndromic sensorineural hearing loss: a HuGE review. [Review] [92 refs]. *Genetics in Medicine* 2002;4(4):258-274.
6. Resendes BL, Williamson RE, Morton CC. At the speed of sound: gene discovery in the auditory system. [Review] [101 refs]. *American Journal of Human Genetics* 2001;69(5): 923-935.
7. Rabionet R, Lopez-Bigas N, Arbones ML et al. Connexin mutations in hearing loss, dermatological and neurological disorders. [Review] [80 refs]. *Trends in Molecular Medicine* 2002;8(5):205-212.
8. Seidman MD, Ahmad N, Bai U. Molecular mechanisms of age-related hearing loss. [Review] [75 refs]. *Ageing Research Reviews* 2002;1(3):331-343.
9. Kemperman MH, Hoefsloot LH, Cremers CW. Hearing loss and connexin 26. [Review] [23 refs]. *Journal of the Royal Society of Medicine* 2002;95(4):171-177.
10. Hone SW, Smith RJ. Genetics of hearing impairment. [Review] [98 refs]. *Seminars in Neonatology* 2001;6(6): 531-541.
11. Petit C. Usher syndrome: from genetics to pathogenesis. [Review] [163 refs]. *Annual Review of Genomics & Human Genetics* 2001;2:271-297.
12. Petit C, Levilliers J, Hardelin JP. Molecular genetics of hearing loss. [Review] [373 refs]. *Annual Review of Genetics* 2001;35:589-646.
13. Tekin M, Arnos KS, Pandya A. Advances in hereditary deafness. [Review] [57 refs]. *Lancet* 2001;358(9287): 1082-1090.

14. Nadol JB, Jr., Merchant SN. Histopathology and molecular genetics of hearing loss in the human. [Review] [53 refs]. *International Journal of Pediatric Otorhinolaryngology* 2001;61(1):1-15.

15. Steel KP, Kros CJ. A genetic approach to understanding auditory function [comment]. [Review] [69 refs]. *Nature Genetics* 2001;27(2):143-149.

16. Kopp P. Pendred's syndrome and genetic defects in thyroid hormone synthesis. [Review] [93 refs]. *Reviews in Endocrine & Metabolic Disorders* 2000;1(1-2):109-121.

17. Grundfast KM, Siparsky N, Chuong D. Genetics and molecular biology of deafness. Update. [Erratum appears in *Otolaryngologic Clinics of North America* 2001 Jun;34(3): vii-viii]. [Review] [82 refs]. *Otolaryngologic Clinics of North America* 2000;33(6):1367-1394.

18. Hutchin TP, Cortopassi GA. Mitochondrial defects and hearing loss. [Review] [101 refs]. *Cellular & Molecular Life Sciences* 2000;57(13-14):1927-1937.

19. Lefebvre PP, Van De Water TR. Connexins, hearing and deafness: clinical aspects of mutations in the connexin 26 gene. [Review] [17 refs]. *Brain Research—Brain Research Reviews* 2000;32(1):159-162.

20. Van Camp G, Smith RJ. Maternally inherited hearing impairment. [Review] [33 refs]. *Clinical Genetics* 2000;57(6):409-414.

21. Kiernan AE, Steel KP. Mouse homologues for human deafness. [Review] [27 refs]. *Advances in Oto-Rhino-Laryngology* 2000;56:233-243.

22. Takasaki K, Balaban CD, Sando I. Histopathologic findings of the inner ears with Alport, Usher and Waardenburg syndromes. [Review] [42 refs]. *Advances in Oto-Rhino-Laryngology* 2000;56:218-232.

23. Usami S, Abe S, Akita J et al. Sensorineural hearing loss associated with the mitochondrial mutations. [Review] [25 refs]. *Advances in Oto-Rhino-Laryngology* 2000;56: 203-211.

24. Kelley PM, Cohn E, Kimberling WJ. Connexin 26: required for normal auditory function. [Review] [34 refs]. *Brain Research—Brain Research Reviews* 2000;32(1):184-188.

SUDDEN SENSORINEURAL HEARING LOSS

Definition

- Loss of >30 dB at three contiguous frequencies that develops within 3 days (strict definition)

Incidence and epidemiology

- 1/5000-10,000/year.
- Male = female.
- Majority of cases between 30-60 years of age.
- 90% Unilateral.

Pathology and pathogenesis

- Evidence supporting a viral etiology includes the following:
  - A variety of viruses can cause a hearing loss that mimics CMV (e.g., CMV, mumps, rubella, parvovirus, adenovirus, influenza).
  - Serologic studies of patients with sudden SNHL report an increase in titers of antibodies against a variety of viral agents; not seen in control populations.
  - A viral prodrome is documented in 25%-30% of cases.
  - Morphologic studies of temporal bones derived from patients with sudden SNHL display atrophy of the organ of Corti, stria vascularis, and tectorial membrane—changes that are similar to those seen in a viral labyrinthitis.
  - MRI scans with paramagnetic enhancement have shown enhancement of the cochlea in patients with sudden SNHL not seen in controls, implying an inflammatory etiology.
  - The beneficial response to corticosteroids also implicates an inflammatory pathology.
- The evidence for a vascular etiology is less compelling and includes the following:
  - Sudden SNHL occurs in cases of:
    - Sickle-cell anemia.
    - Waldenström's macroglobulinemia.
    - Systemic vasculitides.
    - Postcardiac bypass (presumably caused by micro-air embolus).
  - If the pathology was vascular, the apical region of the cochlea with the most tenuous blood supply should be affected most commonly. However, low-frequency hearing loss is *not* the most common manifestation of sudden SNHL (see below).
  - In addition, agents designed to increase cochlear blood supply have not been proved beneficial in the treatment of sudden SNHL.
- Theoretical evidence for rupture of the internal labyrinthine membranes being an etiology (see section on perilymph fistula).

Differential diagnosis

- Congenital
  - Osseous or bony-osseous abnormalities (e.g., Mondini deformity).
- Infection
  - Syphilis.
  - Lyme disease not definitely established as a mediator of hearing loss.
  - HIV (direct effects and opportunistic infections).
  - Bacterial meningitis more common in bilateral disease.
- Neoplasm
  - Acoustic neuroma.
  - Meningioma.
  - Cholesterol granuloma.
  - Cholesteatoma.
- Trauma
  - Barotrauma.
  - Blunt or penetrating trauma.
  - Noise.
- Ototoxins.
- Neurologic disorders
  - Multiple sclerosis (MS).
  - Basilar migraines.
- Psychogenic
  - Conversion disorder.
  - Malingering.

Clinical presentation

- Sudden hearing loss, often noticed upon awakening.
- Tinnitus.
- Vertigo: 40% of patients.

Investigations

- Audiometry
  - Flat (41%).
  - High frequency (29%).
  - Low frequency (17%).
  - Profound (13%).
- Evoked potential audiometry or otoacoustic emissions
  - Indicated when "pseudohypacusis" is suspected.
- Imaging
  - Indicated in all patients to rule out retrocochlear pathology.
- Blood tests
  - Complete blood cell count (CBC) with sedimentation rate.
  - Fluorescent treponemal antibody, absorbed test (FTA-ABS) or microhemagglutination-*Treponema pallidum* (MHA-TP) to rule out otosyphilis.
  - Lyme titers in endemic areas of questionable value.
  - HIV serology in at-risk patients.
  - Thyroid function tests and other metabolic studies (generally unrevealing).
- Lumbar puncture

❑ Indicated in cases of sudden or rapidly progressive BHL to rule out infectious or malignant process.

Treatment

- Corticosteroids (e.g., prednisone 40-60 mg/day × 1-2 weeks) is the only treatment of proven therapeutic efficacy.
- The addition of antiherpetic agents (valacyclovir, acyclovir) appears to have no benefit.
- Treatment with a variety of other agents—including carbogen gas, vasodilators, anticoagulants, antiplatelet drugs, and plasma expanders—have no proven benefit.

Prognosis

- Factors that implicate a poor prognosis for hearing recovery include:
  ❑ Patient age (the older patient has a poorer prognosis for recovery).
  ❑ The presence of vertigo.
  ❑ Severe to profound hearing loss.
- A better prognosis is seen in patients:
  ❑ With flat or midfrequency hearing losses.
  ❑ Who receive prompt administration of steroids.

Selected References from the Recent Literature

1. Nageris BI, Popovtzer A. Acoustic neuroma in patients with completely resolved sudden hearing loss. *Annals of Otology, Rhinology & Laryngology* 2003;112(5):395-397.
2. Fernandez CA, Carceller MA, Garcia JR *et al*. Sudden deafness as a manifestation of the rupture of a cerebral arteriovenous malformation. *Otolaryngology—Head & Neck Surgery* 2003;128(4):592-594.
3. Uri N, Doweck I, Cohen-Kerem R *et al*. Acyclovir in the treatment of idiopathic sudden sensorineural hearing loss. *Otolaryngology—Head & Neck Surgery* 2003;128(4):544-549.
4. Schattner A, Halperin D, Wolf D *et al*. Enteroviruses and sudden deafness. *CMAJ Canadian Medical Association Journal* 2003;168(11):1421-1423.
5. Furuhashi A, Matsuda K, Asahi K *et al*. Sudden deafness: long-term follow-up and recurrence. *Clinical Otolaryngology & Allied Sciences* 2002;27(6):458-463.
6. Zadeh MH, Storper IS, Spitzer JB. Diagnosis and treatment of sudden-onset sensorineural hearing loss: a study of 51 patients. [Review] [15 refs]. *Otolaryngology—Head & Neck Surgery* 2003;128(1):92-98.
7. Lorenzi MC, Bittar RS, Pedalini ME *et al*. Sudden deafness and Lyme disease. *Laryngoscope* 2003;113(2):312-315.
8. Lee H, Sohn SI, Jung DK *et al*. Sudden deafness and anterior inferior cerebellar artery infarction. *Stroke* 2002;33(12):2807-2812.
9. Berrocal JR, Ramirez-Camacho R. Sudden sensorineural hearing loss: supporting the immunologic theory. [Review] [73 refs]. *Annals of Otology, Rhinology & Laryngology* 2002;111(11):989-997.
10. Suckfull M, Wimmer C, Reichel O *et al*. Hyperfibrinogenemia as a risk factor for sudden hearing loss. *Otology & Neurotology* 2002;23(3):309-311.
11. Tucci DL, Farmer JC, Jr., Kitch RD *et al*. Treatment of sudden sensorineural hearing loss with systemic steroids and valacyclovir. *Otology & Neurotology* 2002;23(3):301-308.
12. Kitajiri S, Tabuchi K, Hiraumi H *et al*. Is corticosteroid therapy effective for sudden-onset sensorineural hearing loss at lower frequencies? *Archives of Otolaryngology—Head & Neck Surgery* 2002;128(4):365-367.
13. Chandrasekhar SS. Intratympanic dexamethasone for sudden sensorineural hearing loss: clinical and laboratory evaluation. *Otology & Neurotology* 2001;22(1):18-23.
14. Inoue Y, Kanzaki J, Ogawa K. Vestibular schwannoma presenting as sudden deafness. *Journal of Laryngology & Otology* 2000;114(8):589-592.

PERILYMPH FISTULA (PLF)

Definition

- A communication between the fluids of the inner and middle ear.

Epidemiology

- PLF remains controversial. Although briefly thought to be a relatively common cause of inner ear dysfunction, it is now considered by most authorities to be a rare entity.

Pathology

- A PLF may arise via three basic mechanisms:
1. A *congenital dehiscence* in the otic capsule that may include the round window membrane or the oval window. These congenital dehiscences are typically associated with congenital malformations of the inner ear (e.g., Mondini's), and the fluid emanating from the inner ear is really CSF and not perilymph.
2. *Trauma* to the temporal bone (blunt or penetrating) may dislodge the stapes, producing a PLF. Barotrauma may result in a rupture of the round window membrane or a leak through the oval window.
3. A *spontaneous* fistula is a controversial entity. It has been postulated that increased intracranial pressure (caused by coughing, straining, sneezing) may be transmitted to the inner ear via an intact cochlear aqueduct, rupturing the round window membrane or the stapes footplate. An alternative hypothesis is that such *explosive* trauma results in rupture of the internal labyrinthine membranes. The concept of a spontaneous PLF has not been supported by recent experimental or clinical data.

Clinical presentation

- Current data would support the diagnosis of a possible PLF when a sudden hearing loss and/or vertigo occur immediately subsequent to a traumatic event. The persistence of a fistula would be suggested by fluctuations in hearing and/or vertigo with straining or other provocative maneuvers.

Diagnostic evaluation

- Other than middle ear exploration, there are no definitive diagnostic tests for PLF. Tests that have been suggested include:
  - The reproduction of vertigo and nystagmus when pressure is applied to the ear via pneumatic otoscopy. This test may be augmented by performing pneumatic otoscopy while the patient is undergoing ENG (recording eye movements) or platform posturography (increased sway).
  - An increased SP/AP on ECOG has been suggested as a criterion; however, this test lacks diagnostic accuracy and validation.
  - No biochemical markers have been developed that are specific to perilymph.
  - High-resolution CT scans of the temporal bones are indicated in cases of trauma or when a congenital dysplasia is suspected.
  - Middle ear exploration for evaluation for a spontaneous PLF should be performed using an endoscope passed though a myringotomy. If performed under local anesthesia, the TM should be anesthetized using a topical agent (phenol, EMLA). Injecting the ear canal with local anesthetic should be avoided because it predisposes to false-positive results.

Treatment

- Initial management of a suspected spontaneous PLF, or a PLF sustained from a barotraumas, is bed rest, head elevation, and avoidance of straining.
- If fluctuations in hearing or active vertiginous events persist after 72 hours of conservative management, the middle ear should be explored (as described above).
- If a PLF is strongly suspected or confirmed via exploration, a tympanomeatal flap is elevated and the round window is packed with adipose tissue. Packing the oval window is generally reserved for cases of visualized oval window fistula, because packing the oval window may be complicated by a residual conductive hearing loss.
- A suspected case of traumatic dislocation of the stapes should be explored immediately and the oval window patched with autogenous tissue (e.g., adipose tissue, perichondrium, temporalis fascia, vein). Some authorities would place a stapes prosthesis at the time of the repair.
- Cases of a CSF leak associated with inner ear anomalies generally present with recurrent meningitis and require definitive management with mastoid/middle ear obliteration, closure of the eustachian tube, and closure of the ear canal.

Selected References from the Recent Literature

1. Gehrking E, Wisst F, Remmert S *et al.* Intraoperative assessment of perilymphatic fistulas with intrathecal administration of fluorescein. *Laryngoscope* 2002;112(9): 1614-1618.
2. Gunesh RP, Huber AM. Traumatic perilymphatic fistula. *Annals of Otology, Rhinology & Laryngology* 2003;112(3): 221-222.
3. Kim SH, Kazahaya K, Handler SD. Traumatic perilymphatic fistulas in children: etiology, diagnosis and management. *International Journal of Pediatric Otorhinolaryngology* 2001;60(2):147-153.

4. Maitland CG. Perilymphatic fistula. [Review] [41 refs]. *Current Neurology & Neuroscience Reports* 2001;1(5): 486-491.

5. Rauch SD. Transferrin microheterogeneity in human perilymph. *Laryngoscope* 2000;110(4):545-552.

6. Selmani Z, Pyykko I, Ishizaki H *et al*. Role of transtympanic endoscopy of the middle ear in the diagnosis of perilymphatic fistula in patients with sensorineural hearing loss or vertigo. *ORL Journal of Oto-Rhino-Laryngology & Its Related Specialties* 2002;64(5):301-306.

AUTOIMMUNE INNER EAR DISEASE (AIED)

Definition
Primary AIED
Rapidly progressive (progressing over a period of weeks to months) bilateral SNHL that responds to the administration of immunosuppressives. Note that although this disorder is likely immune-mediated, there is no direct evidence that it is autoimmune

Secondary AIED
Inner ear involvement as a part of multisystemic autoimmune disorder (e.g., Wegener's granulomatosis).

Epidemiology
- Primary AIED is a rare disorder, considerably less common than sudden SNHL.
- Primary AIED occurs in middle-aged adults, 65% of whom are female.
- Inner ear involvement is generally rare in multisystemic autoimmune disorders, with the exception of Wegener's granulomatosis. In this disorder, the middle ear is affected in 30%-50% of patients with approximately 30% of these patients suffering from inner ear involvement.

Pathology and pathogenesis
- Experimental animal studies and human temporal bone studies have yielded the following potential mechanisms of pathogenesis for primary or secondary AIED:
  - An autoimmune labyrinthitis, in which inflammatory cells enter the scala tympani via the spiral modiolar vein.
  - A vasculitis affecting the vessels feeding the inner ear.
  - An antibody-mediated, noninflammatory pathology, in which antibodies mediate direct pathologic effects on cochlear cells, without eliciting an inflammatory response.

Clinical presentation
Primary AIED
- Rapidly progressive (weeks to months) SNHL.
- Ultimately bilateral hearing loss (however, the hearing loss may be unilateral at initial presentation).
- Fluctuating hearing loss.
- Vestibular complaints in 50% of patients.

Cogan's syndrome
- Nonsyphilitic interstitial keratitis, SNHL, vertigo, and tinnitus.
- Other forms of ocular inflammation (e.g., episcleritis and uveitis may occur, in which case the disorder is referred to as *atypical* Cogan's syndrome).

Wegener's granulomatosis
- Multisystemic autoimmune disease.
- Granuloma formation in the upper and lower respiratory tracts.
- Vasculitis, glomerulonephritis.
- Approximately 30% of patients develop middle ear disease; approximately 10% of patients develop SNHL.

Other Autoimmune Diseases Associated with SNHL

A variety of other autoimmune diseases, particularly those associated with vasculitides, have been associated with SNHL

Differential diagnosis
- Sudden SNHL.
- Meniere's disease.
- Otosyphilis.
- Rare:
  - Meningitis.
  - MS.
  - Dural metastases or CNS lymphoma.

Diagnosis
- A multisystemic review of systems is critical to identify symptoms associated with multisystemic autoimmune disease.
- Serologic tests should include:
  - CBC with differential.
  - Electrolytes, Bun, Cr.
  - Sedimentation rate (ESR).
  - Rheumatoid factor.
  - Antinuclear antibodies.
  - Anti-DNA antibodies.
  - Anti-SSA/B.
  - Antiphospholipid antibodies.
  - C3, C4 complement levels.
  - cANCA.
  - FTA-ABS (MHA-TP).
- MRI scan with paramagnetic enhancement can be used.
- Tests designed specifically to identify primary AIED have been identified. The anti-HSP-70 antibody (Western blot) has been the most carefully evaluated: however, even this test lacks the desirable diagnostic accuracy.
- Ultimately, the diagnosis is made based on the clinical presentation together with a response to corticosteroids (see Treatment section).

Treatment
- Corticosteroids are the foundation of treatment.
- *Prednisone* (60 mg) is given for 4 weeks. If there is no response, it is rapidly tapered over 2 weeks. If there is

a response, it is slowly tapered over 8 weeks. Patients may require a maintenance dose.

- *Cyclophosphamide* (1-2 mg/kg/day) has been advocated as a primary or secondary treatment. It carries significant side effects, including myelosuppression, opportunistic infection, cystitis, hair loss, and increased risk of malignancies.

- *Methotrexate* was advocated as a prednisone-sparing drug; however, it has recently been shown not to be effective in the treatment of AIED.

- In some patients, the risks and side effects of immunosuppression outweigh the benefits, and they will elect to forego treatment, let the disorder take its natural course, and ultimately avail themselves of a *cochlear implant*.

Selected References from the Recent Literature

1. Mathews J, Rao S, Kumar BN. Autoimmune sensorineural hearing loss: is it still a clinical diagnosis? *Journal of Laryngology & Otology* 2003;117(3):212-214.

2. Benvenga S, Trimarchi F, Facchiano A. Cogan's syndrome as an autoimmune disease [comment]. *Lancet* 2003; 361(9356):530-531.

3. Wang X, Truong T, Billings PB *et al*. Blockage of immune-mediated inner ear damage by etanercept. *Otology & Neurotology* 2003;24(1):52-57.

4. Staecker H, Lefebvre PP. Autoimmune sensorineural hearing loss improved by tumor necrosis factor-alpha blockade: a case report. *Acta Oto-Laryngologica* 2002;122(6):684-687.

5. Ryan AF, Harris JP, Keithley EM. Immune-mediated hearing loss: basic mechanisms and options for therapy. [Review] [41 refs]. *Acta Oto-Laryngologica—Supplement* 2002;(548): 38-43.

6. Jimenez-Alonson J, Gutierrez-Cabello F, Castillo JL *et al*. Ear involvement in systemic lupus erythematosus patients: a comparative study. J Laryngol Otol 116:103-7. [comment]. *Journal of Laryngology & Otology* 2002;116(9):746.

7. Lunardi C, Bason C, Leandri M *et al*. Autoantibodies to inner ear and endothelial antigens in Cogan's syndrome [comment]. *Lancet* 2002;360(9337):915-921.

8. Lunardi C, Bason C, Leandri M *et al*. Autoantibodies to inner ear and endothelial antigens in Cogan's syndrome. *Lancet* 2002;360(9337):915-921.

9. Kastanioudakis I, Ziavra N, Voulgari PV *et al*. Ear involvement in systemic lupus erythematosus patients: a comparative study. *Journal of Laryngology & Otology* 2002;116(2): 103-107.

10. Tomasi JP, Lona A, Deggouj N *et al*. Autoimmune sensorineural hearing loss in young patients: an exploratory study. *Laryngoscope* 2001;111(11 Pt 1):2050-2053.

11. Kaylie DM, Hefeneider SH, Kempton JB *et al*. Decreased cochlear DNA receptor staining in MRL.MpJ-Fas(lpr) autoimmune mice with hearing loss. *Laryngoscope* 2001 111(7):1275-1280.

12. Salley LH, Jr., Grimm M, Sismanis A *et al*. Methotrexate in the management of immune mediated cochleovestibular disorders: clinical experience with 53 patients. *Journal of Rheumatology* 2001;28(5):1037-1040.

13. Boulassel MR, Deggouj N, Tomasi JP *et al*. Inner ear autoantibodies and their targets in patients with autoimmune inner ear diseases. *Acta Oto-Laryngologica* 2001;121(1):28-34.

14. Ruckenstein MJ, McKown KM, Jacewicz M. Unusual and instructive case of immune-mediated inner ear disease associated with central nervous system vasculitis. *Otolaryngology—Head & Neck Surgery* 2000;122(1):109-111.

TINNITUS

Definition
- The perception of sounds not generated in the external environment.

Objective tinnitus
- 5% of cases.
- Sounds able to be heard by the practitioner.
- Typically pulsatile; may be clicking.

Subjective tinnitus
- 95% of cases.
- May have a variety of sounds (e.g., ringing, chirping, static). Specific nature of the sound not clinically relevant.

Epidemiology
- Affects 40-50 million Americans.
- Men > women.
- Prevalence increases with age.
- Whites > Blacks.
- Southern United States > Northeastern United States.

Pathology and pathophysiology
Objective tinnitus
- Pulsatile tinnitus originates from turbulent blood flow in vessels around the temporal bone. Lesions that can generate such flow patterns include arteriovenous malformations (AVMs) and similar malformations, glomus tumors, carotid stenosis, dehiscent intratemporal carotid artery, and high cardiac output states.
- Pulsatile tinnitus may also be perceived with a normal vasculature in the presence of a conductive hearing loss.
- Benign intracranial hypertension (pseudotumor cerebri) may manifest with bilateral pulsatile tinnitus.
- A clicking tinnitus can be generated by abnormal muscle contractions typically secondary to focal or generalized dystonias (e.g., palatal myoclonus, stapedius muscle contraction).
- A low-pitched hum can be perceived originating from the sigmoid sinus/jugular bulb (e.g., dehiscent or high-riding jugular bulb).

Subjective tinnitus
- Involves tinnitus generation and tinnitus perception.
- Tinnitus generation: resulting from some dysfunction in the auditory tracts.
- May result from central or peripheral dysfunction.
- Many proposed theories to account for tinnitus generation include the following:
  - Tinnitus is associated with hearing loss resulting from *cochlear pathology*. In regions of the cochlea where function is transitioning from normal to abnormal cochlear function, there are regions of hair cell instability. These instabilities may result from altered efferent activation, the goal of which is to optimize cochlear function. Efferent fibers are highly branched, thus activated fibers may synapse on both abnormal and normal cells. In cells that have retained normal to near-normal activities, altered efferent activity may create a state where they are "hypertuned," become unstable, and begin firing spontaneously.
  - Moller has proposed a neural etiology, in which pathologic *afferent fibers* lose their myelin insulation and "cross talk" with each other. In this scenario, a stimulus in one area of the cochlea may lead to discharge in an excess of afferent fibers that is perceived as tinnitus.
  - Others point to a *central* etiology. Support for this hypothesis is garnered from the observation that tinnitus persists in many patients in whom the cochlear nerve is resected. In theory, an alteration in peripheral function leads to a reorganization of central auditory neural pathways. Central changes may include a disinhibition of certain pathways, which, when functioning autonomously, generate a tinnitus signal.
  - Jastreboff maintains that localizing the generation site is not critical to the understanding of tinnitus and its treatment. In his "neurophysiological model," the *perception* of the tinnitus is pathologic. This model is based on a variety of observations, including that when tinnitus-matching experiments are performed, there are no significant differences in the characteristics of the tinnitus experienced by those who are troubled by their tinnitus and those who consider their tinnitus insignificant. Rather, the theory notes that in the 90%-95% of patients who are *not* troubled by their tinnitus, successful *central adaptation* takes place to this chronic, meaningless signal. Those 5%-10% of patients who *suffer* from their tinnitus have undergone a maladaptive central adaptation process, often resulting from adverse psychological associations. Certain patients may be predisposed to this maladaptive response because of the presence of underlying psychopathology.
  - Certain medications, specifically *loop diuretics, salicylicates,* and *quinine* will exacerbate tinnitus.

Clinical presentation
Objective tinnitus
- Patients will present with a specific complaint of hearing a pulsing or clicking sound.
- Auscultation over the mastoid (greater occipital artery-transverse/sigmoid sinus AVM), over the preauricular region, over the eyeball (carotid-cavernous AVM), and in the ear canal (carotid,

petrotympanic vessels) may reveal an audible pulsation.

- Having the patient open his/her mouth without the insertion of a tongue blade may reveal palatal myoclonus.
- Visualization of the TM with a microscope may reveal contractions of the stapedius or tensor tympani.
- Tuning fork tests and/or otoscopy may reveal evidence of a conductive hearing loss.

Subjective tinnitus

- Patients will report a variety of tinnitus "sounds."
- There may be subjective hearing loss, although often the hearing loss will be only in the high frequencies.
- Patients who suffer from their tinnitus will report a variety of complaints, including insomnia, loss of concentration, anxiety, and depression.

Investigations

Pulsatile tinnitus

- Audiogram: rule out conductive hearing loss.
- MRI head with paramagnetic enhancement to rule out a vascular tumor.
- Magnetic resonance angiography (MRA) of head and neck to rule out vascular malformation or occlusion.
- Ophthalmology consult to rule out papilledema associated with pseudotumor.
- Cerebral angiogram if above evaluation is normal and patient wishes to pursue further investigations.

Clicking tinnitus

- Audiogram with manual impedance bridge. While the external ear pressure is held at a constant level, fluctuations in the baseline of the immittance reading may document contractions of the middle ear muscles.
- MRI head with paramagnetic enhancement to rule out a structural cause for a dystonia.

Subjective tinnitus

- Audiogram.
- MRI head with paramagnetic enhancement if the tinnitus is unilateral or the hearing asymmetric.

Treatment

- Treatment of tinnitus is controversial.
- A wide variety of treatments have been advocated, the vast majority of which have not proved to be effective.
- Based on a critical review of the literature, the following can be said about the treatment of tinnitus:
  - Placebo treatment has an acute efficacy of approximately 40%.
  - No medications (with the exception of tricyclic antidepressants [see below]), homeopathic

remedies, or herbal preparations have been shown to be effective.
- Acupuncture is not effective.
- Tricyclic antidepressants may have a role in the treatment of patients with concomitant depression.
- The role of benzodiazepines, selective serotonin reuptake inhibitors (SSRIs) and other newer antidepressants requires further study.
- Electrical stimulation requires further study with more sophisticated devices and better controls.
- Hearing aids may provide effective masking.
- Tinnitus-masking devices may have some limited value in patients without significant hearing loss.
- Tinnitus Retraining Therapy (TRT), as developed by Jastreboff, is a multimodality therapy incorporating counseling, patient education, and a low-level, white-noise tinnitus masker. This treatment is based on sound scientific principles and has shown significant promise in limited trials. Its efficacy requires verification in larger, better-controlled studies, and it has been criticized for not incorporating formal psychological or psychiatric intervention.
- Psychological or psychiatric intervention may be required in the most disturbed patients, because their distress is often complicated by concomitant psychopathology.

Prognosis

- The vast majority (90%-95%) of patients accommodate their tinnitus within 3-6 months of onset.
- A minority experiences significant psychological distress, which is challenging to treat based on regimens currently available.

Selected References from the Recent Literature

1. Eggermont JJ. Central tinnitus. [Review] [55 refs]. *Auris, Nasus, Larynx* 2003;30 Suppl:S7-12.
2. Golz A, Fradis M, Martzu D *et al.* Stapedius muscle myoclonus. [Review] [10 refs]. *Annals of Otology, Rhinology & Laryngology* 2003;112(6):522-524.
3. Cacace AT. Expanding the biological basis of tinnitus: cross-modal origins and the role of neuroplasticity. [Review] [244 refs]. *Hearing Research* 2003;175(1-2):112-132.
4. Andersson G. Psychological aspects of tinnitus and the application of cognitive-behavioral therapy. [Review] [84 refs]. *Clinical Psychology Review* 2002;22(7):977-990.
5. Baguley DM. Mechanisms of tinnitus. [Review] [94 refs]. *British Medical Bulletin* 2002;63:195-212.
6. Waddell A, Canter R. Tinnitus. [Review] [30 refs]. *Clinical Evidence* 2002;(7):481-489.
7. Lockwood AH, Salvi RJ, Burkard RF. Tinnitus. [Review] [49 refs]. *New England Journal of Medicine* 2002;347(12):904-910.
8. Roy D, Chopra R. Tinnitus: an update. [Review] [14 refs]. *Journal of the Royal Society of Health* 2002;122(1):21-23.

9. Sismanis A. Tinnitus. [Review] [50 refs]. *Current Neurology & Neuroscience Reports* 2001;1(5):492-499.

10. Moller AR. Symptoms and signs caused by neural plasticity. [Review] [73 refs]. *Neurological Research* 2001; 23(6):565-572.

11. Marsot-Dupuch K. Pulsatile and nonpulsatile tinnitus: a systemic approach. [Review] [29 refs]. *Seminars in Ultrasound, CT & MR* 2001;22(3):250-270.

12. Sahley TL, Nodar RH. A biochemical model of peripheral tinnitus. [Review] [148 refs]. *Hearing Research* 2001;152 (1-2):43-54.

13. Holgers KM, Erlandsson SI, Barrenas ML. Predictive factors for the severity of tinnitus. [Review] [50 refs]. *Audiology* 2000;39(5):284-291.

14. Weissman JL, Hirsch BE. Imaging of tinnitus: a review. [Review] [49 refs]. *Radiology* 2000;216(2):342-349.

15. Kroener-Herwig B, Biesinger E, Gerhards F *et al*. Retraining therapy for chronic tinnitus. A critical analysis of its status. [Review] [42 refs]. *Scandinavian Audiology* 2000;29(2):67-78.

16. Simpson JJ, Davies WE. A review of evidence in support of a role for 5-HT in the perception of tinnitus. [Review] [68 refs]. *Hearing Research* 2000;145(1-2):1-7.

17. Jastreboff PJ, Jastreboff MM. Tinnitus Retraining Therapy (TRT) as a method for treatment of tinnitus and hyperacusis patients. [Review] [45 refs]. *Journal of the American Academy of Audiology* 2000;11(3):162-177.

18. Henry JA, Meikle MB. Psychoacoustic measures of tinnitus. [Review] [85 refs]. *Journal of the American Academy of Audiology* 2000;11(3):138-155.

19. Kaltenbach JA. Neurophysiologic mechanisms of tinnitus. [Review] [105 refs]. *Journal of the American Academy of Audiology* 2000;11(3):125-137.

20. Moller AR. Similarities between severe tinnitus and chronic pain. [Review] [52 refs]. *Journal of the American Academy of Audiology* 2000;11(3):115-124.

COCHLEAR IMPLANTS

Definition

An implantable prosthesis designed to restore hearing to patients with severe to profound hearing loss by transforming acoustic stimuli to electrical signals that stimulate spiral ganglion neurons.

Indications

Adults

- 18 years old or older.
- Severe to profound bilateral SNHL.
- Postlingual onset of hearing loss.
- No to limited benefit from hearing aids.
- Less than 50% performance in open set test, typically hearing in noise test (HINT) sentences.

Children

- 12 months to 17 years (although younger children have been implanted).
- Profound SNHL.
- No to minimum benefit with hearing aid use of:
  - 3 months in 12-23 month old.
  - 6 months in 2-17 year old.

Technology

1. *Microphone* (behind the ear) captures sound and transmits it to a
2. *Speech processor* worn on the body or behind the ear, which processes sound according to preset software and transmits the processed sound as an electrical signal to the
3. *Transmitter coil*, which is housed with a magnet. This magnet makes contact with a subcutaneous magnet, which is housed with the
4. *Receiver stimulator*, which "receives" the signal from the transmitter coil via this percutaneous connection, and then sends the signal down the
5. *Intracochlear electrode array*, which contains multiple electrodes that directly stimulate the spiral ganglion neurons of the auditory nerve.

Technique/surgery

Many incisions have been used; however, more minimal postauricular incisions have gained favor with most surgeons.

1. Drill a well for the implant approximately 4 cm posterosuperior to the posterior lip of the ear canal.
2. Perform a cortical mastoidectomy.
3. Open the facial recess.
4. Make a cochleostomy just anteroinferior to the round window.
5. Introduce the electrode array, secure it in its well, and then pass it into the cochlea via the cochleostomy.

6. Once the implantation is completed, pack the cochleostomy and facial recess with fascia or muscle.
7. Perform a multilayer closure

Activation of the implant takes place 2-6 weeks postimplantation (to allow for incision healing and decreased edema).

Complications

- *Facial paralysis:* may occur from thermal or direct trauma. It is managed by decompression of the mastoid segment of the nerve.
- *CSF leak:* generally seen in cases of inner ear malformations (e.g., Mondini's) in which there is an incomplete partition between the IAC and the labyrinth. These malformations may require the placement of a special short electrode or may be managed with traditional electrodes. The labyrinth is then packed with fascia. Postoperative bed rest and head elevation are recommended. Lumbar drain can be performed per the discretion of the surgeon.
- *Labyrinthitis ossificans:* a number of conditions, including meningitis and otosclerosis, may cause ossification that prevents passage of the electrode into scala tympani. Management options for this condition include the following:
  - If the ossification is restricted to the basal region, often the scala vestibuli can be opened and the electrode can be passed into this space with good results.
  - If the ossification is restricted to the base, a limited drill-out of the basal turn can be performed, and the electrode then passed into the scala tympani.
  - If the ossification is thought to be focal, based on preoperative CT and or MRI scans, two cochleostomies can be drilled, one proximal and one distal to the obstruction. A "split" electrode can be used, with one segment passed into the proximal cochleostomy, and one into the distal cochleostomy.
  - A complete cochlear drill-out can be performed. The canal is taken down and the ear canal is closed, as is the eustachian tube. The cochlea is drilled out, and the electrode is laid in the bed of the cochlea. The mastoid is obliterated with fat or muscle.
- *Wound dehiscence:* managed with local wound care, as well as topical and systemic antibiotics. Rotation of a local flap may be necessary. Explantation is not usually necessary.
- *Otitis media:* promptly managed with standard oral antibiotics.
- *Meningitis:* Elevated incidence was noted in children postimplant. The risk was particularly elevated in children who underwent implantation with a Clarion device that used a silastic "positioner" to place the electrode closer to the modiolus. The positioner has been withdrawn from the market. Children with

cochlear dysplasias were also at increased risk. Current recommendations are to ensure that all children and adults have been immunized against streptococcus and all children against *H. influenzae*. Perioperative antibiotics are recommended for 1-3 weeks postimplantation.

Selected References from the Recent Literature

1. Barton GR, Bloor KE, Marshall DH *et al*. Health-service costs of pediatric cochlear implantation: multi-center analysis. *International Journal of Pediatric Otorhinolaryngology* 2003;67(2):141-149.
2. Miyamoto RT, Houston DM, Kirk KI *et al*. Language development in deaf infants following cochlear implantation. *Acta Oto-Laryngologica* 2003;123(2):241-244.
3. Tye-Murray N. Conversational fluency of children who use cochlear implants. *Ear & Hearing* 2003;24(1 Suppl):82S-89S.
4. Geers AE, Nicholas JG, Sedey AL. Language skills of children with early cochlear implantation. *Ear & Hearing* 2003; 24(1 Suppl):46S-58S.
5. Bluestone CD. Prevention of meningitis: cochlear implants and inner ear abnormalities. *Archives of Otolaryngology—Head & Neck Surgery* 2003;129(3):279-281.
6. Sennaroglu L, Saatci I, Aralasmak A *et al*. Magnetic resonance imaging versus computed tomography in pre-operative evaluation of cochlear implant candidates with congenital hearing loss. *Journal of Laryngology & Otology* 2002;116(10):804-810.
7. Higgins KM, Chen JM, Nedzelski JM *et al*. A matched-pair comparison of two cochlear implant systems. *Journal of Otolaryngology* 2002;31(2):97-105.
8. Ramsden RT. Cochlear implants and brain stem implants. [Review] [8 refs]. *British Medical Bulletin* 2002;63: 183-193.

CONGENITAL AURAL ATRESIA

Definition
- Congenital malformation of the external auditory canal (EAC) with or without middle ear malformation.
- Intimately associated with microtia.

Epidemiology
- 1/10,000-20,000.
- Unilateral: 70%; bilateral: 30%.
- Nonsyndromal > syndromal.

Pathology and pathogenesis
- Failure of embryogenesis of the external and middle ears occurs during first 30 weeks of gestation.
- The external canal is derived from the ectoderm of the first branchial cleft. Its development is completed by midterm.
- The eustachian tube, middle ear, and mastoid derive from the endoderm of the first branchial arch. Their development is completed by 30 weeks of gestation.
- The malleus head, incus body, and lateral process of the incus derive from the mesoderm of the first branchial arch.
- The manubrium, long process of the incus, and stapes superstructure derive from the mesoderm of the second branchial arch.
- The development of the ossicles is completed by week 26.
- The auricle develops from the six hillocks of this (first and second branchial arches). Its development is completed by week 12.

Clinical presentation
- In general, the more severe the auricular deformity, the more likely will be the presence of a canal deformity.
- The more severe the canal deformity, the more likely will be the presence of the a middle ear deformity.
- A variety of grading systems and scales have been developed.
- In general, these various grading systems evaluate the anatomy, based on physical exam and CT scan, as follows.

Auricle
1. Small, but well formed.
2. Identifiable, but various degrees of anomaly.
3. Absent or rudimentary appendage.

External canal
1. Narrow but intact; TM visible.

2. Tract identifiable.
3. No tract.

Middle ear
1. Size of the middle ear space (normal, decreased, absent).
2. Presence or absence of ossicles.
3. Viable stapes and mobile oval window.

Investigations
- Audiogram.
- CT scan.

Treatment
- The principles of treatment is as follows:
  - Microtia repair precedes canal repair.
  - Bilateral atresias may be repaired at 4-6 years of age.
  - Unilateral atresia repair is generally postponed until the child can play a part in the decision (>13 years old).
  - A patient is not a surgical candidate if the middle ear space is absent or poorly developed.
  - If the oval window/stapes is not identifiable, particular care must be taken during surgery because of the abnormal course of the facial nerve. The nerve often curves anteriorly as it courses inferiorly after the second genu and crosses the middle ear space unprotected by a fallopian canal.
  - Most surgeons currently favor the *anterior approach* for reconstruction:
    - The TMJ is used as the anterior landmark, and the tegmen is used as the superior landmark.
    - These structures are followed medially until the atresia plate in encountered.
    - The atresia plate is then curetted.
    - The abnormal ossicles are either freed or replaced.
    - The TM is reconstructed with temporalis fascia.
    - Split skin is used to line the canal.
    - Care must be taken to reconstruct the anterior sulcus to prevent anterior blunting of the TM.

Complications
- SNHL.
- Vertigo.
- VIIth nerve paralysis.
- Infection.
- Graft failure.
- Failure to maintain closure of the air-bone gap (long-term).
- Restenosis (long-term).

VESTIBULAR DISORDERS

Peripheral Vestibular Disorders

Benign positional vertigo (BPV)

Definition

- A peripheral vestibular disorder characterized by paroxysmal episodes of vertigo, lasting for seconds, elicited by rapid changes in head position.

Incidence and epidemiology

- Most common form of vertigo.
- Most common in fifth to sixth decade of life.
- Female:male ratio = 2:1.
- Etiology:
  - Idiopathic: 50%-65%.
  - Head trauma: 20%.
  - Vestibular neuronitis: 2%-15%.

Pathophysiology and pathology

- Canalolithiasis
  - This is the prevailing theory of pathogenesis.
  - Symptoms originate from free-floating particles within an SCC, typically the posterior canal.
  - When acted on by a force such as gravity, the canalith acts like a plunger, creating endolymph flow and stimulation of the ampullary hair cells.
  - Settling of the debris allows for the cupula to return to the resting position, accounting for the brief duration of symptoms.
  - The delay in movement of the canalith (caused by inertia) after the provoking head position is assumed accounts for the latency seen in symptoms (see below).
- Cupulolithiasis
  - Proposed by Schuknecht, it was thought to be the pathophysiologic mechanism accounting for BPV, until supplanted by the theory of canalolithiasis.
  - BPV is attributed to debris accumulated on the cupula of the posterior canal.
  - It may account for a minority of cases of BPV.

Clinical manifestations

- True rotatory vertigo, lasting seconds, elicited by a rapid change in head position.
- Head movements in a nonaxial plane, such as looking up and rolling over bed.
- Latency of onset = 10 seconds.
- Duration 30-60 seconds.
- The posterior SCC is most commonly affected (>90%). Placing the head in the dependent position with the head turned so the affected ear is facing the floor (Dix-Hallpike maneuver) creates a torsional nystagmus that beats toward the affected ear and a vertical upbeat nystagmus. The vertical component of the nystagmus can be accentuated by having the patient look away from the direction of the torsional nystagmus.
- Returning the patient to an upright position causes a reversal of the torsional nystagmus.
- In 10% of cases, patients will manifest a variant form of BPV:
  - Anterior canal BPV (1%-2% of cases): torsional and *downbeat* nystagmus. Clinical symptoms are identical to those of posterior canal BPV.
  - Horizontal canal BPV (5%): Patients manifest pure horizontal nystagmus when *rolled* to one side while in the supine position with the head flexed at a 30-degree angle.
  - The nystagmus may be geotropic (toward the floor) or ageotropic (toward the ceiling).
    - Geotropic nystagmus is believed to result from canalolithiasis, and ageotropic nystagmus is believed to result from cupulolithiasis.
    - The direction of the nystagmus may change when the patient's head is rolled to the contralateral side. This created a practical problem in deciding which ear is affected. Clinical experience indicates that the nystagmus beats the strongest when the affected ear faces the floor.
- The disorder is typically self limited but may have a duration of days to months.
- It is a recurrent condition with a 50% recurrence within 50 months of the initial presentation.

Investigations

- Patients presenting with typical signs and symptoms generally require no investigations.
- ENG will reveal the classic nystagmus pattern during dynamic positioning testing if the patient has active disease.
- A unilateral caloric weakness may be detected on ENG.
- In persistent cases that do not respond to routine treatment, an MRI of the head with enhancement is required to rule out a posterior fossa neoplasm.

Treatment

- Posterior and anterior canal BPV are effectively treated with the Epley canalith repositioning maneuver (CRP).
- The maneuver begins by placing the patient in the provoking position as in the Dix-Hallpike maneuver. The head is then rotated 90 degrees to the contralateral side, while the neck is maintained in extension. The patient is then further rolled onto his shoulder, so the head completes a 180-degree rotation.

- The maneuver has a 70% success rate after 24-48 hours, and 80% of patients have a resolution of symptoms after 2 weeks.
- There is no need for mastoid oscillation during the maneuver or restrictions in head position after the maneuver.
- The Semont maneuver is an alternative positional maneuver not commonly used in North America.
- Brandt-Daroff exercises, in which the patient alternates lying down on his/her right and left side with his/her head slightly extended and turned to the ceiling, may help prevent recurrence.
- Vestibular rehabilitation physical therapy is effective at alleviating the residual symptoms of lightheadedness and positional imbalance seen in approximately 30% of patients.
- Although rare, patients who fail multiple positioning maneuvers and rehabilitation therapy and who do not have any central disease may require surgical treatment.
- The current surgical treatment of choice is the posterior canal plugging, in which a small fenestration is made in the posterior canal and the canal is plugged with bone pate mixed with fibrin glue. Complications include a temporary conductive hearing loss, temporary acute vertigo, permanent profound hearing loss (5%), and permanent vestibular loss.
- Sectioning of the nerve to the posterior canal that runs in the singular canal (singular nerve section) is technically difficult and may be complicated by a profound hearing loss secondary to violation of the ampulla of the posterior canal or the cochlea.

Meniere's disease
Definition
- An idiopathic inner ear disorder characterized by symptoms of fluctuating, progressive SNHL, recurrent vertigo lasting for hours, and tinnitus and aural fullness in the affected ear.

Epidemiology
- Affects 10-150/100,000 people. Incidence varies depending on the diagnostic criteria used by the investigators.
- Males = females.
- Peak incidence: fifth decade.
- Rare onset before 20 years old and after 70 years old.

Pathology
- The only consistent finding on morphologic analysis is swelling of the endolymphatic fluid compartment (*endolymphatic hydrops*).

Pathogenesis
- The potassium intoxication hypothesis has dominated theories of pathogenesis. It postulates that:
  - Flow of endolymph occurs from base to apex of the cochlea and drains into the endolymphatic sac.
  - An obstruction occurs within the endolymphatic duct system (e.g., a malfunctioning endolymphatic sac, fibrosis within the ducts).
  - Progressive swelling of the endolymphatic compartment (scala media) occurs.
  - The pressure buildup within the scala media ultimately leads to a rupture of Reissner's membrane.
  - Disruption of the barrier between the endolymph and perilymph leads to potassium passing from endolymph to perilymph. This causes a loss in the electrochemical gradient necessary for hair cells to function.
  - At this point, there is dysfunction of the inner ear, resulting in the characteristic vertigo and auditory symptoms
  - Healing of Reissner's membrane restores the endocochlear potential and inner ear function.
  - Recurrence of this process accounts for the episodic symptoms.
  - Although the potassium intoxication–endolymphatic hydrops model remains the best accepted model of Meniere's disease, significant problems with this model include:
    - Endolymphatic flow is radial, not longitudinal down the cochlea.
    - Endolymphatic hydrops is seen in temporal bones derived from patients with a variety of conditions that do not manifest symptoms similar to those seen in Meniere's disease.
    - No significant obstruction in the endolymphatic ducts has been noted in patients with Meniere's disease, compared with control temporal bones.
    - Studies of animal models of hydrops have not been able to correlate the degree and progression of hydrops with auditory dysfunction.

Clinical manifestations
- Meniere's disease is characterized by the clinical symptom complex of:
  - Recurrent, episodic vertigo lasting for hours.
  - Fluctuating, progressive SNHL.
  - Tinnitus in the affected ear.
  - Aural fullness in the affected.
- An attack may be preceded by otalgia.
- The hearing loss involving the low frequencies and the audiogram will manifest one of these patterns:

- ❑ Inverted "V" (low- and high-frequency SNHL).
- ❑ Low-frequency hearing loss.
- ❑ Flat SNHL.
- The hearing loss is progressive, with the maximal SNHL eventually being 65-75 dB.
- The incidence of bilaterality is 45%, although decades may pass before the contralateral ear is affected.
- Vertigo episodes decrease with duration of disease.
- Although the overall course is progressive, the timing of individual periods of exacerbations and remissions is highly variable and capricious.
- Variants of Meniere's disease:
  - ❑ Lermoyez syndrome:
    - A period of increasing aural fullness, hearing loss, and tinnitus that is alleviated with the onset of a vertiginous episode.
  - ❑ Otolithic crisis of Tumarkin:
    - Sudden loss of extensor tone resulting in the patient falling.
    - Seen in patients with established Meniere's disease.
    - No concurrent vertigo or loss of consciousness.
    - Must be differentiated from Vertebrobasilar Insufficiency (VBI) by appropriate imaging studies (MRA) and vascular (transcranial Doppler) studies.
  - ❑ Cochlear Meniere's disease:
    - In some patients, the symptoms at the onset of Meniere's do not include both vertigo and hearing loss.
    - Some patients will manifest only fluctuations in hearing, aural fullness, and tinnitus, which is known as cochlear Meniere's disease.
    - The vast majority of these patients will develop vertigo within 1 year of the onset of the auditory symptoms.
  - ❑ Vestibular Meniere's disease:
    - Patients suffering from recurrent episodes of vertigo lasting for hours in the absence of hearing loss have been referred as having vestibular Meniere's disease.
    - The majority (85%) of these patients do not suffer from Meniere's disease, but rather have migrainous vertigo (see section in central vestibular disorders).
    - A minority of patients will ultimately develop auditory pathology.
    - The remainder are classified as having Recurrent Vestibulopathy (see below).

Investigations

- Audiometric assessment is required to establish the diagnosis.
- Vestibular function tests can provide evidence that supports the diagnosis of a peripheral vestibular lesion and are necessary if one is considering surgical intervention.
- MRI scan with enhancement is required to rule out a retrocochlear lesion.
- A test for tertiary syphilis (FTA-ABS or MHA-TP) is required in all patients.
- Much has been made about abnormal SP/AP ratios measured by ECOG in patients with Meniere's disease. It must be emphasized that:
  - ❑ This test lacks the sensitivity and specificity during the early stages of Meniere's disease to either rule in or rule out the diagnosis.
  - ❑ SP/AP ratios are elevated in well-established cases of Meniere's disease, but once the clinical syndrome has declared itself, the patient is diagnosed with the disease and does not require an ECOG to "confirm" the diagnosis.
  - ❑ Abnormalities in SP/AP ratios do not correlate with the presence of endolymphatic hydrops, as has been shown by numerous animal studies.

Treatment

- The treatment of Meniere's disease remains a controversial area.
- Development of clinical trials for treatments for Meniere's disease is difficult because of:
  - ❑ The capricious nature of the disease, with its spontaneous and unpredictable exacerbations and remissions.
  - ❑ The nonspecific short-term treatment response rate of 60%-80% seen with virtually any intervention for Meniere's disease.

Medical treatment

- Salt-restriction diets and diuretic therapy remain the foundation of medical treatment.
  - ❑ Neither of these treatments has ever been shown to be more effective than placebo in well-designed, controlled clinical trials.
- Vestibular suppressants (e.g., meclizine, diazepam) should be reserved for periods of exacerbation of vertigo. Their chronic use should be avoided,
- No other medications or nonsurgical interventions (e.g., other restriction diets) have ever been shown to be effective for the treatment of Meniere's disease.

Surgical treatment
Endolymphatic sac surgery
Indication

- Hearing-conservation surgery for patients with intractable vertigo from Meniere's disease.

Contraindication

- None.

Technique
1. Perform a cortical mastoidectomy.
2. Remove the bone overlying the posterior fossa dura, anterior to the sigmoid sinus, inferior to the posterior SCC, and posterior to the facial nerve.
3. The endolymphatic sac is found as a duplication of dura in this region. Retract slightly on the posterior fossa dura to allow visualization of the extraosseous portion of the vestibular aqueduct entering its bony canal.
4. A variety of techniques have been described with regard to management of the endolymphatic sac. Although no one technique has proved more effective than another, they include:
   - Simple decompression.
   - Opening the lateral layer of the sac and inserting a shunt (e.g., silastic) to keep the opening patent–endolymphatic-mastoid shunt.
   - Unroofing the sac by removing the lateral layer.
   - Endolymphatic-subarachnoid shunt (rarely performed).

Complications
- Hearing loss: 1%.
- Facial paralysis: 1%.
- CSF leak: 1%.

Efficacy
- Controversy continues to surround the endolymphatic shunt operation, especially regarding its efficacy with respect to a "sham" operation.
- Based on currently available clinical data, the following conclusions can be drawn:
   - Endolymphatic shunt surgery will provide satisfactory vertigo control in 60% of patients over a 5-year period.
   - Endolymphatic shunt surgery will not affect long-term hearing loss.
   - Over a 5-year period, shunt surgery likely provides no better vertigo control than a sham operation (mastoidectomy).

Vestibular nerve section
Indications
- Hearing conservation surgery for patients with intractable vertigo from Meniere's disease.

Contraindications
- Contralateral vestibular loss

Technique
- The vestibular nerve can be cut using any of the following approaches:
   - Middle fossa: generally no longer performed because of increased risk to the facial nerve and

risk of cutting the nerve distal to the take-off point of the branch to the posterior SCC (decreased efficacy).
   - Retrolabyrinthine (via removal of bone overlying the dura between the sigmoid sinus, the labyrinth, and the facial nerve).
   - Suboccipital (retrosigmoid): most commonly performed. The VIIIth nerve is identified and the vestibular branch (superior) is separated from the cochlear branch (inferior).

Complications
- Vertigo (2-3 days).
- Imbalance (3-6 weeks).
- Hearing loss (2%-3%).
- Facial paralysis (<1%).
- Headache.
- CSF leak.
- Meningitis.

Efficacy
- Vertigo is satisfactorily controlled in 95% of patients at 5 years.
- For many years, the vestibular nerve section was considered the treatment of choice for hearing conservation and vertigo control in Meniere's disease. With the advent of gentamicin treatment, it is much less commonly performed.

Labyrinthectomy
Indication
- Intractable vertigo in a patient with Meniere's disease with poor or nonserviceable hearing.

Contraindication
- Contralateral vestibular loss.

Technique
- Mastoidectomy and labyrinthectomy.
- Transcanal labyrinthectomy has been described but is not commonly performed.

Complications
- Complete loss of hearing.
- Vertigo 2-3 days.
- Imbalance: 3-6 weeks.
- Facial paralysis: 1%.

Gentamicin inner ear perfusion
Indication
- Hearing-conservation procedure for patients with intractable vertigo from Meniere's disease

Contraindication
- Contralateral vestibular loss.

Technique

- General technique involves injecting the middle ear with a concentrated solution of buffered gentamicin (27 mg/mL).
- The frequency of injections varies from center to center:
  - The most aggressive technique involves injections 3×/day × 4 days.
  - Most centers inject the solution weekly or once every 2 weeks.
  - The decreased frequency of injection allows for better hearing preservation without significant sacrifice of vertigo control.
- Endpoints for injection vary from center to center and include:
  - One injection and further injections based on recurrence of symptoms.
  - Termination of injections with resolution of symptoms.
  - Termination of injections with hearing loss documented on audiogram.
  - Termination of injections with signs of a vestibular loss on clinical exam (head thrust, spontaneous nystagmus, head shake nystagmus).
  - Termination of injections with significant vestibular loss documented on balance function tests.

Complications

- Vertigo: an acute episode of vertigo may occur 3-5 days after injection.
- Imbalance: may last 1-2 weeks.
- Hearing loss: current protocols result in some hearing loss in fewer than 10% of patients,

Vestibular neuronitis

Definition

- An acute, single episode of vertigo in the absence of hearing loss, lasting for days.

Epidemiology

- Accounts for approximately 5% of cases of vertigo.
- May occur in mini-epidemics.

Pathology

- Degeneration of vestibular nerve afferent fibers.
- Some loss of vestibular hair cells.

Pathogenesis

- This is generally considered to be a viral infection of the vestibular nerve, resulting in degeneration of vestibular nerve axons.
- Some evidence suggests that the pathology is restricted to the superior division of the vestibular nerve.

Clinical presentation

- Acute onset of vertigo, associated with nausea and vomiting.
- Viral prodrome possible.
- Nystagmus consistent with that seen in peripheral vestibular lesion (see section on nystagmus).
- No associated hearing loss or symptoms of CNS dysfunction.

Investigations

- Audiogram is indicated to rule out hearing loss and possible retrocochlear lesion.
- Other investigations generally not required with typical presentation.

Treatment

- Vestibular suppressants.
- Corticosteroids: may decrease duration and severity of episode.
- Vestibular rehabilitation physical therapy if symptoms of imbalance persist after vertigo resolves.

Labyrinthitis

Definition

- Acute onset of single episode of vertigo *and* hearing loss.

Epidemiology

- Considerably less common than vestibular neuronitis.
- Suppurative labyrinthitis secondary to meningitis: most common cause of acquired hearing loss in children.

Pathology

- Inflammatory infiltrate within the labyrinth.
- As the inflammation resolves, residual sensory cell loss and fibrosis, and ultimately, osteoneogenesis within the scalae, occur.

Pathogenesis

- Viral infection within the inner ear.
- Meningitis may result in bacteria spreading to the inner ear via the IAC or cochlear aqueduct.
- Otitis media may allow spread of bacteria to the inner ear via the round or oval window.

Clinical presentation

- In the case of viral labyrinthitis, the presentation is much like vestibular neuronitis with the exception of the presence of hearing loss.
- Acute onset of vertigo and SNHL in the presence of a meningitis or otitis media.

Investigations
- Audiogram.
- MRI with enhancement to rule out a retrocochlear lesion.
- Lumbar puncture if clinical presentation is consistent with meningitis.

Treatment
- Viral labyrinthitis: as per vestibular neuronitis.
- Bacterial labyrinthitis:
  - When secondary to meningitis: as per meningitis, with parenteral steroids.
  - When secondary to otitis media: parenteral antibiotics and steroids, with myringotomy, with or without ventilation tube insertion.

Syphilis
Definition
- Systemic infection by *T. pallidum* may be transmitted via the transplacental route (congenital) or may be acquired through sexual contact.

Epidemiology
- Incidence of syphilis highest in the nonwhite, urban population.
- Increasing incidence in male homosexual population.
- Hearing loss present in 40% of patients with congenital syphilis and in 80% patients with neurosyphilis.

Pathology
- In secondary and tertiary syphilis:
  - Mononuclear inflammatory cells mediate osteitis and bone resorption.
  - Obliterative endarteritis is in surrounding vessels.
  - In severe cases, *gummas*—consisting of lymphocytic infiltrates, vascular occlusion, and central necrosis—are found in the otic capsule.
- In congenital and secondary acquired syphilis, the inner ear and VIIIth nerve may be involved by a diffuse meningoneurolabyrinthitis.

Clinical presentation
- Clinical course of syphilis divided into stages.
- Primary syphilis:
  - Seen in acquired form.
  - Genital chancre.
- Secondary syphilis and early congenital syphilis:
  - Cutaneous and mucosal lesions.
  - Constitutional symptoms.
  - Meningitis in <3% of cases possibly associated with sudden, bilateral hearing loss.
  - Multisystem involvement possible.
  - Hutchinson's triad (seen in congenital syphilis): notched incisors, interstitial keratitis, hearing loss.

- Tertiary syphilis and late congenital syphilis:
  - Gummatous granulomas affecting many organ systems.
  - Inner ear symptoms may be identical to Meniere's disease:
    - *Hennebert's sign:* vertigo and nystagmus with air pressure applied to the middle ear.
    - *Tullio's phenomenon:* vertigo and nystagmus caused by loud noise.
    - Both of these signs may also be seen in Meniere's disease.

Investigations
- In patients suspected of suffering from otogenic syphilis, a test that is accurate for tertiary syphilis—FTA-ABS or MHA-TP—is required.

Treatment
- Intravenous penicillin with or without corticosteroids.
- Hearing loss may progress despite treatment, necessitating cochlear implantation.

Recurrent vestibulopathy
Recurrent vestibulopathy is a rare condition characterized by recurrent vertigo, lasting for hours and not associated with any other inner ear or systemic pathology. It is speculated to result from a recrudescent viral infection. Its course is fairly benign, with acute attacks being much less frequent than those experienced in Meniere's disease. Vertigo is treated with vestibular suppressants.

Barotrauma
Definition
- Labyrinthine dysfunction secondary to exposure of the inner ear to changes in ambient pressure.

Epidemiology
- Rare disorder.
- Diving: most common etiology.
- Other etiologies:
  - Airplane flights.
  - Forceful sneezing.

Pathology, pathogenesis, clinical manifestations, and treatment
Alternobaric vertigo
- Temporary vertigo and/or SNHL experienced during dive or airplane flight.
- Resolves with no sequelae.
- Requires no specific treatment.

Atmospheric inner ear trauma
- Occurs after dive or forceful sneeze.
- Results in vertigo and temporary or permanent SNHL.

- Proposed mechanisms include:
  - Disruption in inner ear metabolic processes.
  - Rupture of the intralabyrinthine membranes.
  - Damage to receptor cells.

Inner ear decompression sickness
- Occurs when diver exposed to too rapid of a decrease in atmospheric pressure (too rapid an ascent); known commonly as "the bends."
- Results from gas bubbles precipitating within the labyrinthine fluids and vessels.
- May result in vertigo and temporary and/or permanent SNHL as a result of ischemic injury.
- Treatment: recompression in hyperbaric chamber.

Perilymph fistula
- See previous section.

Superior canal dehiscence syndrome
Definition
- A newly described syndrome of inner ear dysfunction secondary to dehiscence of bone overlying the superior SCC.

Epidemiology
- Because it is a rare condition, epidemiologic characteristics yet to be defined.

Pathology and pathophysiology
- A dehiscence overlying the superior SCC where it interfaces with the middle fossa dura is presumed to be congenital.
- Some traumatic or otherwise provoking event appears to make this dehiscence symptomatic.
- The dehiscence creates a "third window" in the inner ear. This third window makes the inner ear's vestibular component sensitive to acoustic or other pressure stimuli that cause motion within the inner ear fluids.
- The third window also causes some dissipation of the air conduction sound wave, causing a *cochlear conductive hearing loss* (see below).

Clinical presentation
- Dysequilibrium and vertigo provoked by loud sound or pressure, applied to the affected ear, may also be evoked by straining.
- The nystagmus pattern is characteristic of superior canal stimulation or inhibition, depending on the provocative stimulus.
- The nystagmus is best visualized with Frenzel's glasses or while administering ENG.
- Upbeat and torsional nystagmus may be generated by:
  - Tragal pressure.
  - Pneumatic otoscopy.
  - Low-frequency acoustic stimulus.

  - Straining against pinched nostrils.
  - Straining against a closed glottis.
- Patients also complain of chronic disequilibrium.
- Weber's test will lateralize to the affected ear.

Investigations
- Audiometric assessment reveals the following characteristic findings:
  - A mild to moderate conductive hearing loss in the affected ear.
  - Intact stapedial reflex.
- ENG testing reveals the characteristic nystagmus pattern from superior canal involvement in response to provocative stimuli.
- Absence of vestibular-evoked myogenic potentials (VEMPs)
- CT scan of the temporal bone using a specific high-resolution paradigm will reveal the dehiscence.

Treatment
- Resurfacing or plugging the canal via a middle fossa approach.

Psychogenic dizziness
- Psychogenic dizziness is truly a *chronic anxiety disorder* with superimposed *panic* and/or *phobic* disorders.
- Patients present with vague symptoms of dizziness (i.e., they are unable to define or describe their symptoms of dizziness in precise terms).
- Associated symptoms may include chronic lightheadedness, feeling of detachment from the environment, and fatigue.
- Symptoms tend to be *chronic* and are *worse* in crowded environments with rich visual fields such as shopping malls and grocery stores.
- Patients may describe difficulty driving.
- Symptoms are *better* at home or at rest.
- Symptoms may be reproduced by *hyperventilation*, not by caloric testing.
- Some patients may have had a remote true vertiginous that served as a *trigger* for perpetuating psychiatric disease.
- The key to making this diagnosis is an accurate patient *history*.
- Treatment is with psychiatric intervention, which will typically include anxiolytic treatment with SSRIs with or without benzodiazepines, and psychotherapy (e.g., cognitive behavioral therapy).

Central Vestibular Disorders

Migrainous vertigo
- Recurrent vertigo lasting for minutes to hours.
- No complaints of unilateral auditory dysfunction.
- History of migraines in patient, or strong family history of migraines.

- Most commonly *do not* occur concurrently with headache.
- Less frequently present as true *basilar migraines* characterized by migraine headaches associated with symptoms of brainstem dysfunction (vertigo, decreased hearing, diplopia, dysarthria, dysphagia, etc.).
- More common in females than males (3:1).
- May vary with menstrual cycle.
- May be confused with Meniere's disease ("vestibular Meniere's").
- Generally benign course, with vertigo occurring several times/year.

Treatment
- Infrequent episodes treated with vestibular suppressants.
- Role of migraine abortants, such as the serotonin receptor antagonists, yet to be established.
- More frequent episodes may respond to a migraine prevention (elimination) diet.
- Migraine prophylaxis, such as tricyclic antidepressants.

Multiple sclerosis
- Demyelinating disorder generally presents between 20 and 40 years of age.
- Disease is characterized by multiple neurologic symptoms.
  - Vertigo: presenting symptom in 5% of patients, occurs in 50% of patients during course of disease.
- Patients with MS may develop a variety of nystagmus patterns, including those that can mimic a peripheral vestibular lesion.
- One characteristic nystagmus pattern is internuclear ophthalmoplegia (INO), which may be bilateral in patients with MS.
  - INO results from a lesion in the MLF, resulting in a unilateral deficit in *adduction* and a contralateral *abducting* nystagmus when gaze is directed away from the site of the lesion. Thus the nystagmus only occurs in one eye (dissociated nystagmus).

Vascular Disease

Vertebrobasilar Insufficiency (VBI)
- Caused by recurrent episodes of decreased blood flow in the vertebrobasilar circulation.
- May be due to occlusive lesion (e.g., atherosclerosis), dissection, or decreased cardiac output.
- Manifested by symptoms including:
  - Diplopia.
  - Dysarthria.
  - Dysphagia.
  - Drop attacks.
  - Dizziness (vertigo).
  - Paresthesias.
  - Motor weakness.
- Vertigo may be only symptom in up to 25% of patients with VBI.
- Disorder to be considered in elderly patients with recurrent episodes of vertigo with or without other neurologic symptoms)
  - Note: Two most common causes of recurrent vertigo in the elderly: BPV and VBI.
- Diagnostic work-up includes transcranial Doppler and/or MRA.

Lateral medullar infarct
- Also known as *Wallenberg's syndrome.*
- Results from occlusion of the posterior inferior cerebellar artery (PICA).
- Symptoms include:
  - Vertigo.
  - Ipsilateral limb weakness and ataxia.
  - Ipsilateral facial hemianesthesia.
  - Ipsilateral Horner's syndrome.
  - Ipsilateral IXth and Xth nerve dysfunction (vocal cord paresis/paralysis, decreased gag, palatal weakness).
  - Alterations in contralateral pain and temperature sensation.

Pontine syndrome
- Results from infarction in the distribution of the AICA.
- Vertigo.
- Symptoms include:
  - Ipsilateral hearing loss and tinnitus.
  - Ipsilateral limb weakness and ataxia.
  - Ipsilateral facial hemianesthesia.
  - Ipsilateral Horner's syndrome.
  - Ipsilateral facial paralysis.
  - Contralateral hemibody sensory loss.

Cerebellar infarction
- Usually cardioembolic.
- May manifest with vertigo alone and may mimic a vestibular neuronitis.
- May be differentiated from vestibular neuronitis by the following findings:
  - Gaze-evoked direction changing nystagmus.
  - Failure of fixation to decrease amplitude of nystagmus.
  - Postural instability and falling when walking.

Selected References from the Recent Literature

1. Baloh RW. Episodic vertigo: central nervous system causes. [Review] [32 refs]. *Current Opinion in Neurology* 2002;15(1): 17-21.

2. Becvarovski Z, Bojrab DI, Michaelides EM *et al*. Round window gentamicin absorption: an in vivo human model. *Laryngoscope* 2002;112(9):1610-1613.

3. Belden CJ, Weg N, Minor LB *et al*. CT evaluation of bone dehiscence of the superior semicircular canal as a cause of sound-and/or pressure-induced vertigo. [comment]. *Radiology* 2003;226(2):337-343.

4. Bisdorff AR, Debatisse D. Localizing signs in positional vertigo due to lateral canal cupulolithiasis. *Neurology* 2001;57(6):1085-1088.

5. Carey JP, Minor LB, Peng GC *et al*. Changes in the three-dimensional angular vestibulo-ocular reflex following intratympanic gentamicin for Meniere's disease. *JARO* 2002;3(4):430-443.

6. Dimitri PS, Wall C III, Rauch SD. Multivariate vestibular testing: laterality of unilateral Meniere's disease. *Journal of Vestibular Research* 2001;11(6):405-412.

7. Evans RW, Baloh RW. Episodic vertigo and migraine. *Headache* 2001;41(6):604-605.

8. Haynes DS, Resser JR, Labadie RF *et al*. Treatment of benign positional vertigo using the semont maneuver: efficacy in patients presenting without nystagmus. *Laryngoscope* 2002;112(5):796-801.

9. Kaplan DM, Nedzelski JM, Al Abidi A *et al*. Hearing loss following intratympanic instillation of gentamicin for the treatment of unilateral Meniere's disease. *Journal of Otolaryngology* 2002;31(2):106-111.

10. Li JC, Li CJ, Epley J *et al*. Cost-effective management of benign positional vertigo using canalith repositioning. *Otolaryngology–Head & Neck Surgery* 2000;122(3): 334-339.

11. Mhatre AN, Jero J, Chiappini I *et al*. Aquaporin-2 expression in the mammalian cochlea and investigation of its role in Meniere's disease. *Hearing Research* 2002;170(1-2):59-69.

12. Minor LB, Cremer PD, Carey JP *et al*. Symptoms and signs in superior canal dehiscence syndrome. *Annals of the New York Academy of Sciences* 2001;942:259-273.

13. Minor LB, Carey JP, Cremer PD *et al*. Dehiscence of bone overlying the superior canal as a cause of apparent conductive hearing loss. *Otology & Neurotology* 2003;24(2): 270-278.

14. Ostrowski VB, Kartush JM. Endolymphatic sac-vein decompression for intractable Meniere's disease: long term treatment results. [Review] [38 refs]. *Otolaryngology–Head & Neck Surgery* 2003;128(4):550-559.

15. Ruckenstein MJ. Therapeutic efficacy of the Epley canalith repositioning maneuver. *Laryngoscope* 2001;111(6):940-945.

16. Schwaber MK. Transtympanic gentamicin perfusion for the treatment of Meniere's disease. [Review] [14 refs]. *Otolaryngologic Clinics of North America* 2002;35(2):287-295.

17. Soderman AC, Bagger-Sjoback D, Bergenius J *et al*. Factors influencing quality of life in patients with Meniere's disease, identified by a multidimensional approach. *Otology & Neurotology* 2002;23(6):941-948.

18. Stahl JS, Daroff RB. Time for more attention to migrainous vertigo? *Neurology* 2001;56(4):428-429.

19. Thakar A, Anjaneyulu C, Deka RC. Vertigo syndromes and mechanisms in migraine. *Journal of Laryngology & Otology* 2001;115(10):782-787.

20. Tirelli G, D'Orlando E, Giacomarra V *et al*. Benign positional vertigo without detectable nystagmus. *Laryngoscope* 2001;111(6):1053-1056.

21. Weisleder P, Fife TD. Dizziness and headache: a common association in children and adolescents. *Journal of Child Neurology* 2001;16(10):727-730.

22. Wu IC, Minor LB. Long-term hearing outcome in patients receiving intratympanic gentamicin for Meniere's disease. *Laryngoscope* 2003;113(5):815-820.

TUMORS OF THE EAR AND TEMPORAL BONE

Cancer of the Ear and Temporal Bone

Definition
- Malignant neoplasm of the temporal bone, surrounding soft tissue, and lateral skull base.

Epidemiology
- 6/1,000,000.
- Male = female.
- Mean age at presentation: 50 years old.

Pathology
Epithelial neoplasms
- Squamous cell carcinoma (SCCA): most frequent pathology.
- Basal cell carcinoma: much less frequent.

Tumors of the minor salivary glands: next most common
- Adenocarcinoma.
- Adenoid cystic carcinoma.
- Acinic cell carcinoma.
- Malignant mixed tumor.

Other malignancies
- Sarcomas (rhabdomyosarcoma, chondrosarcoma).
- Chordoma.
- Lymphoma.

Clinical presentation
- Otorrhea (80%): more common in epithelial malignancies.
- Pain (60%): deep boring pain indicates advanced disease.
- Decreased hearing (CHL > SNHL).
- Facial nerve paresis/paralysis (35%).
- Other cranial nerve involvement (20%).

Staging
- No established staging system.
- Patterns of spread from primary site (external canal) (5-year survival: 70%-75%):
  - Middle ear, mastoid, fallopian canal (5-year survival: 60%)
  - TMJ, parotid, infratemporal fossa (5-year survival: 25%)
  - Dura, internal carotid, jugular bulb, petrous apex (5-year survival: 0%)

Surgery
1. Sleeve resection
- Resection of the soft tissue and bone of the ear canal (include posterior aspect of TMJ), leaving TM in place.
- Indicated for tumors of the cartilaginous canal.

2. Lateral temporal bone resection
- Resection of the skin and the soft tissue of the external ear canal, and the contents of the middle ear lateral to the stapes.
- Indicated for tumors of the bony external ear canal not encroaching on the TM.

3. Subtotal temporal bone resection
- An ill-defined operation that involves a lateral temporal bone resection, together with other contents of the temporal bone that may include the:
  - Facial nerve.
  - Squamous portion of the temporal bone.
  - Sigmoid sinus/jugular vein.
  - Labyrinth.
- Indicated for tumors that involve, and extend medial to, the TM.

4. Total temporal bone resection
- Indicated for extensive tumor. Such tumors have very poor prognosis.
- Two techniques have been advocated:
  - *En bloc* resection as proposed by Lewis. This is a difficult operation that has a high complication rate. It involves approaching the temporal bone from above (middle fossa), posteriorly (posterior fossa), and anteriorly (a preauricular approach into the infratemporal fossa with mobilization of the carotid). The final cut, made with a chisel, cuts across the medial aspect of the petrous apex.
  - A more controlled technique has been advocated in which the temporal bone is "drilled out" as it would be for a lateral skull base approach. This approach does not allow for *en bloc* resection but decreases complications.
  - These two approaches seem to offer similar prognoses.

Adjunctive treatments
- Depends on tumor types and extent of tumor.
- Local, regional, or free flaps required for most of the previously described procedures; most common flaps used: the temporalis and the free latissimus dorsi.
- Parotidectomy with or without neck dissection (anterior extension, salivary gland tumor).
- Radiation therapy: for cancers that require more than a lateral temporal bone resection and for cancers that demonstrate aggressive behaviors (e.g., adenoid cystic).
- Chemotherapy: particularly for sarcomas.

Complications
- Wound infection/breakdown.
- CSF leak.
- Facial paralysis.
- Lower cranial nerve paralyses.

- CVA–stroke.
- Death.

Glomus Tumors

Definition
- Vascular, generally benign tumors of the temporal bone.

Epidemiology
- Incidence = 10% that of acoustic neuromas.
- May present at any age; majority within 50-60 years old.
- Sporadic >> familial.
- In sporadic form, male:female = 2-3:1
- Multicentricity:
  - Sporadic form: 7%-8%.
  - Familial form: 25%-30%.
  - Most common combination = glomus tumor + carotid body tumor.

Pathology
- Arise from the glomus bodies of Guild located on the jugular bulb (giving rise to glomus jugulare tumors) and on the Arnold's and Jacobson's nerves (giving rise to glomus tympanicum tumors).
- Tumors arising from this tissue type referred to as paragangliomas or chemodectomas.
- Histologic features: nests of large polyhedral epitheliod cells (chief cells) with a vacuolated cytoplasm and small, oval, hyperchromatic nuclei; nests of cells separated by a fibrous stroma rich in capillaries and venules.
- Overwhelmingly benign.
- Rare, malignant tumors defined by the presence of metastases (that must be distinguished from multicentricity).

Clinical presentation
- Glomus tympanicum tumors
  - Arise on the middle ear, typically off Jacobson's nerve.
  - Often present as an asymptomatic, retrotympanic, red, middle ear mass, noted on routine physical examination.
  - Other associated symptoms: pulsatile tinnitus, hearing loss (conductive > SNHL), otalgia, and otorrhea.
  - May display Brown's sign (blanching with the application of positive pressure on pneumatic otoscopy).
- Glomus jugulare tumors
  - Arise off the jugular bulb.
  - Present with same symptoms as tympanicum tumors; however, involvement of the jugular

foramen leads to cranial nerve involvement, particularly of the lower cranial nerves. Facial nerve less commonly involved. The Vth and VIth nerves rarely involved.

Investigations
- CT scan of the temporal bone
  - Delineates extent of bony erosion (labyrinth, carotid canal, ossicles).
  - Helps distinguish between tympanicum tumors from jugulare tumors because jugulare tumors display erosion of the jugular bulb.
- MRI scan with enhancement
  - Useful in larger tumors to assess intracranial and extratemporal extension, involvement of internal carotid artery, and cavernous sinus.
- Angiography
  - Will confirm diagnosis if other exams are equivocal.
  - Detects multicentricity.
  - Allows for preoperative embolization.

Treatment
- Glomus tympanicum tumors are managed via surgical resection:
  - Transcanal.
  - Transmastoid (canal wall up with facial recess, canal wall down).
- The management of glomus jugulare tumors is controversial:
  - Radiation therapy is the treatment of choice in some centers:
    - Radiation treatment induces a vasculitis that denies a tumor its blood supply.
    - It achieves control rates of close to 90% over 10 years.
    - Treatment protocols involve 35-45 Gray.
    - Radiation therapy offers excellent control rates with minimal complications. There is rarely an exacerbation in symptoms of cranial nerve dysfunction. Rather, improvement in cranial nerve function after radiation is seen in a significant number of patients.
  - Surgical therapy:
    - The development of lateral skull base approaches has allowed the resection of jugulare tumors for cure.
    - Embolization is used within 24 hours of the surgery.
    - The Fisch infratemporal fossa approach type A is the most common surgical technique is used:
1. Make an upper cervical incision and expose the carotid artery, jugular vein, lower cranial nerves, and facial nerve.

2. Perform a mastoidectomy.
3. Identify and decompress the facial nerve.
4. Take down the canal wall.
5. Denude the sigmoid sinus of bone all the way to jugular bulb.
6. Mobilize the facial nerve anteriorly.
7. Identify the carotid artery in the carotid canal.
8. Identify the tumor.
9. Either ligate or pack the sigmoid.
10. Ligate the jugular vein.
11. Resect the tumor and pack the inferior petrosal sinuses.
12. Pack the eustachian tube, close the ear canal, and ablate the mastoid with temporalis or fat.
13. Intracranial extension may be addressed by opening the posterior fossa dura.
    - The surgery may be modified by mobilizing only the descending portion of the facial nerve, or skeletonizing it without mobilization in the case of smaller tumors
    - An extended facial recess approach may be used instead of taking the canal wall down, thus preserving hearing.
    - Surgical approaches offer cure as opposed to control; however, they are often complicated with increased lower cranial nerve palsies, resulting in vocal cord paralysis and aspiration. Facial nerve paralysis may be temporary or permanent.

Tumors of the Cerebellopontine Angle (CPA)

Definition
- The CPA is CSF-filled space bordered by the brainstem medially, the cerebellum posteriorly, the lower cranial nerve bundles inferiorly, and the posterior face of the temporal bone laterally.

Incidence and epidemiology
- *Vestibular schwannomas* (acoustic neuromas [Ans]) are:
  - The most common neoplasm involving the CPA.
  - Affects 10 adults/million/year.
  - Acoustic neuromas account for 6% of intracranial tumors.
  - They are most commonly sporadic (95%), with 5% of cases being bilateral and caused by neurofibromatosis type II (NF2) (see section on genetic hearing loss).
  - The mean age of presentation of sporadic acoustic neuromas is 50 years old.
  - The mean age of presentation of NF2 is 30 years old.
- *Meningiomas* are the second most common neoplasm affecting the CPA.
  - They account for approximately 15% of intracranial neoplasms, with approximately 5% of

these lesions involving the CPA (approximately 10% of CPA lesions).
- Other rare tumors of the CPA include:
  - Epidermoids (5%).
  - Facial nerve and lower cranial nerve schwannomas (neuromas) (1%-2%).
  - Lipomas.
  - Primary brain neoplasms (gliomas, astrocytomas, ependymomas).
  - Metastatic lesions.

Pathology
Acoustic neuromas
- A schwannoma arising from the vestibular branch of the VIIIth cranial nerve.
- Equal incidence of arising from superior and inferior branch of the vestibular nerve.
- May arise at zone of transition between central and peripheral myelin—Obersteiner-Redlich zone—or from Schwann cells in the region of Scarpa's ganglion.
- Schwannomas demonstrate two morphologic patterns:
  - Antoni A pattern: densely packed cells with spindle-shaped nuclei; may form "whirled patterns," which are referred to as Verocay bodies
  - Antoni B pattern: less dense, vacuolated pleomorphic cells more common in larger tumors.
- Morphology of NF2 lesions and sporadic acoustic neuromas are the same.
- NF2 is associated with a mutation in a tumor suppressor gene located on the long arm of chromosome 22 (the NF2 gene). This mutation may also be seen in sporadic cases (40%).
- Secondary factors influence growth rate, including:
  - Growth factors: nerve growth factor (NGF), platelet-derived growth factor (PDGF), fibroblast growth factor (FGF).
  - Hormones.

Meningiomas
- Arise from cap cells that cluster at the tips of arachnoid villi.
- Grow along the dura along the posterior face of the IAC, involving the CPA, posterior fossa, and clivus.

Epidermoids
- Arise from congenital epithelial rests within the temporal bone or CPA.
- Consist of a stratified squamous lining surrounding desquamated keratin.
- Slow-growing tumors presenting in the second to fourth decade.
- Tend to envelop neural and vascular structures and project within brainstem fissures and sulci (making them very difficult to resect).

- May extend superiorly through the tentorium cerebelli into the middle fossa.

Clinical presentation
Acoustic neuromas
- Hearing loss with or without tinnitus: 95%; may result from:
  - Direct neural compression, or
  - Vascular compression within the IAC causing a cochlear hearing loss.
  - Approximately 10% (3%-25%) present with sudden SNHL.
- Vestibular dysfunction: 60%
  - Vertigo: 20%-30%.
  - Ataxia: 40%, peripheral vs. central.
  - Vth nerve (numbness, pain): 10%-20%.
  - VIIth nerve: 5%-15%
  - Diplopia (VIth nerve): 2%.
  - Lower cranial nerves: 3%.
  - Headaches:
    - 20% medium size tumors.
    - 40% large tumors.
    - Caused by hydrocephalus in a minority of cases.

Meningiomas
- Present with similar symptoms as acoustic neuromas, but with a slightly different distribution:
  - 60% present with hearing loss.
  - Facial pain: 60%
- Tumors possibly quite large before the encroach on the IAC creating symptoms, thus these patients have higher incidence of cerebellar compression.

Epidermoids
- As per acoustic neuromas.
- Have a higher incidence of facial paralysis.
- Facial nerve neuromas
  - Neuromas may present anywhere along the course of the facial nerve.
  - Intratemporal facial nerve neuromas distal to the IAC may present with conductive hearing loss, facial spasm, and facial weakness.
  - Tumors within the IAC present with symptoms similar to those seen in acoustic neuromas but with a higher incidence of *facial spasm*.

Investigations
Audiogram
- Classic presentation: asymmetric SNHL with poor speech discrimination score.
- Audiogram may display:
  - Rollover: poorer speech discrimination with increased intensity.
  - Reflex decay of the stapedius reflex.
- ABR (see section on audiology):
  - Absent waveform.

- Wave I the only identifiable waveform.
- Prolonged latency of wave V (most common):
  - IT5.
  - Absolute V.
  - I-V interval.
- Note: For many years, ABR was the screening test of choice for diagnosis of acoustic neuromas, a role that has now been supplanted by MRI. Currently its only value in the evaluation of a patient with an acoustic neuroma or similar tumor is prognostic; the poorer the waveforms, the poorer the prognosis for hearing preservation.

Vestibular function tests
- Not required for the work-up of these patients.
- May have a limited role in the prognosis for hearing preservation.
  - Some claim that an abnormal caloric test portends for a better prognosis for hearing preservation than does normal caloric testing. In a small tumor, an abnormal caloric may indicate that the tumor originates from the superior vestibular nerve and therefore will be easier to resect with hearing preservation than an inferior vestibular nerve tumor.

MRI scan with paramagnetic enhancement
- Investigation of choice for the screening for and evaluation of a CPA tumor:
  - Schwannomas will display displacement of CSF on T2-weighted images and enhancement on T1-weighted enhanced images.
  - Schwannomas may demonstrate a cystic component.
  - Meningiomas tend to be more heterogenous than schwannomas.
  - Meningiomas will enhance, often revealing a "dural tail" along the posterior face of the temporal bone.
  - Epidermoids are heterogenous tumors, hyperintense on T2 imaging, and will not enhance.

Treatment: acoustic neuromas
Conservative
- Many patients over the age of 60-65 years old will not require intervention.
- Only 30% of these tumors will display aggressive growth patterns (>2 mm/year) that will necessitate intervention.
- A MRI scan should be obtained 6 months after the first scan to ensure that no aggressive growth has taken place. After that, a MRI scan can be performed at a 1-year interval. The duration between subsequent scans can be extended.
- This approach can be maintained as long as the tumor does not encroach on the brain, causing

pathology secondary to brainstem or cerebellar compression.
- Similarly, small tumors (<2–3 mm), regardless of the age of the patient, should be observed to ensure that they are not artifactual and not growing.

Radiation therapy
- The role of radiation therapy in the management of acoustic neuromas remains controversial.
- Focused-beam radiation therapy, provided by gamma-knife or linear accelerator, may slow or arrest tumor growth.
- Issues that have not been thoroughly evaluated are:
  - Whether radiation actually alters the biologic growth rates of these slow-growing tumors.
  - The optimal treatment protocol.
  - The risk of malignant degeneration.
  - The failure rate and risks of postradiation surgery.
- Currently, radiation therapy appears to offer similar rates of hearing preservation, slightly less facial paralysis, and a slightly greater incidence of Vth nerve pathology, when compared with surgery.
- Surgery does "cure" the tumor, whereas radiation treatment does not.
- Radiation therapy does not cause surgical complications such as CSF leak, meningitis, and headache.

Surgery
- Surgical resection, in experienced hands, remains the treatment of choice for acoustic neuromas.
- The choices of surgical approaches are as follows:
  - Middle fossa (subtemporal) approach:
    - Used for small, generally intracanalicular tumors, measuring up to 1-1.5 cm.
    - Performed through a small temporal craniotomy.
    - The temporal lobe is retracted and the floor of the middle fossa is exposed. The IAC runs parallel to the EAC and bisects the angle formed by the greater petrosal nerve and the arcuate eminence. Most surgeons currently identify the IAC at its most medial portion and then extend the dissection laterally.
    - Advantages:
      - Superior hearing preservation rates.
      - More rapid recovery.
      - Low risk of CSF leak.
      - Low incidence of postoperative pain.
    - Disadvantages:
      - Limited exposure of the CPA and posterior fossa, so its use is generally restricted to small tumors.
      - Bony dissection comes right down on the facial nerve, making the risk of temporary facial paresis/paralysis slightly higher.

- Retraction on the temporal lobe may increase CNS morbidity.
- Suboccipital (retrosigmoid) approach:
  - This is the "workhorse" approach that can be used for any size tumor with or without hearing preservation.
  - Perform a suboccipital craniotomy inferior to the transverse sinus and posterior to the sigmoid sinus.
  - Retract the cerebellum, exposing the brainstem, CPA, and tumor.
  - Remove the posterior, superior, and inferior components of the bone surrounding the IAC.
  - Incise the dura and debulk the tumor.
  - Dissect the tumor off the facial nerve, the cochlear nerve (if possible), and the brainstem.
  - Advantages:
    - It is standard approach for neurosurgeons, so they are familiar with the anatomy from this perspective
    - It offers a wide exposure of the posterior fossa.
    - The hearing can be preserved with this approach:
  - Disadvantages:
    - A slightly poorer hearing preservation rate than the middle fossa approach for small tumors.
    - An inability to directly visualize the most lateral portion of the IAC (the fundus), although this can be overcome via the use of an endoscope.
    - Increased incidence of postoperative headache.
    - Retraction on the cerebellum, increasing the risk of hemorrhage, hematoma, and stroke.
    - A slight increase in the incidence of CSF leak in some series.
- Translabyrinthine approach:
  - This approach offers the most direct exposure of the CPA.
  - Perform a cortical mastoidectomy.
  - Denude the sigmoid of bone from the sinodural angle to the bulb.
  - Remove the bone overlying the posterior fossa dura.
  - Perform a labyrinthectomy.
  - Skeletonize the IAC.
  - Incise the dura of the IAC and the posterior fossa.
  - Resect the tumor.
  - Close the space with an abdominal fat graft.
  - Advantages:
    - The most direct approach to the CPA.
    - No need for retraction of the cerebellum.
    - Full visualization of the IAC.

○ Identification of the facial nerve from the brainstem to the labyrinthine component.
○ Perhaps a slightly lower risk of CSF leak.
○ Deceased incidence of postoperative headaches when compared with a suboccipital approach.
- Disadvantages:
  ○ Hearing is sacrificed.
  ○ Exposure of the brainstem can be limited, especially with a high jugular bulb and/or an anterior sigmoid sinus. However, in experienced hands, this should not be a limitation.
  ○ The neurosurgeon must become comfortable with the different perspective of the brainstem offered by this approach.
- Complications of surgery
  - Hearing loss
    - The most important predictor of hearing preservation is tumor size. Tumors above 1.5-2.0 cm have a low rate of hearing preservation.
    - Secondary predictors of hearing preservation include:
      ○ The status of the ABR configuration (as discussed previously)
      ○ The nerve of origination of the tumor, with tumors originating off the superior vestibular nerve having a somewhat better hearing preservation rate.
  - Facial paralysis
    - Incidence directly related to tumor size.
    - Tumors under 1.5 cm will have a permanent rate of paralysis of less than 5%.
  - Vertigo and imbalance
    - Vertigo is usually present for 3 days.
    - Imbalance may persist for weeks and is best addressed with vestibular rehabilitation physical therapy.
  - CSF leak: approximately 15%.
  - Meningitis: approximately 15%.
  - Temporal lobe or cerebellar edema, stroke, or hematoma
    - Fortunately rare today, but can be devastating and fatal.
- Notes on resection of other tumor types:
  - Meningiomas are resected using the same principles.
  - Large meningiomas involving the clivus may require a combination of approaches to accomplish a resection.
  - Epidermoids are extremely difficult to completely resect because of their insinuation around vital structures. They are, therefore, highly prone to recurrence.

□ Lipomas generally should not be resected because they cause little morbidity but have a significant incidence of neural pathology as a consequence of resection.

TUMORS OF THE PETROUS APEX

Definition
- The petrous apex is a pyramidal structure with the following borders:
  □ Medial: clivus.
  □ Lateral: labyrinth and the IAC.
  □ Anterior: internal carotid artery.
  □ Posterior: dura, posterior fossa, superior petrosal sinus.

Epidemiology
- Tumors of the petrous apex are rare.
- The vast majority are cholesterol granulomas.

Pathology
- *Cholesterol granuloma:* cyst containing cholesterol crystals, surrounded by giant cells and chronic inflammation, contained within a thick fibrous tissue.
- *Epidermoid:* see section on epidermoids in CPA tumors.
- *Mucocele:* benign collection of mucoid secretions.
- *Chondrosarcoma*
- *Chondroma:* malignant embryonal tumor derived from the notochord, site of origin is typically the clivus.
- *Neuromas:* trigeminal, facial.

Pathogenesis
- Cholesterol granuloma:
- Classic hypothesis
  □ Well-pneumatized petrous apex becomes obstructed by mucosa in the middle ear and mastoid.
  □ Obstruction creates a vacuum, with the decreased pressure resulting in hemorrhage from the mucosal lining of the petrous apex.
  □ Anaerobic breakdown of blood leads to precipitation of cholesterol crystals.
  □ The crystal creates a foreign body reaction and a slowly expanding cyst.
- Alternative hypothesis (Jackler)
  □ Pneumatization of the petrous apex leads to expansion into the marrow containing spaces in the petroclival region.
  □ The highly vascular bone marrow has a propensity to hemorrhage into the petrous apex cells.
  □ Blood accumulation in petrous cells obstructs outflow into the middle ear/ mastoid.

- From this point the pathogenesis is identical to that described for the classic theory.

Clinical presentation
- Cholesterol granuloma
  - Pain (hemifacial, retro-orbital).
  - Headache.
  - Diplopia.
  - Other.
  - Otalgia.
  - Vertigo.
  - Hearing loss.
  - Facial paralysis.
- Epidermoid
  - Hearing loss.
  - Facial paralysis.
  - Vertigo.
  - Pain.

Treatment
Cholesterol granulomas
Drainage
1. Infracochlear technique
   - Postauricular incision.
   - Ear canal transected.
   - TM elevated posteriorly, inferiorly, and anteriorly; pedicled to the malleus and superiorly.
   - Hypotympanic bone drilled down.
   - Air cell tract between jugular (posterior), carotid (anterior), and cochlea (superior) followed medially.
   - Cholesterol granuloma opened and drained to the middle ear.
   - Stent may be placed to try to prevent closure.
2. Infralabyrinthine
   - Postauricular incision.
   - Cortical mastoidectomy.
   - Retrofacial, infralabyrinthine cell tract followed medially.
   - Boundaries: facial nerve (anterior), posterior SCC (superior), and jugular bulb (inferior).
   - Cholesterol granuloma opened and drained into mastoid.

Resection
Translabyrinthine/transcochlear
- If no hearing present.

Middle fossa
- If hearing is intact.
- Risk of laceration to the facial nerve.

Advantage of drainage procedures
- Nondestructive.
- Lower complication route.
- Infracochlear approach offers:

- Shorter more direct route.
- More direct drainage.
- Greater risk to more vital structures.

Complications
- Closure and reaccumulation (treated by reopening tract).
- SNHL.
- Vertigo.
- Facial paralysis.
- Damage to carotid.
- Damage to jugular bulb.

Epidermoids
- Resection via middle fossa or translabyrinthine/transcochlear route.
- Epidermoids prone to recurrence because of their insinuation around nerves and into sulci of brain.

Selected References from the Recent Literature

1. Al Mefty O, Teixeira A. Complex tumors of the glomus jugulare: criteria, treatment, and outcome. *Journal of Neurosurgery* 2002;97(6):1356-1366.
2. Barrs DM. Temporal bone carcinoma. [Review] [63 refs]. *Otolaryngologic Clinics of North America* 2001;34(6):1197-1218.
3. Baser ME, DG RE, Gutmann DH. Neurofibromatosis 2. [Review] [56 refs]. *Current Opinion in Neurology* 2003;16(1): 27-33.
4. Battista RA, Wiet RJ. Stereotactic radiosurgery for acoustic neuromas: a survey of the American Neurotology Society. [Review] [47 refs]. *American Journal of Otology* 2000;21(3): 371-381.
5. Brackmann DE, Owens RM, Friedman RA et al. Prognostic factors for hearing preservation in vestibular schwannoma surgery. [Review] [24 refs]. *American Journal of Otology* 2000;21(3):417-424.
6. Brackmann DE, Toh EH. Surgical management of petrous apex cholesterol granulomas. *Otology & Neurotology* 2002;23(4):529-533.
7. Breau RL, Gardner EK, Dornhoffer JL. Cancer of the external auditory canal and temporal bone. [Review] [24 refs]. *Current Oncology Reports* 2002;4(1):76-80.
8. Fish BM, Huda R, Dundas SA et al. B-cell lymphoma of the external auditory meatus. *Journal of Laryngology & Otology* 2002;116(1):39-41.
9. Friedmann I, Graham MD. The ultrastructure of cholesterol granuloma of the middle ear: an electron microscope study. The Journal of Laryngology and Otology, 1979; Vol. 93, pp. 433-442. *Journal of Laryngology & Otology* 2002;116(11): 877-881.
10. Gillespie MB, Francis HW, Chee N et al. Squamous cell carcinoma of the temporal bone: a radiographic-pathologic correlation. [comment]. *Archives of Otolaryngology–Head & Neck Surgery* 2001;127(7):803-807.
11. Ho SY, Kveton JF. Acoustic neuroma. Assessment and management. [Review] [52 refs]. *Otolaryngologic Clinics of North America* 2002;35(2):393-404.

12. Hu J, Liu S, Qiu J. Embryonal rhabdomyosarcoma of the middle ear. *Otolaryngology–Head & Neck Surgery* 2002;126(6):690-692.

13. Jackler RK, Cho M. A new theory to explain the genesis of petrous apex cholesterol granuloma. *Otology & Neurotology* 2003;24(1):96-106.

14. Jackson CG. Glomus tympanicum and glomus jugulare tumors. [Review] [80 refs]. *Otolaryngologic Clinics of North America* 2001;34(5):941-970.

15. Jackson CG, McGrew BM, Forest JA *et al*. Lateral skull base surgery for glomus tumors: long-term control. *Otology & Neurotology* 2001;22(3):377-382.

16. Knegt PP, Ah-See KW, Meeuwis CA *et al*. Squamous carcinoma of the external auditory canal: a different approach. *Clinical Otolaryngology & Allied Sciences* 2002;27(3): 183-187.

17. Lim LH, Goh YH, Chan YM *et al*. Malignancy of the temporal bone and external auditory canal. *Otolaryngology–Head & Neck Surgery* 2000;122(6):882-886.

18. Miman MC, Aktas D, Oncel S *et al*. Glomus jugulare. *Otolaryngology–Head & Neck Surgery* 2002;127(6):585-586.

19. Miura M, Sando I, Orita Y *et al*. Histopathologic study of the temporal bones and Eustachian tubes of children with cholesterol granuloma. *Annals of Otology, Rhinology & Laryngology* 2002;111(7 Pt 1):609-615.

20. Moody SA, Hirsch BE, Myers EN. Squamous cell carcinoma of the external auditory canal: an evaluation of a staging system. *American Journal of Otology* 2000;21(4): 582-588.

21. Mosnier I, Cyna-Gorse F, Grayeli AB *et al*. Management of cholesterol granulomas of the petrous apex based on clinical and radiologic evaluation. *Otology & Neurotology* 2002;23(4): 522-528.

22. Murphy MR, Selesnick SH. Cost-effective diagnosis of acoustic neuromas: a philosophical, macroeconomic, and technological decision. [Review] [29 refs]. *Otolaryngology–Head & Neck Surgery* 2002;127(4):253-259.

23. Nyrop M, Grontved A. Cancer of the external auditory canal. *Archives of Otolaryngology–Head & Neck Surgery* 2002;128(7): 834-837.

24. Pellet W, Regis J, Roche PH *et al*. Relative indications for radiosurgery and microsurgery for acoustic schwannoma. [Review] [117 refs]. *Advances & Technical Standards in Neurosurgery* 2003;28:227-282.

25. Roland PS, Eston D. Stereotactic radiosurgery of acoustic tumors. [Review] [37 refs]. *Otolaryngologic Clinics of North America* 2002;35(2):343-355.

26. Rosenberg SI. Natural history of acoustic neuromas. [Review] [55 refs]. *Laryngoscope* 2000;110(4):497-508.

27. Sato K, Takahashi H, Yao K *et al*. Cancer of the ear: a report of 22 patients. *Acta Oto-Laryngologica–Supplement* 2002;(547): 97-99.

28. Shuto J, Ueyama T, Suzuki M *et al*. Primary lymphoma of bilateral external auditory canals. *American Journal of Otolaryngology* 2002;23(1):49-52.

29. Soon SL, Bullock M, Prince ME. Ceruminous adenocarcinoma: a rare tumour of the external auditory canal. *Journal of Otolaryngology* 2001;30(6):373-377.

30. Stipkovits EM, Graamans K, Vasbinder GB *et al*. Assessment of vestibular schwannoma growth: application of a new measuring protocol to the results of a longitudinal study. [Review] [23 refs]. *Annals of Otology, Rhinology & Laryngology* 2001;110(4):326-330.

31. Watabe-Rudolph M, Rudolph KL, Averbeck T *et al*. Telomerase activity, telomere length, and apoptosis: a comparison between acquired cholesteatoma and squamous cell carcinoma. *Otology & Neurotology* 2002;23(5):793-798.

32. Weber PC, Patel S. Jugulotympanic paragangliomas. [Review] [38 refs]. *Otolaryngologic Clinics of North America* 2001;34(6):1231-1240.

33. Wolfe SG, Lai SY, Bigelow DC. Bilateral squamous cell carcinoma of the external auditory canals. *Laryngoscope* 2002;112(6):1003-1005.

34. Yeung P, Bridger A, Smee R *et al*. Malignancies of the external auditory canal and temporal bone: a review. *ANZ Journal of Surgery* 2002;72(2):114-120.

FACIAL PARALYSIS

Congenital

Bilateral

Möbius syndrome
- Rare congenital/genetic syndrome: autosomal dominant with variable expressivity.
- Bilateral facial paralysis.
- Abducens palsy: unilateral or bilateral.
- Deformity of the extremities.

Myotonic dystrophy
- Familial disorder.
- Progressive weakness and atrophy of the muscles of the head and neck.

Unilateral
- Typically originates from birth trauma.
- Results from pressure on the extratemporal facial nerve by the maternal sacrum or, rarely, by obstetrical forceps.
- Prognosis excellent for complete recovery within 5 weeks of birth.

Acquired

Trauma
- See section on temporal bone trauma.

Infection
Bacterial
- See section on otitis media.

Viral
Ramsay Hunt syndrome
Definition
- Recrudescent herpes (varicella) zoster infection involving the sensory and/or motor components of the facial nerve.

Epidemiology
- 3%-12% of cases of facial paralysis in adult.
- 5% in children.
- Second-most common cause of acquired facial paralysis.

Clinical Manifestations (in order of frequency)
- Severe otalgia.
- Vesicular eruption on concha and external ear canal (may also be on palate and anterior tongue).
- Facial paralysis.
- SNHL.
- Vertigo.

Pathology
- Diffuse inflammatory infiltrate along facial nerve, likely originating in region of geniculate ganglion.

Pathogenesis
- Varicella zoster virus remains dormant in the non-neuronal satellite cells that surround the nerve cell bodies in the geniculate ganglion.
- At the time of recrudescence, the virus replicates and is released into the extracellular space; from here it is taken up by the *sensory* cell bodies of the geniculate ganglion. It is then transmitted to the skin by the *sensory* cell axons.

Investigations
- An audiogram is indicated in cases of suspected SNHL.
- Facial nerve testing is generally not helpful because the management is medical.

Treatment
- Valacyclovir 1 g tid × 10-14 days or famciclovir 500 mg tid × 10 days.
- Prednisone 40-60 mg/day decreases postherpetic neuralgia and may improve facial nerve function.
- Antibiotic/steroid eardrops may be of some benefit to prevent bacterial superinfection in the external ear.
- Ophthalmology consultation for herpetic or exposure keratitis.

Prognosis
- The vast majority of patients obtain complete or near complete recovery of the facial nerve. Fifty percent of cases may have some evidence of residual facial nerve dysfunction.

Bell's palsy
Definition
- An acute-onset, typically unilateral, facial paralysis that may be associated with other cranial nerve dysfunction.

Epidemiology
- Most common form of facial paralysis.
- Accounts for 60%-75% of cases of facial paralysis.
- Incidence = 20-30/100,000.
- Male = female.
- History of recurrence = 10%.
- More common in pregnancy (3× rate of nonpregnant female, even more common in preeclampsia).
  - Typically occurs in third trimester or postpartum.
  - Prognosis is same as for nonpregnant females.

Pathology

- Demyelination of the facial nerve occurs throughout its intratemporal course.
- Pathology may be more severe in the intralabyrinthine segment and at the meatal foramen.
- Lymphocytic infiltrate may be noted along the course of the nerve.

Pathogenesis

- Current evidence supports the hypothesis that a recrudescent herpes simplex type 1 infection results in facial nerve edema and a compromise in the vascular supply in the region of the labyrinthine segment of the fallopian canal. The result of this process is Wallerian degeneration of the nerve.

Clinical manifestations

- Acute onset (within 48 hours) of facial paralysis.
- Usually unilateral.
- Commonly associated with pain, which may be severe; pain typically retroauricular and may radiate anteriorly.
- May be associated with other signs of cranial nerve dysfunction, including:
  - Facial numbness.
  - Hyperacusis.
  - Dysfunction of cranial nerves IX and X and C2.
  - *Most common* associated finding: hypesthesia or dysesthesia of cranial nerves V and IX.
- Recurrence rate = 10% (higher in diabetics).
- Complete paralysis = 70%.
- Careful physical exam must be performed to rule out presence of:
  - Otologic disease.
  - Parotid neoplasm.
  - Motor and sensory neurological deficits.
  - Fissured tongue (Melkersson-Rosenthal).
  - Facial edema (Melkersson-Rosenthal).

Investigations

- In the face of a typical presentation, investigations are not generally required.
- ENOG and volitional EMG provide information as to prognosis and to possible indications for surgery (see below). If patient has ENOG amplitude <90% of control side *and* absence of volitional movement on EMG, the prognosis for full recovery is less favorable.
- Signs that further work-up is necessary include:
  - Bilateral simultaneous facial paralysis (may be indicative of systemic disease).
  - Loss of spontaneous facial movements (CNS disease).
  - Multiple cranial nerve deficits (may be associated with CNS disease or Bell's palsy)
  - No signs of recovery 3-6 weeks after onset (? neoplasm).
  - Full or almost full recovery not achieved in 3-6 months (? neoplasm).
  - Presence of facial twitch or spasm prior to onset of paralysis (? neoplasm).
  - Selective sparing of motor branches of the facial nerve (? neoplasm).
  - Slow progression of the paralysis over 3 weeks or more (? neoplasm).

Treatment

- Supportive care for eye.
- Prednisone 40-60 mg/day × 2 weeks.
- Antiherpetic agent (as for Ramsay Hunt).
- Role for surgical intervention.
  - Most controversial aspect of management.
  - Recent evidence suggests that in the subpopulation with the poorest prognosis (complete paralysis, ENOG <90% of control, no volitional EMG), a facial nerve decompression may be beneficial. The decompression must be performed via a middle fossa approach and focus on the intralabyrinthine and perigeniculate portions of the nerve.

Disorders Associated with Bilateral Simultaneous Facial Paralysis

- Guillain-Barré syndrome:
  - Progressive ascending motor paralysis.
  - Typically follows a viral infection.
- Bell's palsy (as above, bilateral simultaneous occurs in 0.3% of patients with this disorder).
- Multiple idiopathic cranial nerve neuropathies.
- Encephalitis of the brainstem.
- Benign intracranial hypertension:
  - Typically manifests with headache, visual disturbance, and pulsatile tinnitus.
  - Cranial nerve VI the most frequent cranial nerve involved.
  - Facial nerve rarely involved.
- Syphilis
  - Presentation with bilateral facial paralysis mandates performance of a FTA-ABS (or MHA-TP).
- Leukemia
- Lyme disease
  - *Ixodes* tickborne spirochete (*Borrelia burgdorferi*).
  - Reservoir white-footed mouse and white-tailed deer.
  - Three stages:
    - Stage 1
      - Erythema migrans (enlarging, annular erythematous skin lesions that shift in location).

- ○ Fever, malaise, arthralgias.
- ○ Regional lymphadenopathy.
  - Stage 2
    - ○ Weeks to months after onset.
    - ○ Characterized by neurological abnormalities, including meningitis, cranial nerve neuropathies, and peripheral neuropathies.
    - ○ Facial paralysis: unilateral (more common) or bilateral.
  - *Stage 3*
    - ○ Months to years after onset.
    - ○ Arthritis.
    - ○ Recurrent meningitis.
    - ○ Neurologic deficits.
  - ❑ Treatment:
    - Doxycycline, ceftriaxone.
- Sarcoidosis
  - ❑ Noncaseating granulomatous disease most typically involving the lungs.
  - ❑ Other findings: liver dysfunction, arthralgias, weakness and fatigue, and elevated calcium levels.
  - ❑ Facial nerve involved in 5% of cases (more commonly unilateral).
  - ❑ Variant of sarcoidosis: uveoparotid fever (Heerfordt's disease), which consists of:
    - Uveitis.
    - Parotitis.
    - Low-grade fever.
    - Cranial nerve dysfunction: most commonly involved facial nerve (50% of cases).
- Meningitis.
- Prepontine or pontine tumor.
- Therefore, a patient presenting with a bilateral facial paralysis requires:
  - ❑ Syphilis and lyme serology.
  - ❑ ACE.
  - ❑ MRI head with enhancement.
  - ❑ Lumbar puncture.

Progressive Paralysis

- Suggestive of a CNS or temporal bone neoplasm.
- Neoplasms that more commonly present with facial paralysis include:
  - ❑ Facial nerve schwannoma (neuroma).
  - ❑ Metastatic lesion to CPA.
  - ❑ Acoustic neuroma.
  - ❑ Primary CNS tumor (typically malignant).
  - ❑ Cholesteatoma (epidermoid) of the petrous apex.
  - ❑ Cholesterol granuloma.
  - ❑ Fibrous dysplasia of the temporal bone.
  - ❑ Glomus jugulare tumor.

Miscellaneous Disorders

Melkersson-Rosenthal Syndrome

- Recurrent facial edema.
- Recurrent facial paralysis.
- Fissured tongue.
- Other symptoms include:
  - ❑ Headache.
  - ❑ Granular cheilitis.
  - ❑ Vth nerve neuralgia.
  - ❑ Other lower cranial nerve dysfunction.
  - ❑ Cervical dysautonomia.
- Unknown etiology.
- Supportive treatment.

HIV

- A neurotropic virus that can cause facial paralysis at any stage of infection.

The House Brackmann Scale for the Evaluation of Facial Nerve Function/Recovery

- Grade I: Normal facial function.
- Grade II: Mild dysfunction:
  - ❑ Slight weakness is noted on close inspection. The patients may have a slight synkinesis.
  - ❑ Normal symmetry and tone is noted at rest.
  - ❑ Forehead motion is moderate to good, complete eye closure is achieved with minimal effort, and slight mouth asymmetry is noted.
- Grade III: Moderate dysfunction:
  - ❑ An obvious but not disfiguring difference is noted between both sides. A noticeable but not severe synkinesis, contracture, or hemifacial spasm is present.
  - ❑ Normal symmetry and tone is noted at rest.
  - ❑ Forehead movement is slight to moderate, complete eye closure is achieved with effort, and a slightly weak mouth movement is noted with maximum effort.
- Grade IV: Moderately severe dysfunction:
  - ❑ An obvious weakness and/or disfiguring asymmetry is noted.
  - ❑ Symmetry and tone are normal at rest.
  - ❑ No forehead motion is observed. Eye closure is incomplete, and an asymmetric mouth is noted with maximal effort.
- Grade V: Severe dysfunction:
  - ❑ Only a barely perceptible motion is noted.
  - ❑ Asymmetry is noted at rest.
  - ❑ No forehead motion is observed.
  - ❑ Eye closure is incomplete and mouth movement is only slight.
- Grade VI: Total paralysis:
  - ❑ Gross asymmetry is noted.
  - ❑ No movement is noted.

Selected References from the Recent Literature

1. Redaelli de Zinis LO, Gamba P, Balzanelli C. Acute otitis media and facial nerve paralysis in adults. *Otology & Neurotology* 2003;24(1):113-117.

2. Buyukavci M, Tan H, Akdag R. An alarming sign for serious diseases in children: bilateral facial paralysis. *Pediatric Neurology* 2002;27(4):312-313.

3. Mori T, Nagai K, Asanuma H. Reactivation of varicella-zoster virus in facial palsy associated with infectious mononucleosis. *Pediatric Infectious Disease Journal* 2002;21(7):709-711.

4. Benecke JE, Jr. Facial paralysis. [Review] [27 refs]. *Otolaryngologic Clinics of North America* 2002;35(2):357-365.

5. Terzis JK, Noah EM. Möbius and Möbius-like patients: etiology, diagnosis, and treatment options. *Clinics in Plastic Surgery* 2002;29(4):497-514.

6. Kuhweide R, Van de Steene V, Vlaminck S, Casselman JW. Ramsay Hunt syndrome: pathophysiology of cochleovestibular symptoms. [Review] [43 refs]. *Journal of Laryngology & Otology* 2002;116(10):844-848.

7. Kalish RA, Kaplan RF, Taylor E *et al*. Evaluation of study patients with Lyme disease, 10-20-year follow-up. *Journal of Infectious Diseases* 2001;183(3):453-460.

8. Yetiser S, Tosun F, Kazkayasi M. Facial nerve paralysis due to chronic otitis media. *Otology & Neurotology* 2002;23(4):580-588.

9. Kvestad E, Kvaerner KJ, Mair IW. Otologic facial palsy: etiology, onset, and symptom duration. *Annals of Otology, Rhinology & Laryngology* 2002;111(7 Pt 1):598-602.

10. Sasaki MG, Leite PG, Leite AG *et al*. Bilateral peripheral facial palsy secondary to lymphoma in a patient with HIV/AIDS: a case report and literature review. *Brazilian Journal of Infectious Diseases* 2002;6(1):50-54.

11. Sherman JD, Dagnew E, Pensak ML *et al*. Facial nerve neuromas: report of 10 cases and review of the literature. [Review] [43 refs]. *Neurosurgery* 2002;50(3):450-456.

12. Toelle SP, Boltshauser E. Long-term outcome in children with congenital unilateral facial nerve palsy. *Neuropediatrics* 2001;32(3):130-135.

13. Suzuki F, Furuta Y, Ohtani F *et al*. Herpes virus reactivation and gadolinium-enhanced magnetic resonance imaging in patients with facial palsy. *Otology & Neurotology* 2001;22(4):549-553.

14. Furuta Y, Kawabata H, Ohtani F *et al*. Western blot analysis for diagnosis of Lyme disease in acute facial palsy. *Laryngoscope* 2001;111(4 Pt 1):719-723.

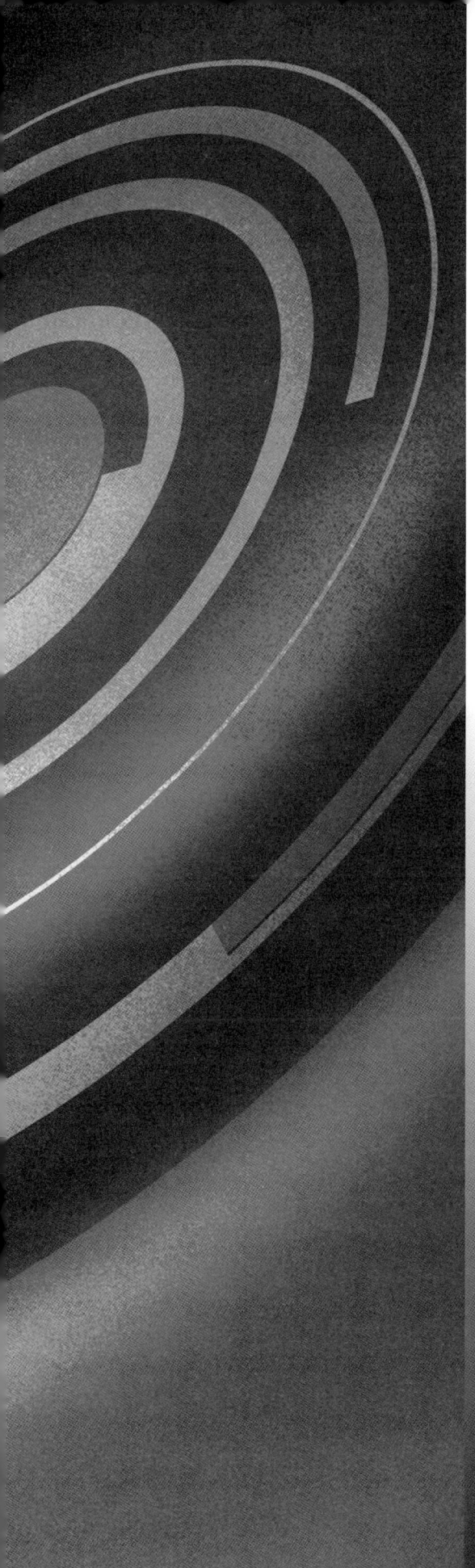

Rhinology

PHYSIOLOGY OF THE NOSE

Nasal airway
- Surface area is 150 cm².
- Air is humidified and warmed.
- Airway resistance is altered through congestion and decongestion.

Nasal blood vessels
- Resistance vessels (arterioles and precapillary sphincters) control blood flow.
- Exchange vessels (capillaries) filter and absorb fluid.
- Capacitance vessels (veins, venous sinusoids) control blood volume.
- Sensory innervation occurs via CN V1 and CN V2.

Sympathetic Vasomotor Control
- Vasoconstriction (norepinephrine, avian pancreatic polypeptide, and neuropeptide Y).

Parasympathetic Vasomotor Control
- Secretion (acetylcholine, vasoactive intestinal peptide).

Nasal glands and secretion
- Mucus produced by goblet cells and submucosal glands.
- Parasympathetic control.

Mucociliary function
- Pseudostratified ciliated respiratory epithelium, mucous blanket, and mucus-producing glands.
- Moist surface for humidification and cleaning of inspired air.
- Cilia beat at rate of 800-1000 strokes/minute.
- Mucous blanket moves 3-35 mm/min.
- Mucous blanket has two layers:
  - Periciliary fluid—serous
  - Viscoelastic mucous layer
- Nasal mucus: 95% water; 3% glycoprotein (mucin); 2% salts, immunoglobulins (IgA), lysozymes, and lactoferrin.
- Mucus cleared posteriorly in nose towards pharynx where swallowed.
- Mucus cleared in the direction of ostia in sinuses.

Nasal airway resistance
- Greatest contribution made by anterior nasal airway.
- Three functional regions:
  - Nasal vestibule (external nasal valve).
  - Internal nasal valve: 1.3 cm posteriorly from nares; narrowest, highest-resistance segment (50% of total nasal resistance).
  - Nasal cavum: posterior to piriform aperture.

- Major sites for regulation of airway resistance are dilator nares muscles and venous sinusoids of turbinates.

Nasal cycle
- Intrinsic variability of nasal airway resistance presents, in at least 40% of people.
- Cycle lasts 2-6 hours.
- One side of nose congests while the opposite decongests.

Olfaction
- Requires airflow through nose.
- **CN I and CN V** fibers.
- CN I mediates most smells:
  - Made up of 40 olfactory nerve bundles.
  - From olfactory epithelium into brain via cribriform plate.
- CN V mediates somatosensory sensations:
  - Perception of pungent odors (ammonia, hot peppers).
  - At high concentrations, most odorants also stimulate CN V.

Olfactory epithelium
- Pseudostratified columnar.

Location
- Superior septum, cribriform plate, superior and middle turbinates.

Cell types
- Bipolar receptor neurons, synapse in olfactory bulb:
  - Each receptor cell expresses a single receptor gene.
  - Approximately 1000 types of receptors exist in vertebrate olfactory epithelium.
  - Each receptor cell responds electrophysiologically to more than one type of odorant molecule.
- Microvillar cells: neuronal cells, unknown function
- Sustentacular cells: insulate bipolar cells from each other, regulate mucus composition, deactivate odorants.
- Basal cells (horizontal and globose): can regenerate olfactory fibers.
- Bowman gland cells: produce mucus.

Mechanism of olfaction
- Odorant carried into olfactory cleft, adsorbed onto mucus.
- Odorant-binding proteins (OBPs) facilitate binding to receptor cells.
- Binding initiates G-protein (cAMP-dependent) cascade, resulting in cell depolarization.
- Synapse onto secondary neurons at glomeruli located within olfactory bulb.

- Further integration/processing.
- Projection onto primary olfactory cortex (antolfactory nucleus, prepiriform cortex, lateral entorhinal cortex, periamygdaloid cortex, and amygdala).
- Secondary olfactory cortex in orbitofrontal region.

Anosmia

Definitions
- Anosmia: inability to detect any odor sensation.
- Hyposmia: decreased sensitivity to some or all odorants.
- Dysosmia: distorted perception of smell.
- Phantosmia: perception of an (usually) unpleasant odor when no odor is present.

Etiology
- Obstructive
  - Intranasal polyposis.
  - Chronic sinusitis.
  - Allergic rhinitis.
  - Intranasal tumor.
- Sensorineural loss
  - Prior upper respiratory infection.
    - Causes scarring of olfactory epithelium.
    - Influenza virus: produces necrosis of pseudostratified ciliated columnar epithelium.
  - Head trauma (20%-30%) of severe head trauma results in olfactory loss.
    - Results from shearing olfactory nerve filaments through cribriform plate.
    - May also cause anosmia via obstruction, cerebral ischemia, or intracranial hemorrhage.
  - Iatrogenic—subsequent to neurosurgical procedures or sinus surgery
- Idiopathic Smell Dysfunction
  - Comprise 19%-26% of patients with olfactory dysfunction.
- Congenital
  - Kallmann's syndrome (anosmia and hypogonadism).
- Systemic diseases
  - Multiple sclerosis.
  - Parkinson's disease.
  - Huntington's chorea.
  - Epilepsy (specifically temporal lobe affecting unilateral nostril).
  - Alzheimer's (plaques and neurofibrillary tangles in anterior olfactory nuclei).
  - AIDS dementia.
  - Schizophrenia.
- Nutritional deficiencies
  - Pellagra.
  - Pernicious anemia.
  - Korsakoff's psychosis.

Evaluation
- Nasal endoscopy.
- CT scan.
- MRI (best for CNS etiology).
- Psychophysical testing.
  - The Smell Identification Test is a convenient method for the psychophysical evaluation of smell function. It provides the patient with four test booklets, each with 10 scratch-and-sniff odorants. Each odorant has a list of four possible answers, and the patient must choose one answer before moving on to the next odorant. The results are then compared with norms established for the patient's age and sex. Based on the results of these tests, the patient's results may be classified as normal, mild, moderate, or severe hyposmia, anosmia, or probable malingering.

Treatments
Obstructive
- Steroids (short-course systemic [e.g., prednisone 40-60 mg p.o. × 1 week] followed by topical steroid spray for minimum of 1 month) for allergic rhinitis or nasal polyps.
- Surgical resection

Traumatic
- Allow olfactory neuroepithelium to regenerate (15%-39%).

Sensory deficits of unknown etiology
- Vitamins A and B and Zinc have been advocated for use in patients with anosmia with sensory receptor failure; however, the efficacy of these treatments has not been established.

Selected References from the Recent Literature

1. Apter AJ, Gent JF, Frank ME. Fluctuating olfactory sensitivity and distorted odor perception in allergic rhinitis. *Archives of Otolaryngology—Head & Neck Surgery* 2000;125:1005-1010.
2. Ogawa T, Rutka J. Olfactory dysfunction in head injured workers. *Acta Oto-Laryngologica—Supplement* 2000;540:50-57.
3. Potagas C, Dellatolas G, Ziegler M *et al.* Clinical assessment of olfactory dysfunction in Parkinson's disease [see comments]. *Movement Disorders* 2000;13:394-399.
4. van Dam FS, Hilgers FJ, Emsbroek G *et al:* Deterioration of olfaction and gustation as a consequence of total laryngectomy. *Laryngoscope* 1999;109:1150-1155.
5. Sugiura M, Aiba T, Mori J, Nakai Y. An epidemiological study of postviral olfactory disorder. *Acta Oto-Laryngologica—Supplement* 2000;538:191-196.
6. Dawes PJ. Clinical tests of olfaction. *Clinical Otolaryngology & Allied Sciences* 2000;23:484-490.
7. Cullen MM, Leopold DA. Disorders of smell and taste. *Medical Clinics of North America* 2000;83:57-74.

8. Spielman AI. Chemosensory function and dysfunction. *Critical Reviews in Oral Biology & Medicine* 2000;9:267-291.

9. Delank KW, Stoll W. Olfactory function after functional endoscopic sinus surgery for chronic sinusitis. *Rhinology* 2000;36:15-19.

10. Jones N, Rog D. Olfaction: a review. *Journal of Laryngology & Otology* 2000;112:11-24.

11. Martzke JS, Kopala LC, Good KP. Olfactory dysfunction in neuropsychiatric disorders: review and methodological considerations. *Biological Psychiatry* 2000;42:721-732.

12. Cowart BJ, Young IM, Feldman RS, Lowry LD. Clinical disorders of smell and taste. *Occupational Medicine* 2000;12: 465-483.

13. Vowles RH, Bleach NR, Rowe-Jones JM. Congenital anosmia. *International Journal of Pediatric Otorhinolaryngology* 2000;41:207-214.

14. Doty RL, Yousem DM, Pham LT *et al.* Olfactory dysfunction in patients with head trauma. *Archives of Neurology* 2000;54:1131-1140.

15. Mott AE, Cain WS, Lafreniere D *et al.* Topical corticosteroid treatment of anosmia associated with nasal and sinus disease. *Archives of Otolaryngology—Head & Neck Surgery* 2000;123:367-372.

16. Yousem DM, Geckle RJ, Bilker WB *et al.* Posttraumatic olfactory dysfunction: MR and clinical evaluation. *American Journal of Neuroradiology* 2000;17:1171-1179.

17. Golding-Wood DG, Holmstrom M, Darby Y *et al.* The treatment of hyposmia with intranasal steroids. *Journal of Laryngology & Otology* 2000;110:132-135.

18. Downey LL, Jacobs JB, Lebowitz RA. Anosmia and chronic sinus disease. *Otolaryngology—Head & Neck Surgery* 2000;115: 24-28.

19. Nordin S, Murphy C, Davidson TM *et al.* Prevalence and assessment of qualitative olfactory dysfunction in different age groups. *Laryngoscope* 2000;106:739-744.

20. Apter AJ, Mott AE, Frank ME, Clive JM. Allergic rhinitis and olfactory loss. *Annals of Allergy, Asthma, & Immunology* 2000;75:311-316.

21. Duncan HJ, Seiden AM. Long-term follow-up of olfactory loss secondary to head trauma and upper respiratory tract infection. *Archives of Otolaryngology—Head & Neck Surgery* 2000;121:1183-1187.

EPISTAXIS

Anatomy

Nose supplied by branches of the *external carotid artery* and *internal carotid artery*.

Branches of the External Carotid

- Facial artery via superior labial artery: anterior septum and ala.
- Internal maxillary artery:
  - Sphenopalatine: posterior and anterior nasal cavity.
  - Greater palatine artery (via descending palatine): posteroinferior nasal cavity.

Internal Carotid (via Ophthalmic)

- Anterior ethmoid artery: anterior nasal cavity.
- Posterior ethmoid artery: posterior nasal cavity.

  Little's area (i.e., Kiesselbach's plexus), located on the anterior septum, consists of converging vessels from branches of the internal and external carotid systems, with 90% of all nosebleeds occurring in this area. Posterior bleeds typically involve the sphenopalatine artery. Ethmoid arteries are more likely to be involved secondary to maxillofacial trauma.

Etiology
Local
- Trauma (maxillofacial, nose picking, cocaine).
- Foreign bodies.
- Infection.
- Iatrogenic (surgery).
- Neoplasms of the nasal cavity or nasopharynx.
- Chemical toxins (heavy metals such as mercury, chromium, and phosphorous; sulfuric acid; ammonia; gasoline; glutaraldehyde).

Systemic disorders
- Arteriosclerosis associated with hypertension.
- Osler-Weber-Rendu disease (hereditary hemorrhagic telangiectasia): autosomal dominant disease in which contractile elements are lacking in the vessel walls. Mucosal telangiectasias cause severe recurrent nosebleeds, often requiring repeated laser coagulation of vessels or skin grafting of the nasal cavity.
- Hematologic disorders: hemophilia, leukemia, multiple myeloma, immune thrombocytopenia purpura (ITP), polycythemia vera.
- Drugs: NSAIDs, aspirin, warfarin; chemotherapeutic agents causing to thrombocytopenia.
- Vitamin deficiency: Vitamins C or K deficiency.

Treatment
- Safeguard airway, breathing, and circulation.
- Medical:
  - Remove all clots from nose and localize site of bleeding.
  - Apply topical vasoconstrictors and anesthetics via spray and pledget (e.g., cocaine 4%, 4% lidocaine with 1% oxymetazoline, or 4% lidocaine with 1% phenylephrine).
  - Attempt to visualize bleeding site with anterior rhinoscopy or rigid endoscopy.
  - Bleeding can be controlled by:
    - Applying firm pressure to the anterior nose.
    - Chemical cautery with silver nitrate if bleeding is superficial.
    - Electrical cautery, which is particularly useful when combined with endoscopy.
    - Placement of anterior packs (Vaseline-coated gauze, expandable sponge [e.g., Merocel], balloon catheter), which stops most bleeding. Bilateral packing may be required.
    - Placement of posterior packs in cases of severe bleeding not controlled by anterior packs. Posterior packs are placed in the nasopharynx. They do not generally tamponade bleeding themselves but provide a buttress against which an anterior pack may be placed.
    - Transoral injection via the greater palatine foramen has been reported to be successful in some posterior bleeds emanating from the sphenopalatine artery.
- Interventional radiology: angiography with embolization of branches of the external carotid artery. Typically performed for epistaxis refractory to medical therapy and packing.
- Surgical:
  - Ligation of branches of internal maxillary artery (using Caldwell-Luc approach to expose and remove posterior antral wall).
  - Ligation of anterior and posterior ethmoidal arteries. May be performed together with internal maxillary artery ligation or after failure of embolization.
  - Ligation of the sphenopalatine artery via a transnasal, endoscopic approach.
  - Ligation of external carotid artery; typically performed as an emergency procedure.
  - Laser photocoagulation for Osler-Weber-Rendu syndrome. Can use Nd-YAG, KTP, or Argon lasers and coagulate from periphery to central portion of lesion.
  - Septal dermatoplasty in patients with Osler-Weber-Rendu syndrome. The septal mucosa is removed and the cartilage resurfaced with skin grafts.

Complications

Complications of Epistaxis

- Hypotension.
- Hypoxia.
- Anemia.
- Aspiration (pneumonitis).

Complications from packing

- Sinus effusions and sinusitis from blocked sinus ostia.
- Middle ear effusions by blocked eustachian tube (posterior packs).
- Toxic shock syndrome *(Staphylococcus aureus)*.
- Dysphagia
- Aspiration
- Periods of nocturnal hypoventilation, hypoxia, and hypercapnia have been associated with posterior packs (nasopulmonary reflex).
- Septal perforation.
- Arrhythmias (cocaine or lidocaine overdose).

Complications from embolization

- Groin hematoma or bleeding.
- Facial pain and hypersensitivity.
- Skin slough.
- Internal carotid artery (ICA) intimal injury.
- Facial paralysis.
- Cerebrovascular accident (CVA).
- Myocardial infarction (MI).

Complications from surgical ligation

- Facial hypoesthesia/paresthesia.
- Sinusitis.
- Skin slough.
- Synechia.
- Oroantral fistula.
- MI.
- Blindness (trauma to the optic nerve during posterior ethmoid ligation).

Selected References from the Recent Literature

1. Barlow DW, Deleyiannis WB, Pinczower EF. Effectiveness of surgical management of epistaxis at a tertiary care center. *Laryngoscope* 1997;107:21-24.
2. Bent JP, Wood BP. Complications resulting from treatment of severe posterior epistaxis. *Journal of Laryngology & Otology* 1999;113:252-254.
3. Bergler W, Riedel F, Baker-Schreyer A *et al*. Argon plasma coagulation for the treatment of hereditary hemorrhagic telangiectasia. *Laryngoscope* 1999;109:15-20.
4. Cullen MM, Tami TA. Comparison of internal maxillary artery ligation versus embolization for refractory posterior epistaxis. *Otolaryngology—Head & Neck Surgery* 1998;118:636-642.
5. El-Guindy A. Endoscopic transseptal sphenopalatine artery ligation for intractable posterior epistaxis. *Annals of Otology, Rhinology & Laryngology* 1998;107:1033-1037.
6. Frikart L, Agrifoglio A. Endoscopic treatment of posterior epistaxis. *Rhinology* 1998;36:59-61.
7. Lennox PA, Harries M, Lund VJ, Howard DJ. A retrospective study of the role of the argon laser in the management of epistaxis secondary to hereditary haemorrhagic telangiectasia. *Journal of Laryngology & Otology* 1997;111:34-37.
8. Lim SM, Lane RJ. Recurrent epistaxes in hereditary haemorrhagic telangiectasia. *Journal of the Royal Society of Medicine* 1997;90:271-273.
9. London SD, Lindsey WH. A reliable medical treatment for recurrent mild anterior epistaxis. *Laryngoscope* 1999;109:1535-1537.
10. Monte ED, Belmont MJ, Wax MK. Management paradigms for posterior epistaxis: A comparison of costs and complications. *Otolaryngology—Head & Neck Surgery* 1999;121:103-106.
11. Moreau S, De R, Babin E *et al*. Supraselective embolization in intractable epistaxis [review] [45 cases]. *Laryngoscope* 1998;108:887-888.
12. Pollice PA, Yoder MG. Epistaxis: a retrospective review of hospitalized patients. *Otolaryngology—Head & Neck Surgery* 1997;117:49-53.
13. Pringle MB, Beasley P, Brightwell AP. The use of Merocel nasal packs in the treatment of epistaxis. *Journal of Laryngology & Otology* 1996;110:543-546.
14. Pritikin JB, Caldarelli DD, Panje WR. Endoscopic ligation of the internal maxillary artery for treatment of intractable posterior epistaxis. *Annals of Otology, Rhinology & Laryngology* 1998;107:85-91.
15. Shinkwin CA, Beasley N, Simo R *et al*. Evaluation of Surgicel Nu-knit, Merocel and Vasolene gauze nasal packs: a randomized trial. *Rhinology* 1996;34:41-43.
16. Snyderman CH, Goldman SA, Carrau RL *et al*. Endoscopic sphenopalatine artery ligation is an effective method of treatment for posterior epistaxis. *American Journal of Rhinology* 1999;13:137-140.
17. Stangerup SE, Dommerby H, Siim C *et al*. New modification of hot-water irrigation in the treatment of posterior epistaxis. *Archives of Otolaryngology—Head & Neck Surgery* 1999;125:686-690.
18. Tan LK, Calhoun KH. Epistaxis. *Medical Clinics of North America* 1999;83:43-56.
19. Tseng EY, Narducci CA, Willing SJ, Sillers MJ. Angiographic embolization for epistaxis: a review of 114 cases. *Laryngoscope* 1998;108:615-619.
20. Winstead W. Sphenopalatine artery ligation: an alternative to internal maxillary artery ligation for intractable posterior epistaxis. *Laryngoscope* 1996;106:667-669.

RHINITIS

Allergic Rhinitis

Incidence and Etiology
- Incidence: 15 million patients.
- Onset: most commonly 12-15 years of age.
- Strong genetic predilection; demonstrated by early elevation of serum IgE in cord blood; mother's history more significant.
- Environmental effects secondary to early exposure to allergen.

Pathogenesis
- Primary exposure to inhaled allergen leads to IgE generation. The F_c component of the IgE antibody then binds to inflammatory cells such as mast cells.
- Secondary exposure to antigens leads to antigen binding to, and cross-linking of, the IgE antibodies bound to mast cell surface. This leads to degranulation of the mast cell and a release of a variety of inflammatory mediators, some of which are preformed with others generated *de novo* upon antigen binding. These factors include histamine, eosinophilic chemotactic factor, prostaglandins, leukotrienes, bradykinin, platelet-activating factor, and tumor necrosis factor α (TNFα). Nasal itching is provoked by histamine and prostaglandins. Sneezing and rhinorrhea are triggered by histamine and leukotrienes. Nasal congestion results from vasodilation and increased capillary permeability and which are caused by histamine, kinins, leukotrienes, and TNFα. These effects, caused by inflammatory mediators, are known as the early phase response and occur within the first hour of antigen exposure.
- A late phase response, mediated by inflammatory cells recruited by inflammatory mediators, occurs 2-8 hours after the initial response. Eosinophils, basophils, and mast cells are the primary mediators of this response.

Clinical manifestations
- Symptoms include nasal obstruction, rhinorrhea, and itching of eyes, nose, and palate.
- Physical exam reveals:
  - Pale blue, edematous turbinates.
  - Thin, clear nasal secretions.
  - "Allergic salute" in children.
  - Allergic "shiners" secondary to chronic, nonspecific vascular congestion.
  - Possible periorbital swelling and lid edema.
- May be associated with other atopic symptoms, such as eczema or asthma.
- Secondary manifestations include sinus infection, serous otitis media, and nasal polyps.

Investigations
Allergy testing
- Screening for inhalant allergy.
  - Use history to modify initial battery of allergens to expose to the patient.
  - All inhalant allergy is produced by IgE.
  - *In vitro* tests (using patient's blood).
    - These tests depend on the identification of allergen-specific IgE in the serum. This gives a direct, quantitative measurement of the degree of sensitivity to the allergen. RAST and ELISA are good for inhalant allergy, insect sting allergy, and some food allergy.
      - RAST (radio-allergosorbent test): incubate patient's serum in a tube with a disk on which allergen is adhered. IgE binds when specific to the allergen. Wash off nonspecific IgE, then incubate with radiolabeled anti-IgE. Wash off unbound IgE, and measure the amount of remaining radioactivity with a gamma counter.
      - ELISA (enzyme-linked immunosorbent assay): Uses an enzyme-activated marker instead of radioactivity, resulting in a color change that can be quantified with a colorimeter, with a fluorometer, or by luminescence.
      - Dipstick test: performed on the patient's serum, which is mixed with allergens to produce color variation similar to a pH strip.
      - PRIST (paper radio-immunosorbent test): measures the total IgE in the serum (not antigen specific). It is of historical interest only but led to the other immunotechniques.
      - Basophil histamine release test: measures the amount of histamine released by basophils after exposure to specific antigens.
    - Main advantages: obtaining a quantitative, objective measure of IgE directed against a specific antigen; ability to test patients who are highly allergic and might have an anaphylactic response to skin testing; and lack of interference with concurrent medications.
    - Main disadvantages: expense, potential lack of correlation of IgE levels with patient's *in vivo* allergic symptoms, and variability in the quality of performance of the test.
    - The results of these tests must be used cautiously, because there are false-positive tests. However, given a positive test and a clinical history of allergy to the specific antigen, one can presume that allergy exists. SET and the *in vitro*

tests allow for quantitation and therefore can be used to define a starting point for immunotherapy.

In vivo screens (provocation or skin tests [simple, rapid, low cost, high sensitivity]):

- ○ Scratch test: apply small drop to skin, scratch through surface of skin. Not used often because of high false-positive and false-negative rates.
- ○ Prick test: lift upper layers of skin with sharp needle and release, then drop antigen extract, read in 20 minutes. Results rated 0 to 4+, compared with a negative control. Most commonly used as a panel of eight, including positive and negative controls (histamine and glycerin).
- ○ Intradermal test: used after prick test is negative. Inject antigen at 1:100 mg/mL to form a wheal.
- ○ Skin endpoint titration (SET): Intradermal testing using serially increased concentrations as the test progresses. Negative wheal is an initial 4-mm diameter wheal that gets no bigger than 5 mm. Positive wheal is 2 mm more than prior negative wheal. Two successive positive wheals confirm the diagnosis and end the test.
  - ▼ Odd responses: *flash response* (several negative wheals followed by an unusually large wheal). Does not represent a true endpoint for testing; patient must return for repeat testing.
  - ▼ Plateau response: negative results followed by positive results that do not increase in size. Once an increase occurs, it is arbitrarily designated the endpoint.
  - ▼ Hourglass response: Rare, because higher concentrations are the starting point, but one can see an initially higher wheal, which first decreases and then increases with increasing concentrations.
- ○ Nasal testing: rarely used diagnostically.
- ○ Bronchial challenge testing: Expose those previously defined as having allergies to a specific antigen, and perform pulmonary function tests (PFTs) to assess reactivity.
- • Intradermal testing: delivers a fixed, known quantity of antigen.
- • Nasal (mucosal) testing: examined for eosinophils. This is no longer considered pathognomonic.
- ■ Screening for food allergy.
  - ○ Tests, although used, are not sensitive, and one must rely more heavily on the history alone.

- ○ Treatment: elimination of the possible offending antigen for 5-7 days.
- ■ Testing protocol.
  - ○ Patients should eliminate antihistamines for 48 hours and, if possible, tricyclic antidepressants for 4 days prior to testing.
  - ○ Must verify positive response to histamine and negative response to glycerine to accurately perform tests.

Treatment
Avoidance
Best approach for reduction of symptoms.

Pharmacotherapy
Antihistaminics H$_1$ class
- ■ Indications
  - ○ Itching, nasal discharge, sneezing, **not congestion (Box 1).**
- ■ Adverse effects
  - ○ First generation: sedation, dry mouth, urinary retention.
  - ○ Second generation: with liver dysfunction, lethal ventricular arrhythmias.
- ■ Contraindications
  - ○ Astemizole: concurrent therapy with macrolides or antifungal agents (inhibitors of cytochrome P450).

Decongestants (pseudoephedrine, phenylpropanolamine)
- ■ Indication
  - ○ Congestion, often used in conjunction with antihistamines.
- ■ Adverse effects
  - ○ Anxiety, insomnia, irritability, headache, palpitations, decreased urinary flow, constipation.
- ■ Contraindications
  - ○ Hypertension, coronary artery disease, concurrent use of MAO-inhibitors.

Corticosteroids
- ■ Topical (beclomethasone, flunisolide).

Box 1. Antihistaminics H$_1$ Class

FIRST GENERATION	SECOND GENERATION
Brompheniramine (Dimetane)	Astemizole (Hismanal)
Chlorpheniramine (Chlor-Trimeton)	Cetirizine (Zyrtec)
Diphenhydramine (Benadryl)	Fexofenadine (Allegra)
Promethazine (Phenergan)	Loratadine (Claritin)
Hydroxyzine (Atarax)	Desloratadine (Clarinex)
Clemastine (Tavist)	

- Indications
  - Sneezing, nasal itching, rhinorrhea, reactive mucosal edema.
- Adverse effects
  - Nasal burning, sneezing, epistaxis, septal perforation.
- Intraturbinal injection: biannual injection that may alleviate symptoms year round.
  - Indication
    - Failure of methods mentioned previously.
  - Adverse effect
    - Blindness, therefore currently not generally advocated.
- Oral (prednisone).
  - Indication
    - Treatment of severe nasal allergy of short duration.

Cromolyn sodium (intranasal cromolyn 4%)

- Indications
  - Sneezing, rhinorrhea, nasal congestion, ocular irritation.
- Adverse effects (rare)
  - Bronchospasm, wheezing, laryngeal edema, joint swelling.

Anticholinergics (ipratropium bromide nasal spray)

- Indication
  - Rhinorrhea.
- Adverse effect
  - Dry mouth.

Topical antihistamines: azelastine (Astelin). This drug inhibits histamine and other inflammatory mediators. It has a rapid onset of action (30 minutes) with a 12-hour duration of action. It has been shown to be approximately as effective at controlling nasal symptoms as oral antihistamines, but not quite as effective as topical nasal steroids. It does not address extranasal allergic symptoms.

- Indication
  - As per oral antihistamines, may also help nasal congestion.
- Adverse effects
  - It is absorbed systemically with 40% bioavailability. Main side effects are bitter aftertaste, drowsiness, and headache.

Montelukast: Leukotriene antagonist
Indications

- Allergic rhinitis, will relieve symptoms of:
  - Congestion.
  - Sneezing.
  - Itching.
  - Discharge.
- Approximately as effective as loratidine.
- Less effective than topical corticosteroids.

Contraindications

- Caution in cases of severe liver disease.

Adverse effects

- Serious, but rare: angioedema, anaphylaxis, hepatic eosinophilic infiltration, Churg-Strauss syndrome.
- Common: headache, abdominal pain, cough, fever, fatigue, elevated liver function tests, pruritis, urticaria.

Immunotherapy

- Indications
  - Pharmacotherapy insufficiently controls symptoms, produces undesirable side effects, or interferes with patient's lifestyle.
  - Appropriate avoidance measures of indoor allergens are not feasible or do not provide adequate relief of symptoms.
  - Inability to avoid allergen, particularly with multiple offending agents.
  - Prolonged use of, or inability to wean from, pharmacotherapy.
  - Failure of, or contraindication to, pharmacotherapy.
  - Proven IgE-mediated atopic disease.
  - Patient history of allergic rhinitis for at least two seasons (seasonal), or 6 months per year (perennial).
  - Positive skin tests or serum-specific IgE that correlate with rhinitis symptoms. Discontinuation if no improvement after 2 years.
- Contraindication
  - Potentially unreliable patient.
- Advantages
  - Potentially curative (only such option).
  - Between 80% and 90% able to discontinue therapy after 3-5 years.
- Disadvantage
  - Expensive (cost may actually be less over a lifetime in carefully selected patients).

Basis for immunotherapy

- Repeated exposure to the immune system facilitates minimizing of the immune response.
- Large doses of antigen administered parenterally suppress IgE formation.
- It stimulates the formation of allergen-specific IgG-blocking antibodies that compete for IgE target sites.
- There is decreased basophil and lymphocyte reactivity.
- Small doses of antigen actually increase IgE production.

Technique
Skin end-point titration (SET)

- Use of progressively increasing intradermal injections to determine the presence of atopic disease as well as a safe starting dose.

Radioallergosorbent testing (RAST)

- Levels of specific IgE may be used to calculate safe starting dose.

Steps

1. Administer antigen 1-2× / week until a response is noted.
2. Administer antigen weekly for 1 year.
3. Administer antigen every other week for the second year.
4. Administer antigen every 2-3 weeks for the third year.
5. Adjust the dosage of antigen to obtain the desired effects.

Complications

Anaphylaxis

- Allergic emergency (an average of one fatality per year).
- Treatment of anaphylaxis
  - Epinephrine (0.5 mL subcutaneously 1/1000 epinephrine).
  - Call for help.
  - Supplemental oxygen.
  - Secure airway.
  - IV access.
  - Volume expansion (normal saline or Ringer's lactate).
  - Dopamine: if pressure not responsive to volume expansion (2-50 μg/kg/min).
  - Antihistamine (diphenhydramine: Benadryl 50 mg iv).
  - Corticosteroid (methylprednisolone 125 mg iv/im).
  - H_2 blocker (e.g., cimetidine 300 mg iv/im).
  - Heparin.

Results of immunotherapy

In general: 50% improve, 25% no change, 25% worse.

Nonallergic Rhinitis

Viral

Protection

- Several endogenous factors protect the nasal mucosa. The submucosal glands produce mucus that entraps viruses. Cilia of the mucosal epithelium propel the mucus into the nasopharynx, where it is swallowed, thereby preventing the microorganisms from penetrating the nasal mucosa. In addition, nasal glands produce enzymes, antibodies, and protective proteins that inactivate or kill many viruses.

Viruses

- In all, over 200 different species are implicated in viral rhinitis. Rhinovirus is the most common culprit. The influenza viruses produce a more debilitating illness; there may be necrosis of the ciliated epithelial layer of the mucosa along with systemic symptoms. Secondary bacterial superinfections may occur.

Therapy

- There is no specific therapy, only symptomatic relief.

Bacterial

Rhinoscleroma

- Seen in Africa, Central and South America, and India.
- Etiology: *Klebsiella rhinoscleroma*.
- Characterized by three clinical stages: (1) rhinitis, (2) infiltrative, and (3) nodular. Large, red, tumor-like masses are seen in the nodular phase. These masses possess *Mikulicz's cells* (large clear cells containing the bacilli), and *Russell bodies* (eosinophilic plasma cells with prominent nuclei).
- Treatment: Streptomycin or tetracycline for 4-6 weeks or until two biopsies are negative. Surgery may be required to treat scarring.

Leprosy

- Etiology: *Mycobacterium leprae*.
- Clinical manifestations:
  - Tuberculoid leprosy: small anesthetic patches on nasal mucosa with few associated bacteria on biopsy.
  - Lepromatous leprosy: diffuse mucosal involvement with nodular lesions heavily infiltrated with bacteria and nasal discharge. May erode bone and cartilage, leading to septal perforation and nasal collapse.
- Treatment: Dapsone.

Tuberculosis

- Nasal involvement rare, usually secondary to pulmonary involvement. Manifests as nodular or ulcerative lesions on mucosa.

Syphilis

- Etiology: *Treponema pallidum*.
- Clinical manifestations:
  - Primary: chancre on external nose or vestibule.
  - Secondary: rhinitis.
  - Tertiary: gummas, which are nodular, firm, and red. Invade mucous membranes, bone, and cartilage, leading to septal perforations and nasal collapse.

Fungal

Rhinosporidiosis

- Seen in India and Africa.
- Etiology: *Rhinosporidium seeberi*.
- Clinical manifestations: raspberry polyp = a bleeding polyp studded with sporangia.
- Treatment: Dapsone and excision of polyp.

Vasomotor Rhinitis

- Perennial rhinitis in which no specific allergen can be identified.

Symptoms

- Chronic rhinitis and obstruction; sneezing less common.
- May be provoked by a variety of nonspecific stimuli (e.g., temperature change, humidity change, fatigue, stress).
- Thought to result from a dysautonomia of the nasal mucosal parasympathetic innervation (acetylcholine, substance P, vasoactive intestinal peptide).

Treatment

- Topical steroids, ipratropium bromide. Vidian neurectomy via a variety of routes may be effective in the short term.

Drug-Induced Rhinitis

- *Rhinitis medicamentosa*
  - Results from rebound vasodilation and mucosal edema after chronic application of topical decongestants (oxymetazoline, xylometazoline, phenylephrine). As mucosa becomes less sensitive to vasodilators, increased dose of the drug is used with shorter durations of vasoconstriction, creating a vicious cycle. The presence of the preservative benzalkonium chloride in the spray seems to exacerbate the condition.
  - Prevention: Restrict use of topical decongestants to 3-5 days.
  - Treatment of established rhinitis medicamentosa is difficult. Topical and systemic steroids are usually instituted. Ipratropium bromide spray may be used as an adjunct to the steroids. Another strategy is having the patient desensitize one side of the nasal cavity and then the other. These patients often have a phobic response to nasal obstruction, and psychiatric intervention may be helpful.
- Antihypertensives
  - Guanethidine, hydralazine, and prazosin (α blockers) cause vasodilation and nasal obstruction. Reserpine and methyldopa deplete norepinephrine stores, leading to unopposed cholinergic stimulation. Beta blockers may also cause rhinitis.
- Aspirin intolerance: leads to rhinorrhea, nasal polyposis, and asthma.
- Birth control pill (see below).

Pregnancy

- Estrogen is believed to have a variety of effects on the nasal mucosa, including increased acetylcholine production caused by acetylcholinesterase inhibition, increased glandular hyperactivity, and increased acid mucopolysaccharide content of the ground substance. The condition typically worsens in the third trimester. Similar effects may be seen as the result of birth control pill administration and estrogen replacement therapy.
- Treatment: Topical corticosteroids are the mainstays of treatment. Antihistamines may also be prescribed. Vasoconstrictors are permitted but should be used with caution. Systemic steroids may be used safely in the third trimester.

Hypothyroidism

- Myxedema, resulting in edema of the nasal mucosa, may cause nasal obstruction.

Gustatory rhinitis

- Reflex cholinergic discharge triggered by sensory receptors on the palate, causing nasal secretion, flushing, tearing, and/or sweating.
- Treatment: ipratropium bromide nasal spray prior to meal.

End-stage vascular atony of chronic allergic or inflammatory rhinitis

- Secondary to prolonged and profound parasympathetic stimulation of the nasal vascular system leading to permanent loss of vascular tone. Analogous to varicose vein.

Rhinitis of no airflow

- Seen in laryngectomy/choanal atresia/adenoid hypertrophy.
- The vascular bed of the nose loses its tone and the turbinates become boggy and swollen when the nasal mucosa is excluded from reciprocating the flow of air.

Compensatory hypertrophic rhinitis

- When an excess space is created in the nasal cavity, one or more turbinates will hypertrophy to fill this space. This effect has been postulated to protect the nose from excess nasal airflow with its drying and cooling effects.

Eosinophilic and basophilic nonallergic rhinitis

- A clinical condition of unknown etiology in which symptoms suggest allergic rhinitis but IgE test and skin test for appropriate allergens are negative. Cytology of nasal mucosa determines the conditions. Nasal steroids provide dramatic improvement.

Atrophic Rhinitis (Ozena)

- Pathology and pathophysiology: End stage of prolonged infection and/or overly aggressive resection of intranasal structures (turbinates). Results in chronic inflammation, leading to atrophy and fibrosis of the nasal mucosa and an overly patent nasal cavity. The epithelium becomes squamous or cuboidal.
- Clinical findings: The secretory glands produce a scant, thick mucus that forms crusts and, at times, obstructive casts. There is frequent bacterial superinfection *(Klebsiella ozena)* contributing to the foul smell of the nasal contents. Patients will complain of nasal obstruction, yet clinical examination reveals a wide patent airway.
- Treatment: Mild cases are treated with aggressive humidification and lubrication of the nasal cavity. Crusts are debrided. Severe cases may require a Young procedure, in which one nostril is surgically closed for 6-12 months, after which the closure is reversed and the other nostril is closed for a similar duration of time.

Systemic disorders

- Superior vena cava syndrome: Characterized by periorbital erythema/edema, nasal stuffiness, headache, and progressive facial swelling. All head and neck vasculature is distended. Chest radiograph will show a mass encroaching on the vena cava in 97% of all cases.
- Horner's syndrome: Unilateral hyperemia, swelling, hypersecretion, miosis, and nasal obstruction. Caused by interference with sympathetic innervation.
- Cirrhosis.
- Uremia.

Selected References from the Recent Literature

1. Allergic rhinitis in childhood. *Allergy* 1999;54 Suppl 55:7-34.
2. Baraniuk JN. Mechanisms of rhinitis. *Allergy & Asthma Proceedings* 1998;19:343-347.
3. Benninger MS, Anon J, Mabry RL. The medical management of rhinosinusitis. *Otolaryngology—Head & Neck Surgery* 1997;117:S41-S49
4. Bousquet J. Antihistamines in severe/chronic rhinitis. *Clinical & Experimental Allergy* 1998;28 Suppl 6:49-53.
5. Chand MS, MacArthur CJ. Primary atrophic rhinitis: a summary of four cases and review of the literature. *Otolaryngology—Head & Neck Surgery* 1997;116:554-558.
6. Cook PR. Allergic rhinitis. Outcomes of immunotherapy on symptom control. *Otolaryngologic Clinics of North America* 1998;31:129-140.
7. Ferguson BJ. What role do systemic corticosteroids, immunotherapy, and antifungal drugs play in the therapy of allergic fungal rhinosinusitis? *Archives of Otolaryngology—Head & Neck Surgery* 1998;124:1174-1178.
8. Ferguson BJ. Cost-effective pharmacotherapy for allergic rhinitis. *Otolaryngologic Clinics of North America* 1998;31:91-110.
9. Gerth van Wijk RG, de Graaf-in 't Veld C, Garrelds IM. Nasal hyperreactivity. *Rhinology* 1999;37:50-55.
10. Graf P, Hallen H, Juto JE. The pathophysiology and treatment of rhinitis medicamentosa. *Clinical Otolaryngology & Allied Sciences* 1995;20:224-229.
11. Graf P. Rhinitis medicamentosa: aspects of pathophysiology and treatment. *Allergy* 1997;52:28-34.
12. Jiang RS, Hsu CY, Chen CC *et al.* Endoscopic sinus surgery and postoperative intravenous aminoglycosides in the treatment of atrophic rhinitis. *American Journal of Rhinology* 1998;12:325-333.
13. Jones NS. Current concepts in the management of paediatric rhinosinusitis. *Journal of Laryngology & Otology* 1999;113:1-9.
14. Kips J. Mechanisms of mucosal inflammation in the nose and lungs. *Allergy* 1999;54 Suppl 50:37-38.
15. LaForce C. Use of nasal steroids in managing allergic rhinitis. *Journal of Allergy & Clinical Immunology* 1999;103:S388-S394
16. Lanza DC, Kennedy DW. Adult rhinosinusitis defined. *Otolaryngology—Head & Neck Surgery* 1997;117:S1-S7
17. Lemanske RFJ. A review of the current guidelines for allergic rhinitis and asthma. *Journal of Allergy & Clinical Immunology* 1998;101:S392-S396
18. Levenson T, Greenberger PA. Pathophysiology and therapy for allergic and nonallergic rhinitis: an updated review. *Allergy & Asthma Proceedings* 1997;18:213-220.
19. Lieberman P. Management of allergic rhinitis with a combination antihistamine/anti-inflammatory agent. *Journal of Allergy & Clinical Immunology* 1999;103:S400-S404
20. Lundback B. Epidemiology of rhinitis and asthma. *Clinical & Experimental Allergy* 1998;28 Suppl 2:3-10.
21. Lusk RP, Stankiewicz JA. Pediatric rhinosinusitis. *Otolaryngology—Head & Neck Surgery* 1997;117:S53-S57
22. Mabry RL. Allergy for rhinologists. *Otolaryngologic Clinics of North America* 1998;31:175-187.
23. Malling HJ. Immunotherapy as an effective tool in allergy treatment. *Allergy* 1998;53:461-472.
24. Meltzer EO. Treatment options for the child with allergic rhinitis. *Clinical Pediatrics* 1998;37:1-10.
25. Naclerio R, Solomon W. Rhinitis and inhalant allergens. *JAMA* 1997;278:1842-1848.
26. Sanico A, Togias A. Noninfectious, nonallergic rhinitis (NINAR): considerations on possible mechanisms. *American Journal of Rhinology* 1998;12:65-72.
27. Scadding G. Pharmacological modulation of the allergic response: different modes of action. *Allergy* 1999;54 Suppl 50:39-42.
28. Scadding GK. Clinical assessment of antihistamines in rhinitis. *Clinical & Experimental Allergy* 1999;29 Suppl 3:77-81.
29. Shehata MA. Atrophic rhinitis. *American Journal of Otolaryngology* 1996;17:81-86.
30. Winther B, Gwaltney JMJ, Mygind N, Hendley JO. Viral-induced rhinitis. *American Journal of Rhinology* 1998;12:17-20.
31. Young MC. Rhinitis, sinusitis, and polyposis. *Allergy & Asthma Proceedings* 1998;19:211-218.

RHINOSINUSITIS

Acute Bacterial Rhinosinusitis (ABS)

Definition
- Inflammation of the paranasal sinuses of a presumed bacterial etiology (no evidence of any allergic mechanisms) lasting less than 4 weeks.
- Exacerbation of chronic sinusitis, resulting in a worsening in the character of symptoms or the appearance of new constitutional symptoms.

Etiology and pathogenesis
- Most common predisposing cause of acute bacterial sinusitis is recurrent viral URI. Approximately 0.5% cases of viral URI are complicated by bacterial sinusitis.
  - Other predisposing factors include allergy, foreign body, dental procedure, and barotrauma.
  - Iatrogenic factors have also become increasingly more important: mechanical ventilation, nasogastric tubes, nasotracheal tubes, and nasal packing (epistaxis and procedures).
  - Less common causes of ABS include trauma and mucosal edema associated with pregnancy.

Microbiology
- Studies have shown that *Streptococcus pneumoniae* and *Haemophilus influenzae* cause 70% of community-acquired acute sinusitis in adults.
- In recent years the prevalence of ß-lactamase-producing organisms has increased, with reports as high as 52% for *H. influenzae*.
- Usually associated with dental infections, anaerobic organisms including *Fusobacterium, Peptostreptococcus,* and *Bacteroides* account for about 6%-10% of cases.
- In children, the pathogens responsible for ABS are similar to those for adults, with the exception of *Moraxella catarrhalis*, which has been implicated in approximately 20% of acute sinusitis in children.

Symptoms
- In the early phase of the illness, the symptoms of acute sinusitis may be difficult to distinguish from those of the common cold or allergic rhinitis.
- Certain symptoms common to ABS affect any of the sinuses: headache, facial pain, and elevation of temperature and heart rate.
- The location of facial pain will vary and is related to the sinus involved.
- Depending on the patency of the ostia, purulent nasal discharge may or may not be present.
- Less frequent symptoms include postnasal drip with cough or hoarseness, vague headache, halitosis, and anosmia.

- Children are less likely to complain of facial pain or headache. Persistent nasal congestion and cough (>7 days), high fever, purulent nasal discharge, and the presence of mild periorbital edema probably represent sinusitis.

Signs
- Tenderness to palpation may be evident over the affected sinus.
- Nasal mucous membranes are red and edematous; middle turbinate may be red and swollen; uncinate process may be prominent.
- Pus may emanate from the middle meatus or the sphenoethmoid recess on nasal endoscopy.

Treatment
- Forty percent of ABS will resolve spontaneously. Antibiotics should still be used, because they are believed to facilitate recovery from the acute episode as well as to prevent complications and progressive mucosal changes that may result in chronic sinusitis.
- Many investigators still promote ampicillin or amoxicillin as first-line antimicrobials, despite increased incidence of β-lactamase–producing organisms. Other antibiotics to consider in light of patient allergy, cost, and previous effectiveness include TMP Sulfa, Cefaclor, cefuroxime, and azithromycin.
- Choice is usually empiric, although culture-based antimicrobial selection is preferred.
- When β-lactamase–producing organisms are suspected or confirmed on culture, recommendations include amoxicillin with clavulanate, TMP-SUL, and cefuroxime, a quinolone (in adults).
- Typical treatment course is 10-14 days.
- Changing antibiotic to cover β-lactamase–producing organisms should be considered if the patient reports no symptom resolution after 48-72 hours, especially if the patient is a child.
- Antibiotic therapy should continue for a minimum of 7 days after resolution of symptoms.

FUNGAL RHINOSINUSITIS

Definition and classification
Fungal sinusitis is categorized as:
1. Invasive.
2. Chronic invasive.
3. Mycetoma.
4. Allergic fungal sinusitis.

Aspergillus is the most common reported species associated with fungal sinusitis.

Incidence and etiology

- **Invasive:** Invasive fungal sinusitis is almost always confined to the patient with decreased host immune defenses such as:
  - Transplantation (bone marrow, liver, lung).
  - Diabetes mellitus.
  - Immune deficiency (immunoglobulin deficiency, HIV, systemic prednisone).
  - Immunodeficiency secondary to chemotherapy.
  - Leukemia.
- **Chronic invasive fungal sinusitis** is rare. Patients who live in or have visited Africa (particularly Sudan) are disproportionally represented by this entity.
- **Mycetomas:** Fungal balls are common and grow in the wet, moist cavities of the paranasal sinuses, (typically maxillary) irrespective of the immunologic status of the host. If the host is immunocompromised, the contained fungal infection may become invasive. *Aspergillus* is the most common organism (hence the name *Aspergilloma*).
- **Allergic fungal sinusitis:** Noninvasive fungal infection of the sinus, with eosinophil-mediated allergic response causing the symptoms.

Microbiology

- **Invasive:** The fungus can be seen within the tissue as well as invading it. Biopsy of the suspected tissue for pathology and culture is critical to making the diagnosis. Cultures should be obtained prior to initiation of systemic antifungals. **It is critical that the diagnosis, once suspected, be made as quickly as possible.**
  - **Mucor:** presents as a broad ribbon (10-15 mm), irregular and nonseptated. The hyphae of mucormycosis can be seen invading the vessel wall, leading to thrombosis of the vessel. The most virulent and common species is *Rhizopus oryzae*. *Mucormycosis* has earned the reputation as the most acutely fatal fungal infection known to humans. It grows rapidly, and widespread invasion is observed within 24 hours. *Mucor* has a propensity for vascular invasion and obliteration that leads to ischemia. Its growth is facilitated by acidotic conditions, and as the fungus grows, it facilitates its propagation by this vascular invasion, which leads to ischemia. The use of hyperbaric oxygen in this setting is theoretically attractive because it reduces the ischemia and acidosis, but no controlled studies have shown its efficacy. Patients with diabetes (especially diabetic ketoacidosis) are particularly at risk because of the acidic environment.
  - **Aspergillus:** presents as narrow hyphae with regular septation and 45 degrees branching. Cultures are important for distinguishing

Aspergillus species from less common pathogenic fungal species that are also septated. *Aspergillus* species are the most frequent species found in those with invasive fungal sinusitis. *Aspergillus fumigatus* is the most common species responsible for invasive disease in the United States. *Aspergillus* species can be angioinvasive, but it is not the obliterative invasion seen with mucormycosis.

- **Chronic invasive fungal sinusitis:** pathogenic organism is almost always *Aspergillus flavus*. The histologic picture is a granuloma in which giant cells contain the hyphae.
- **Mycetomas:** A variety of fungal species cause mycetomas and include *A. flavus, A. fumigatus*, and *Mucor*. There is no associated invasion of mucosa, blood vessels, or bone.
- **Allergic fungal sinusitis:** Histopathology reveals the allergic mucin to contain necrotic inflammatory cells, eosinophils, and Charcot-Leyden crystals (a by-product of eosinophil degranulation). In this allergic mucin are hyphae elements, best appreciated with fungal stains. *Aspergillus* is the most common organism involved. There is no invasion in this disease entity.

Clinical manifestation

- **Invasive:** Invasive fungal sinusitis is suspected when an immunocompromised patient develops fever as well as localization of symptoms to the paranasal sinus area, such as orbital swelling, facial pain or paresthesias, or nasal congestion. Nasal endoscopy may reveal **necrosis** of the nasal mucosa, indicative of **mucormycosis,** and, rarely, actual hyphae. Clinically, the areas of invasion are black and necrotic. However, only edema and changes indistinguishable from nonfungal causes of sinusitis are more common. Anesthesia of the nasal mucosa or cheeks, independent of topical anesthetics, is suspicious for invasive fungus. The oral cavity should always be examined for invasion through the hard palate from the sinuses. If the diagnosis is suspected, sinus CT is obtained. CT changes are usually indistinguishable from bacterial sinusitis, although they may show bony erosion or soft tissue invasion. Unfortunately, abnormal imaging studies are common in this compromised population. Up to 42% of patients with leukemia in one series had abnormal sinus radiographs.
- **Chronic invasive fungal sinusitis:** Patient may be immunocompromised and may present with painless proptosis or orbital apex syndrome. The disease course is variable (see below).
- **Mycetomas:** Symptoms are indistinguishable from chronic sinusitis and include nasal obstruction, chronic rhinitis, facial pain, and/or a fetid nasal

discharge. Alternatively, the mycetomas may be asymptomatic and discovered incidentally.

- **Allergic fungal sinusitis:** Clinically, patients with allergic fungal sinusitis are often atopic and develop nasal polyps. Chronic intractable sinusitis is common. One third may have asthma, which is usually mild. Many of the patients have had multiple polypectomies. On sinus CT, bony erosion is common, and the inspissated mucus (brown or greenish-black material with the consistency of peanut butter or cottage cheese) causes a heterogeneous soft tissue density. Another finding on CT scan may be a focus of hyperdense with surrounding hypodense mucoid material. Immunologic testing reveals increased systemic levels of IgE and IgG to the specific fungus, with total IgE levels being extremely high.

Treatment

- **Invasive:** Therapy of invasive fungal sinusitis requires reversal of the underlying predisposing condition, appropriate systemic antifungal therapy, and surgical debridement. Of these, the most important is **reversal of the underlying cause of immunocompromise.** The survival rates of patients with invasive mucormycosis reflect the variance in the ability to reverse the underlying predisposing cause. Invasive fungal sinusitis in the immunocompetent is exceedingly rare and generally less fulminant, but lethal. Treatment of patients with invasive fungal sinusitis is systemic amphotericin B. Nephrotoxicity is the major dose-limiting toxicity and can be reduced with sodium loading. Fever, chills, nausea, and hypotension frequently accompany the first few doses. These toxicities may be reduced with the use of lipophilic amphotericin B delivered through liposomes. These liposomes have an affinity for the reticuloendothelial system and therefore bypass toxicities otherwise imparted to other tissues. Other choices for antifungal therapy include itraconazole, ketoconazole, fluconazole, and miconazole.
- **Chronic invasive fungal sinusitis:** In some patients surgical exenteration and debridement is curative, and in others the disease is relentless despite multiple therapies, including systemic antifungal drugs (amphotericin B and imidazole), and surgery and may end in blindness, cerebral extension, or death.
- **Mycetomas:** Therapy includes conservative surgical removal. There is no need for antifungal therapy.
- **Allergic fungal sinusitis:** Therapy and prognosis of those with allergic fungal sinusitis is independent of the fungal species cultured. Treatment includes conservative, nonmutilating surgical removal of the nasal polyps and inspissated allergic mucin. The mucin is tenacious, and microdebridement can facilitate the removal. Adjuvant systemic steroids (begun perioperatively) in conjunction with surgery can result in cure. Recurrent disease is common. Therapy with amphotericin B, with its attendant toxicity, is not indicated. The role of immunotherapy has yet to be established.

 CHRONIC RHINOSINUSITIS

Definition

- Inflammation of paranasal sinuses:
  - Acute: <4 weeks.
  - Subacute: 4-12 weeks.
  - Chronic: >12 weeks.

Incidence and etiology

- Acute sinusitis affects approximately 30 million people per year. Inadequate treatment of acute sinusitis is the most common cause of chronic sinusitis.
- Risk factors for the development of chronic sinusitis include:
  - Allergic rhinitis.
  - Nonallergic, chronic rhinitis.
  - Aspirin sensitivity.
  - Nasal polyposis.
  - Immunodeficiency disease syndromes.
  - Anatomic abnormalities.
  - Cystic fibrosis.
  - Immotile cilia syndromes.

Pathogenesis

- Changes in sinus function/physiology predispose to development of sinusitis:
  - Patency of sinus ostium.
  - Ciliary function.
  - Quality of nasal gland secretion.

Bacteriology

- See Box 2.

Clinical manifestations
Signs and symptoms

- Eight weeks of persistent signs and symptoms in adult (12 weeks in child).

Major

- Nasal obstruction.
- Nasal discharge (mucopurulent).
- Postnasal drip.
- Facial pressure.
- Facial pain.
- Anosmia/hyposmia.

Box 2. Bacteriology of Chronic Rhinosinusitis

AEROBES

Staphylococcus aureus
Streptococcus pneumoniae
Haemophilus influenzae

ANAEROBES

Prevotella
Porphyromonas
Fusobacterium
Bacteroides

---

*Pediatric chronic sinusitis is less likely to involve anaerobic organisms.

Minor

- Halitosis.
- Cough.
- Fever.

Physical examination may demonstrate:

- Mucopurulent discharge emanating from sinuses.
- Mucosal changes consistent with allergic (pale, boggy) or chronic infectious (erythematous) pathology.
- Anatomic lesions obstructing drainage of the sinuses (deviated septum, concha bullosa, synechiae).
- Nasal polyposis.

Investigations

- Nasal endoscopy: detect anatomic abnormalities, sinus culture.
- Allergy testing.
- CT scan: recommended after good course of medical treatment.
- Sweat chloride (consider in children with appropriate coexistent symptoms).
- Nasal ciliary biopsy (consider in children with appropriate coexistent symptoms).
- Maxillary sinus lavage: for culture, not for definitive treatment.

Treatment

Medical: Mainstay of Treatment

- Prolonged use of antibiotics (4 weeks): requires second-line antibiotics (e.g., amoxicillin/clavulanate, cefuroxime, broad-spectrum quinolone). Antibiotics may change based on culture, with some patients requiring IV therapy. Anaerobic coverage (e.g., metronidazole, clindamycin) has also been advised by some authorities.
- Adjunctive medical therapy should include:
  - Oral corticosteroids that then can be supplanted by topical nasal steroid.
  - Oral decongestants and mucolytics.
  - Nasal irrigations (saline or gentamicin solution).
  - Immunotherapy for atopy.
  - Attempt to address any systemic immune-compromise.

Surgical therapy

- Instituted with persistent symptoms and radiologic changes despite aggressive medical therapy (see following sections).

 ## SINUS MUCOCELE

Classification and Incidence

- Mucoceles are classified primarily by their site of origin (in descending incidence): frontal, ethmoid, maxillary, sphenoid. They can occur spontaneously, postsurgery, or posttrauma. When they become acutely infected, they are termed *mucopyoceles.*

Etiology and pathogenesis

- Sinus mucoceles are chronic cysts of the paranasal sinuses that are lined by normal respiratory epithelium: pseudostratified columnar with goblet cells. Over several years, mucus production in the cyst continues, gradually filling the affected sinus and, over time, causing bony remodeling and erosion. Two pathogenic theories of mucocele formation have been hypothesized: (1) the normal sinus drainage pathway becomes permanently blocked, causing mucous stasis and accumulation (e.g., frontal sinus mucocele), or (2) local factors cause a minor salivary gland duct to become blocked and gradually accumulate mucous (e.g., maxillary mucous retention cyst). In postsurgical mucoceles, a small area of respiratory epithelium is trapped by scar or is otherwise prevented from draining, leading to mucocele formation over time.

Clinical manifestations

- Mucoceles grow slowly and mainly cause symptoms because of mass effect (Table 1).

TABLE 1. Clinical Manifestations of Sinus Mucocele

Location	Symptoms	Signs
Frontal	Diplopia	Proptosis, eye pushed down and out
Ethmoid	Diplopia, nasal obstruction	Hypertelorism
Maxillary	Cosmetic	Cheek asymmetry
Sphenoid	Visual field changes, headache	Proptosis (rare)

- Diagnosis depends on clinical suspicion and signs/symptoms described previously, and it is confirmed by radiology. Mucoceles often are round or oval and exhibit bony remodeling, but they are difficult to differentiate from solid masses on CT scan. MRI scanning normally shows a nonenhancing cyst with the contents hyperintense on T2-weighted scans.
- Acute infection of a mucocele may cause fever, chills, cellulitis, rapid expansion of the mucocele, or local infectious complications, including meningitis or periorbital abscess.

Treatment

- Many mucoceles can be treated adequately endonasally by wide marsupialization under endoscopic guidance. Because mucoceles are lined by normal respiratory mucosa, provision of a mucous drainage pathway is adequate treatment. If the mucocele or bony remodeling is causing either cosmetic or functional deficits, complete excision with immediate or delayed reconstruction can be undertaken.
- Frontal mucoceles following sinus obliteration are especially difficult. The best scenario is a mucocele that can be marsupialized endoscopically, with the creation of an adequate, permanent drainage pathway.

This is often impossible because of the mucocele location. A second option is to reopen the osteoplastic flap, completely excise the mucocele, and reobliterate the sinus. Extensive mucoceles occasionally require cranialization of the sinus. Close follow-up with regular imaging is essential in all patients with obliterated sinuses in order to diagnose postoperative mucoceles while still small. Mucopyoceles often require long courses of IV antibiotics or emergency drainage procedures as well as appropriate treatment of local complications.

Selected References from the Recent Literature

1. Sethi DS. Isolated sphenoid lesions: diagnosis and management. *Archives of Otolaryngology—Head & Neck Surgery* 1999;120(5):730-736.
2. Makeieff M, Gardiner Q, Mondain M, Crampette L. Maxillary sinus mucocoeles—10 cases—8 treated endoscopically. *Rhinology* 1998;36(4):192-195.
3. Lund VJ. Endoscopic management of paranasal sinus mucocoeles. *Journal of Laryngology & Otology* 1998;112(9):840-844.
4. Har-El G, Balwally AN, Lucente FE. Sinus mucoceles: is marsupialization enough? *Archives of Otolaryngology—Head & Neck Surgery* 1997;117(6):633-640.
5. Marks SC, Latoni JD, Mathog RH. Mucoceles of the maxillary sinus. *Archives of Otolaryngology—Head & Neck Surgery* 1997;117(1):18-21.

ENDOSCOPIC SINUS SURGERY

One must have a systematic method of examination, which includes a history, physical examination and endoscopy, and radiologic assessment. Careful examination, selection, patient education, and counseling as well as good follow-up examinations are important to achieve a good outcome.

Indications

- Patients with documented recurrent acute sinusitis refractory to medical management (patients with allergic components will do less well).
- Chronic sinusitis refractory to maximal medical management.
- Unresponsive, obstructive nasal polyposis.
- Extramucosal fungal sinusitis.
- Removal of foreign body.
- Antral-choanal polyp.
- Mucoceles.
- Periorbital abscess.
- Control of epistaxis.
- Excision of selected tumors (e.g., inverting papilloma).
- Transnasal decompression of thyroid orbitopathy.
- Repair of CSF rhinorrhea.
- Intranasal dacryocystorhinostomy.
- Repair of choanal atresia.
- Management of small anterior skull base tumors.
- Decompression of the optic nerve.

Contraindications

- Absence of defined osteomeatal abnormality.
- Osteomyelitis.
- Inaccessible lateral frontal sinus disease.
- Frontal sinus disease accompanied by stenosed internal os.
- Threatened intracranial or intraorbital disease (relative contraindication).

Preoperative Workup

History

A history must include one of the indications listed previously if surgery is to be considered:

- Rule out allergic disease and optimize allergy management before surgery is approached.
- Ask specifically about asthma or wheezing associated with infections as well as sensitivity to aspirin (Samter's triad = asthma, aspirin sensitivity, nasal polyps).
- Perform sweat chloride test on pediatric patients to rule out cystic fibrosis.
- For pediatric patients with recurrent sinusitis and pulmonary infections, consider biopsy of nasal cilia to rule out immotile cilia syndrome, particularly in

the presence of situs inversus (Kartagener's syndrome).
- Rule out migraines, tension headaches, and TMJ arthritis.
- Rule out dental infections, ozena, and nasal crusting.
- Control hypertension to minimize intraoperative and postoperative bleeding.
- Stop ASA, NSAIDs prior to surgery.
- Optimize asthma therapy, usually adding a tapering course of steroids perioperatively.

Comprehensive nasal endoscopy

1. Administer topical decongestants and anesthetics (lidocaine/phenylephrine or cocaine)
2. Use a 30-degree scope initially.
3. Visualize inferior turbinate, inferior meatus, nasopharynx, eustachian tubes, and possibly nasolacrimal duct, looking for mucopus in the following regions:
   - Nasolacrimal duct orifice (possible pneumatized agger nasi).
   - Under torus tubarius (anterior ethmoidal, maxillary or frontal disease).
   - Above eustachian tube (usually from sphenoethmoidal recess draining the posterior ethmoid or sphenoid sinus region).
4. Reinsert between middle and inferior turbinates to sphenoethmoidal recess (the opening of the sphenoid sinus can be seen).
5. On withdrawal of telescope, roll superiorly and laterally into anterior middle meatus (viewing bulla, hiatus semilunaris, infundibular opening, and uncinate).

Radiographic evaluation

Obtain coronal CT scans of sinuses (preferably during quiescent phase of disease; 3-mm coronal thin-cut perpendicular to hard palate). MRI scans can distinguish tumors from trapped fluid or mucus.

1. Assess for the extent of disease, mucosal thickening, air-fluid levels, bony expansion, erosion, or dehiscence.
2. Assess for abnormalities of anatomy:
   - Middle meatal abnormalities (paradoxical middle turbinate, large concha bullosa, lamellar cells).
   - Ethmoidal infundibulum (laterally rotated uncinate, Hailer cells).
   - Maxillary sinus (atelectasis, hiatus semilunaris, large bulla ethmoidalis).
   - Frontal recess (narrow internal os); agger nasi cells.
3. Rule out metallic-like densities or diffusely increased densities within soft tissues, indicating a fungal process.
4. Perform checklist to plan surgical approach:
   - Shape of skull (medially downsloping or flat), particularly in the region of the fovea ethmoidalis.

- Relative thickness of skull and presence of bony dehiscences.
- Vertical height of the posterior ethmoid labyrinth relative to posteromedial roof of maxillary sinus and presence of Onodi cells.
- Relationship of carotic artery and optic nerve to sphenoid sinus.
- Atelectasis of uncinate process.
- Atelectasis of maxillary process.

Endoscopic evaluation of the pediatric patient

1. Exam is often difficult to perform.
2. Postoperative care and debridement often will not be tolerated and may require anesthesia.
3. Adenoidal obstruction should be considered as a source of chronic nasal discharge.
4. Inferior meatal window should be considered initially to avoid middle meatal scarring.

Technique

This technique is used in endoscopic sinus surgery of the ethmoid, sphenoid, and maxillary sinuses.

A. Injection

1. Using a 1% lidocaine solution with 1:100,000 epinephrine, inject the following areas:
- Anterior edge of middle turbinate.
- Lateral nasal wall.
- Superior aspect of the inferior turbinate.
2. Pack the nose with 4% cocaine-soaked cotton pledgets for 10 minutes.

B. Examination

1. Inspect the nose using a 4-mm, 0-degree telescope.
2. Locate the septum, turbinate, posterior choana, and adenoids.
3. Identify the middle turbinate and medially displace it using a Freer elevator.
4. Delineate the uncinate process.

C. Infundibulotomy

1. Place a sickle knife as close as possible to the superior attachment of the uncinate process.
2. With a sawing action, move the knife from the antero-superior position to the postero-inferior position following the curvature of the uncinate.
3. Displace the uncinate medially, taking care not to violate the lamina papyracea.
4. Using small Blakesley forceps, grasp the uncinate at its superior margin and twist infero-medially until it detaches.

D. Ethmoidectomy

1. After the uncinectomy, identify the ethmoid bulla. Enter it using gentle blunt dissection with a suction tip or Blakesley forceps. The anterior ethmoidal artery lies just antero-superior to the ethmoid bulla.
2. Under direct visualization with telescope, exenterate the anterior ethmoid cavity and identify the basal lamella (this demarcates the anterior from the posterior ethmoids and represents the attachment of the middle turbinate to the lateral wall.
3. Remove any diseased mucosa or polyps from the posterior ethmoids.
4. Identify the fovea ethmoidalis and the lamina papyracea to confirm position.

E. Sphenoidectomy

1. Perform a blunt, gentle dissection with a suction tip in the infero-medial aspect of the posterior wall of the posterior ethmoids. Important landmarks include:
- Posterior attachment of the superior turbinate.
- The arch of the posterior choana.
- The superior aspect of the nasal septum.
2. After entering the sphenoid, enlarge the sphenoidotomy with Kerrison forceps or a "mushroom punch."
3. In general, do not perform a dissection within the sphenoid sinus; only gentle removal of polyps, debris, and fungal material should be performed.
4. An alternative technique is to trim the inferior portions of the superior turbinate and identify the natural ostium of the sinus medial to the turbinate. The natural ostium is then enlarged using curettes or punches.

F. Maxillary antrostomy

1. Use a 4-mm, 30-degree scope to improve visualization. The maxillary sinus ostium can usually be readily seen after the uncinate process has been removed.
2. After identifying the ostium, cannulate it with an olive-tip, 3-mm, short, curved suction.
3. Alternatively, if the ostium cannot be identified readily, use a double-ended maxillary sinus ostium seeker prior to cannulation.
4. Enlarge the ostium posteriorly into the posterior fontanel using the Greunwald cutting forceps.
5. Perform anterior enlargement with back-biting cutting forceps.
6. Enlarge the ostium eight to ten times its normal size.
7. Take care to avoid the sphenopalatine artery posteriorly and the lacrimal duct anteriorly.
8. Inspect the maxillary sinus with the 30- and 70-degree telescopes.
9. Remove any polyps, cysts, or diseased mucosa with up-biting forceps or giraffe forceps.
10. A variety of packs may be used to prevent the formation of postoperative synechiae, including the use of Kennedy packs in the middle meatus.

Endoscopic Approaches to the Frontal Sinus

A. Endoscopic frontal sinusotomy

The superior aspect of the uncinate process should be removed. In about 65% of cases this attaches to the lamina papyracea, with the frontal recess being medial to the site of attachment. This increases the medial-to-lateral diameter of the frontal recess. Resection of the posterosuperior wall of the agar nasi allows for increased antero-posterior diameter of the recess.

Complications of frontal sinusotomy

- Stenosis: a major problem that has plagued this procedure. It is best addressed by making a wide aperture at the time of initial surgery. Stents have been disappointing in avoiding this complication.
- CSF leak.

B. Modified (endoscopic) Lothrop procedure

- This is generally a second-line procedure.
- Perform endoscopic frontal sinusotomy as described above, removing the superior aspect of the uncinate and the posterosuperior agger nasi cells. Mark the location of the frontal recess with a K-wire. Remove the superior septum and drill from nose into sinus, staying anterior to the posterior table of the frontal sinus.

C. Draf procedures

- Draf I: Remove anterosuperior ethmoid cells.
- Draf II: Remove floor of frontal sinus to level of septum.
  Note: Draf I and II are procedures essentially performed in endoscopic frontal sinusotomy.
- Draf III: Equivalent to Lothrop procedure.

Intranasal Complications

General Complications

- Complications occur in 2%-12% of patients.
- **Prevention via:**
  - **Preoperative means**
    - Thorough history.
    - Careful exam.
    - Medical management, including short steroid course and antibiotics.
  - **Intra-operative means**
    - CT scan in operating room.
    - Adequate vasoconstriction and hemostasis to provide unobstructed view.
    - Review of landmarks.
    - Frequent palpation of orbit.

Minor complications

- **Minor epistaxis**
  - Polyposis, which leads to increased bleeding.
  - Control with topical and local injection of vasoconstrictors.
  - Preoperative treatment with antibiotics and steroids.
  - Packing.
  - General anesthesia, which causes vasodilation and may increase bleeding.
- **Synechia formation**
  - Most common complication.
  - Most common locations: between middle turbinate and lateral nasal wall and in frontal recess.
- Prevention of synechia formation can be accomplished by:
  - Mucosal preservation, minimal turbinate manipulation, and frequent postoperative debridement.
  - Routine resection of middle turbinates; controversial because it may lead to lateralization of remaining turbinate.
  - Use of nasal packs, including Gelfilm, Telfa, and Merocel, as spacers.
  - Medialization of middle turbinate via suture, packing, and mucosal scoring, which may prevent lateralization of turbinate if it has become "floppy" during the procedure.
- **Osteal stenosis**
  - Stenosis of frontal recess, which occurs in 12% of patients undergoing frontal sinus surgery
  - Avoiding trauma to the frontal sinus recess and meticulous postoperative care.
- **Postoperative sinusitis**
- **Hyposmia, anosmia, possibly due to:**
  - Interference with air flow to olfactory nerve.
  - Damage to olfactory nerve.
  - Damage to olfactory pathway.
- **Dental pain/hypesthesia.**

Major complications:

- **Major epistaxis**
- Arterial bleed from anterior ethmoidal, sphenopalatine, internal carotid.
- Carotid artery injury: may be avoided by preoperative determination of carotid to sphenoid sinus relationship (dehiscent carotid in up to 20%).
- If injury to the internal carotid artery does occur, it should be managed as follows:
  - Nasal packing.
  - External compression of carotid.
  - Controlled hypotension.
  - Neurosurgery consultation.
  - Intraoperative arteriogram; however, if patient is unstable, the carotid should be ligated.
  - Balloon occlusion under EEG surveillance: if no EEG lateralization, carotid should be ligated; if lateralization occurs, bypass should be attempted.

Orbital Complications

Minor complications of FESS occur in 2%-21% of patients. Major complications occur in 0.75%-8% of patients.

Minor complications
- Periorbital ecchymosis.
- Periorbital emphysema.

Major complications
- Major complications include:
  - Orbital hematoma.
  - Blindness.
  - Diminished visual acuity.
  - Diplopia.
  - Symptomatic epiphora.
- Frequent examination and palpation of the orbit intraoperatively will demonstrate any defects of the lamina, in which case the orbital contents will prolapse into the ethmoid sinus cavity with gentle palpation of the globe.
- Early recognition of orbital complications is critical. Intraoperative or postoperative ophthalmoplegia, proptosis, ecchymosis, or relative change in pupil size may indicate intraorbital trauma or hemorrhage and warrant immediate evaluation. **Early consultation with an ophthalmologist is indicated.**

Diagnosis and Management

Orbital Hematoma
- Orbital hematoma occurs because of entry through the lamina papyracea and can occur whether or not the periorbita is injured. With violation of the periorbita, the risk of orbital hematoma with blood retention in the retrobulbar space is increased.
- The most common cause of orbital hemorrhage is from trauma to the orbital veins lining the lamina papyracea. The hematoma that develops from violation of the ethmoid arteries is rarer, and progresses more rapidly, than a venous hemorrhage.
- Orbital hematoma is postseptal and is manifested by proptosis, conjunctival changes such as chemosis, and pupillary changes (mydriasis).
- Intraorbital hemorrhage discovered **intraoperatively** should be treated with removal of nasal packing, immediate ethmoidectomy, and orbital decompression with lateral canthotomy and/or splitting of the periorbita to relieve pressure from the hematoma.
- When hemorrhage is noted **postoperatively**, a careful ophthalmologic baseline examination and subsequent serial examination should be obtained. Nasal packing

should be removed, which will sometimes suffice. If visual acuity continues to deteriorate despite IV Decadron (0.1-0.5 mg/kg) and mannitol (0.5-1.0 mg/kg), an external ethmoidectomy for orbital decompression is indicated to control the bleeding (usually from the anterior or posterior ethmoid artery). Sudden and rapid hemorrhage into the orbit warrants immediate external ethmoidectomy and orbital decompression. A lateral canthotomy and cantholysis of the lower lid can be performed at the bedside if the patient cannot return to the operating room immediately and if vision is deteriorating. Orbital massage to relieve orbital pressure transiently is controversial and contraindicated in patients with previous eye surgery, such as lens implants, retinal detachment repair, or glaucoma surgery.
- In situations of retrobulbar or retroorbital hematoma, the retina can tolerate extreme pressures (hence vascular supply compromise to optic nerve and ischemia) for only 60-90 minutes. In case of an arterial hemorrhage, the time is limited to 15-30 minutes. Neural tissue is extremely sensitive to ischemia.

Diplopia
Postoperative diplopia may be a result of direct or indirect trauma to the extraocular muscles (most commonly, medial rectus and the superior oblique) or cranial nerves, or it may result from the effects of local anesthetics. Anesthetic effects will resolve within a few hours. Nerve injury may recover in 6-12 months if the nerve is not severed. Nerve injury is treated with prisms or strabismus surgery. Muscle injury may be detected by CT scanning and typically will require ophthalmologic surgical repair, which is often difficult.

Blindness
Blindness in the absence of orbital hemorrhage or increased ocular pressure may indicate direct or indirect trauma to the optic nerve, in which case the patient will have a positive Marcus Gunn pupil or "efferent pupillary defect" on the swinging flashlight test. Nasal packing should be removed. If there is no sustained improvement with high-dose steroids, external sphenoethmoidectomy and optic nerve decompression should be considered. The optic nerve sheath may be split to decompress the nerve further and to drain a perineural hematoma.

Damage to orbital wall
If there is dehiscence of, or trauma to, the medial wall of the orbit, patients should not have any positive pressure mask ventilation after extubation from surgery and should absolutely avoid nose blowing for several days postoperatively to prevent subcutaneous emphysema of the orbit. If this should occur, it will typically resolve spontaneously in approximately 1 week.

Damage to the lacrimal system

Obstruction of the lacrimal system resulting in epiphora may occur in the early or late postoperative period and typically is a result of trauma to the nasolacrimal duct from over-resection of the anterior edge of the maxillary sinus os. Many of these injuries may be asymptomatic if the tears drain into any part of the nasal cavity. This complication is unusual if the os is not widened past the anterior attachment of the middle turbinate and if any bone encountered on widening the os is left alone. If this poses a persistent problem, a dacryocystorhinostomy (DCR) would be indicated.

Intracranial Complications

CSF leak (0.2%-1.0%)

- Most commonly occurs where anterior ethmoid artery penetrates lateral lamella of cribriform plate. If a CSF leak is recognized during surgery, then:
  - Attempt intraoperative repair with fascia, fat, mucoperiosteum flap, Gelfoam packing, and fibrin glue.
  - Place lumbar drain.
  - Administer meningitis prophylaxis antibiotics.
  - Perform early postoperative CT to rule out hemorrhage.
- If CSF leak is suspected during postoperative follow-up, it can be detected by:
  - Nasal endoscopy.
  - Coronal CT scan, looking for dehiscence of the anterior table.
  - Intrathecal injection, radioactive tagged serum albumin collected on nasal pledgets (good for detection, not localization).
  - Intrathecal fluorescein and blue light endoscopy,
  - Check of rhinorrhea for beta-2-transferrin.

Management

- Surgical repair, extracranial approach initially (see below).

Meningitis

Typically secondary to CSF leak.

- Symptoms: Fever, headache, drowsiness, confusion, neck stiffness.
- Diagnosis: Lumbar puncture.
- Treatment: High-dose IV antibiotics with good blood-brain barrier penetration.

Brain abscess

- Symptoms: Drowsiness, confusion, headache, fever, nausea, vomiting, seizure.
- Diagnosis: CT or MRI scan, lumbar puncture (LP).
- Treatment: Neurosurgical drainage, systemic antibiotics, evaluation and treatment for CSF leak.

Intracranial hemorrhage/stroke

- Symptoms: New onset of neurologic symptoms in absence of signs of infection.
- Diagnosis: CT or MRI scan.
- Treatment: Neurosurgery consult to rule out need to evacuate intracranial blood.

Cranial hemorrhage (internal carotid artery injury)

Exceedingly rare complication resulting from violation of the carotid in the lateral sphenoid wall.

Management

- Nasal packing with manual compression of ipsilateral cervical internal carotid artery (ICA).
- Controlled hypotension.
- Carotid angiography with EEG surveillance with balloon occlusion proximal and distal to tear.
- If balloon occlusion leads to no neurologic sequelae and controls bleed, no further treatment is necessary.
- If balloon occlusion leads to no neurologic sequelae but fails to control bleeding, ligation of the internal carotid artery is indicated.
- If balloon occlusion leads to significant neurologic symptoms or EEG changes, the balloon is deflated and left in place. A Swan-Ganz catheter is then placed to allow for controlled hypervolemic therapy to optimize cerebral blood flow.

Selected References from the Recent Literature

1. Anand VK, Osguthorpe JD, Rice D. Surgical management of adult rhinosinusitis. *Otolaryngology–Head & Neck Surgery* 2000;117:S50-S52
2. Casiano RR, Livingston JA. Endoscopic Lothrop procedure: the University of Miami experience. *American Journal of Rhinology* 2000;12:335-339.
3. Dursun E, Bayiz U, Korkmaz H *et al.* Follow-up results of 415 patients after endoscopic sinus surgery. *European Archives of Oto-Rhino-Laryngology* 2000;255:504-510.
4. Folker RJ, Marple BF, Mabry RL, Mabry CS. Treatment of allergic fungal sinusitis: a comparison trial of postoperative immunotherapy with specific fungal antigens. *Laryngoscope* 2000;108:1623-1627.
5. Halvorson DJ, Dupree JR, Porubsky ES. Management of chronic sinusitis in the adult cystic fibrosis patient. *Annals of Otology, Rhinology & Laryngology* 2000;107:946-952.
6. Jones NS. Current concepts in the management of paediatric rhinosinusitis. *Journal of Laryngology & Otology* 2000; 113:1-9.
7. Kennedy DW, Senior BA, Gannon FH *et al.* Histology and histomorphometry of ethmoid bone in chronic rhinosinusitis. *Laryngoscope* 2000;108:502-507.
8. Kennedy DW, Senior BA. Endoscopic sinus surgery. A review. *Otolaryngologic Clinics of North America* 2000;30: 313-330.
9. Lusk RP, Stankiewicz JA. Pediatric rhinosinusitis. *Otolaryngology–Head & Neck Surgery* 2000;117:S53-S57.

10. Marple BF, Mabry RL. Comprehensive management of allergic fungal sinusitis. *American Journal of Rhinology* 2000;12:263-268.

11. Metson R, Gliklich RE. Clinical outcome of endoscopic surgery for frontal sinusitis [see comments]. *Archives of Otolaryngology—Head & Neck Surgery* 2000;124:1090-1096.

12. Nguyen QA, Leopold DA. Current concepts in the surgical management of chronic frontal sinusitis. [Review] [80 refs]. *Otolaryngologic Clinics of North America* 2000;30: 355-370.

13. Sabini P, Josephson GD, Reisacher WR, Pincus R. The role of endoscopic sinus surgery in patients with acquired immune deficiency syndrome. *American Journal of Otolaryngology* 2000;19:351-356.

14. Seiden AM, Stankiewicz JA. Frontal sinus surgery: the state of the art. [Review] [48 refs]. *American Journal of Otolaryngology* 2000;19:183-193.

15. Senior BA, Kennedy DW, Tanabodee J *et al*. Long-term impact of functional endoscopic sinus surgery on asthma. *Otolaryngology—Head & Neck Surgery* 2000;121:66-68.

16. Senior BA, Kennedy DW, Tanabodee J *et al*. Long-term results of functional endoscopic sinus surgery. *Laryngoscope* 2000;108:151-157.

17. Weber R, Draf W, Keerl R *et al*: Endonasal microendoscopic pansinusoperation in chronic sinusitis. II. Results and complications. *American Journal of Otolaryngology* 2000;18: 247-253.

OPEN APPROACHES TO THE PARANASAL SINUSES

Caldwell-Luc

The Caldwell-Luc operation was first described by George Caldwell in 1893 and Henry Luc in 1897 for the treatment of chronic maxillary sinusitis. The procedure (as originally described) involved performing a maxillary antrostomy through the canine fossa, stripping the diseased mucosa from the maxillary sinus, and creating an inferior meatal antrostomy to allow for longer-lasting drainage. As endoscopic sinus surgery techniques have improved, the indications for the Caldwell-Luc procedure have decreased. However, there are still many valid indications for this procedure as the treatment of benign maxillary sinus lesions or as an approach to structures surrounding the maxillary sinus.

Indications
- Maxillary sinus lesions
  - Chronic maxillary sinusitis with or without polyposis (especially in patients with impaired mucociliary function).
  - Maxillary sinus disease refractory to endoscopic surgery.
  - Antrochoanal polyp.
  - Maxillary sinus foreign bodies (displaced tooth roots).
  - Maxillary sinus mycetoma (fungus balls).
  - Benign maxillary sinus tumors.
  - Symptomatic maxillary mucocele.
- Approaches to the pterygomaxillary space
  - Internal maxillary artery ligation (for posterior epistaxis).
  - Vidian neurectomy (for vasomotor rhinitis).
  - Biopsy of skull base lesions.
- Approach for repair of facial fractures
  - Tripod, orbital floor, zygomatic arch fractures.
  - Le Fort fractures.
- Other
  - Oroantral fistula.
  - Osteoradionecrosis or osteomyelitis of maxilla.
  - Orbital decompression for Grave's ophthalmopathy (Walsh-Ogura technique).

Contraindications
- Uncontrolled bleeding disorder.
- Usually not performed in pediatric patients; due to possibility of damaging permanent dentition.
- Aplastic maxillary sinus.

Technique
1. Infiltrate gingivobuccal sulcus with local anesthetic with epinephrine.
2. Decongest nasal mucosa with cocaine-soaked pledgets.
3. Incision made in gingivobuccal sulcus from lateral incisor to the first or second molar (leave sufficient mucosa inferiorly to facilitate closure).
4. Incise periosteum and elevate soft tissues overlying the maxillary sinus in a subperiosteal plane to expose the canine fossa.
5. Identify and preserve infraorbital nerve.
6. Enter maxillary sinus with osteotome at a level superior to the roots of the canine and premolar teeth.
7. Remove additional bone with Kerrison rongeur as needed to view the abnormality.
8. Remove irreversibly diseased mucosa, tumor, polyps, or cyst. (Take care when working posteriorly to avoid violating the thin maxillary sinus wall and injuring the maxillary artery. Also take care when working superiorly to prevent injury to the orbital floor and infraorbital nerve.)
9. Create a nasoantral window under the inferior turbinate and enlarge with forward and backbiting forceps.
10. Cavity may be packed with antibiotic impregnated gauze.
11. Close incision with interrupted chromic sutures.

Complications
- Common
  - Hemorrhage or cheek edema/ecchymosis.
  - Persistent facial pain (18%).
  - Tooth or gum pain or numbness (17%).
  - Recurrent disease (12%).
  - Facial paresthesias or numbness (9%).
  - Dacryocystitis (3%).
  - Oroantral fistula (1.5%).
  - Devitalized teeth (<1%).
  - Facial asymmetry (<1%).
- Uncommon
  - Globe, orbital floor, or extraocular muscle injury.
  - Orbital hematoma, proptosis, or blindness.
  - Internal maxillary artery injury.
  - Superior alveolar nerve injury.
  - Loss of teeth on operated side (delayed complication).

OPEN APPROACHES TO THE FRONTAL SINUS

General Indications
- Chronic frontal sinusitis that has not responded to conservative therapy, including endoscopic sinus surgery.
- Chronic frontal sinusitis complicated by:
  - Persistent pain (orbital or frontal).

❑ Intracranial extension of disease.
❑ Orbital extension of disease: mucocele or pyocele.
❑ Osteomyelitis of the frontal bone.

Lynch Frontal Sinus Operation

Developed in 1920, consists of a frontal ethmoidectomy, removal of the middle turbinate, and resection of the entire floor of the frontal sinus.

Advantages
- Simplest form of the frontal sinus operations.
- Can be performed rapidly in patients who are poor medical risks.

Disadvantages
- Cosmetic result often not pleasing.
- Recurrent infection not uncommon.
- Significant incidence of mucocele and pyocele formation after this operation.
- Difficult to maintain continuity between nasal cavity and frontal sinus.

Riedel Operation

- Consists of removing the anterior wall and floor of the frontal sinus, thus offering wide exposure.
- Sinus can be completely obliterated when antero-posterior diameter is small.
- Disfiguring procedure and offers a percentage of cure not much higher than the Lynch procedure.

Classical Lothrop Operation

- Unilateral or bilateral anterior ethmoidectomy and middle turbinectomy, along with removal of interfrontal septum
- Large opening from frontal sinuses into the nasal cavity made by connecting the two nasofrontal orifices and resecting part of the superior nasal septum.
- Effective in eradicating bilateral chronic frontal sinus disease.
- Operation technically difficult.
- Ineffective when the antero-posterior diameter of the frontal sinus is narrow.

Killian Operation

- Modification of the Reidel procedure with attempt to preserve supraorbital rim.
- Often unsatisfactory cosmetic result and difficult to revise.

Anterior Osteoplastic Frontal Sinus Operation with Adipose Obliteration

- An inferiorly hinged trap door is fashioned from the anterior wall of the frontal sinus.
- Direct access to the entire contents of the frontal sinus is possible, along with an excellent view of the nasofrontal orifice
- Intrasinus disease can be removed with ease, and revisions of previous frontal surgery can be performed.
- Adequate drainage from the frontal sinus to the intranasal space can be established, or the frontal sinuses can be completely obliterated by implanting adipose tissue
- It is very successful in the treatment of chronic frontal sinus disease.
- Facial deformity and low morbidity with minimal postoperative care are rare.

 EXTERNAL SPHENOETHMOIDECTOMY

Indications
- Patients with chronic rhinosinusitis in whom the normal anatomic landmarks have been distorted.
- Acute ethmoid and frontal sinusitis complicated by orbital or periorbital abscess.
- Biopsy or some orbital, ethmoid, frontal, or sphenoid sinus lesions.
- Repair of CSF leak.
- Combined with frontal craniotomy for en bloc removal of anterior skull base mass.

Contraindications
- Medical illness.

Technique
1. Administer general anesthesia.
2. Perform Lynch or Chiari incision (angle blade in direction of hair follicles).
3. Incise the skin and subcutaneous tissues down to periosteum.
4. Identify and ligate the angular artery and vein.
5. Take down the attachment of medial canthal tendon.
6. Lateralize the lacrimal sac.
7. Retract the orbital contents laterally.
8. Remember to relax pressure on the orbit every 45-60 seconds (to prevent vasovagal reaction).
9. Locate and ligate anterior ethmoid artery: about 20 mm posterior to posterior lacrimal crest; in frontoethmoid suture line.
10. Locate and ligate the posterior ethmoid artery, about 10 mm behind anterior ethmoid artery. The optic

foramen is 5 mm behind the posterior ethmoid artery.

11. The frontoethmoid suture line identifies the level of the anterior cranial fossa floor.

12. Excise the lacrimal fossa and bone.

13. Continue anteriorly to open the agar nasi cell, proceed posteriorly to open the anterior and posterior ethmoids, then proceed to the sphenoid.

Complications

- Recurrent disease.
- Bleeding.
- Epiphora.
- Frontal sinusitis.
- CSF leak.
- Intracranial hemorrhage.
- Optic nerve trauma.
- Blindness.
- Retrobulbar hemorrhage.
- Transient diplopia secondary to trochlear dislodgment.
- Hypertrophic scar formation.
- Scar band/web formation.

 FRONTAL SINUS OBLITERATION

Indications

- Gold standard for chronic frontal sinusitis refractory to conservative therapy or to previous surgical attempts.
- Mucoceles.
- Pyoceles.
- Frontal bone osteomyelitis with bone necrosis.
- Benign frontal sinus tumors.
- Orbital or intracranial extension of frontal sinus disease.
- Anterior table fracture with injury to the nasofrontal ostium.

Contraindications

- Small hypoplastic frontal sinuses that do not extend into frontal bone.

Technique

Unilateral

1. With a 6-ft Caldwell view preop, cut out a template of the sinus from the radiograph, including interfrontal septum and supraorbital rim; autoclave the template; use as a template for bony cuts.

2. Perform ipsilateral tarsorrhaphy.

3. Inject the incision line above the upper margin of the eyebrow.

4. Carry the incision down to the periosteum, beveling away from hair follicles.

5. Incise the periosteum superiorly, laterally and medially, leaving the inferior margin intact; elevate away

to avoid damage from bony cuts.

6. Bevel 30 degrees toward the sinus with a saw. Complete bone incision with an osteotome and mallet, and pry away the flap from the sinus.

7. Remove diseased mucosa with a Freer elevator and Blakesley forceps. Burr inner cortical bone to ensure complete removal of mucosa and to provide a bed to supply harvested fat.

8. Harvest fat from LLQ abdominal incision to avoid confusion with appendectomy scar.

9. Obliterate the sinus with fat completely, return the flap to position, and close periosteal incisions with 4-0 Vicryl.

10. Close the wound in three layers (frontalis, subcutaneous, and skin), and apply a light-pressure dressing.

Bilateral

1. Perform template procedure as described previously.

2. Make the incision coronal (for those with hair) or brow or mid-forehead (in those who are balding).

3. Elevate the skin flap in the same plane as described previously, using hemostatic Raney clips around the wound edge.

4. Place the template over the frontal periosteum and incise as described previously, with a horizontal incision across nasal process.

5. Incise the bone as described previously, transect the intersinus septum from above, and elevate the flap.

6. Remove the tissue as described previously, and burr down the intersinus septum.

7. Obliterate the sinus with fat, and replace the bone as described previously. Miniplates may be necessary if unstable.

8. Close as described previously.

Complications

- Fracture or injury to the posterior table:
  - Dural tears.
  - CSF leaks.
  - Frontal lobe injury.
  - Meningitis.
  - Brain abscess.
- Fracture of the floor of the sinus or orbital roof:
  - Extraocular muscle injury (diplopia).
  - Globe injury.
  - Hemorrhage (blindness).
- Supraorbital nerve injury (paresthesia, hypoesthesia, or anesthesia to forehead) if transected. Often transient from retraction.
- Loss of frontalis function.
- Hematoma or seroma.
- Wound infection.
- Anosmia (trauma to cribriform plate and olfactory nerve).

CSF RHINORRHEA ORIGINATING FROM THE ANTERIOR CRANIAL FOSSA

Anatomy: Anterior Cranial Fossa or Anterior Skull Base

- Borders
  - Anterior: Frontal crest and posterior wall of frontal sinus.
  - Posterior: lesser wing of sphenoid.
  - Medial: cribriform plate.
  - Lateral: frontal bone.
  - Superior: frontal lobes, olfactory bulb.
  - Inferior: orbital plates of frontal bone, cribriform plate.

Classification of CSF Leak

- Traumatic
  - Accidents account for 80% of all cases (male:female ratio = 4:1).
  - 2%-3% of head-trauma patients develop CSF leak.
  - Intracranial and extracranial surgery causes 16% of cases.
- Atraumatic
  - Adults (<30 years old; female:male ratio = 2:1).
  - Can occur with elevated or normal intracranial pressure
    - High pressure
      - Tumor: may erode skull base or obstruct CSF flow.
      - Hydrocephalus.
    - Normal pressure
      - Congenital cranial base defect (with or without meningocele or meningoencephalocele).
      - Osteomyelitis: Pott's tumor.
      - Idiopathic: may result from transient Valsalva maneuver or straining.
    - Empty sella syndrome
      - Absent *diaphragm sella* (congenital).
      - Pituitary atrophy or degeneration.

CSF Rhinorrhea

Sites

- Most common site is roof of ethmoid and cribriform plate (in region of olfactory fibers).
- May also occur at medial skull base associated with anterior ethmoid artery.
- May be evident immediately or after several weeks posttrauma.
- May be associated with dural herniation.
- Rhinorrhea secondary to trauma with fracture of posterior table of the frontal sinus typically associated with extensive brain injury.

Diagnosis
Signs and symptoms

- Clear rhinorrhea (55% in first 48 hours, 70% by day 7 posttrauma), usually ipsilateral.
- Hyposmia and anosmia in 60%-80%.
- Headache with pneumocephalus (20%).
- Meningitis as initial symptom (risk of developing meningitis in first 3 weeks is 3%-11%) present in 20%.
- Rhinorrhea when upright and tilted back: suggests origin in frontal or ethmoid sinuses, or cribriform plate. Rhinorrhea when upright and tilted forward: suggests origin in sphenoid sinus.

Investigations
Nasal discharge

- Halo sign: Place drop of fluid onto filter paper. The blood will remain in the center and the CSF will migrate peripherally, forming one or more clearer rings.
- Glucose >30 mg/mL suggestive, but normal nasal secretions can have high glucose content.
- Electrophoresis for β_2-transferrin.

Radiologic studies

- Metrizamide cisternography (agent is opaque on CT scan): Inject subarachnoid space, then use fine-cut CT scan of the skull base to demonstrate site of extracranial extravasation (20%-80% success).
- Intrathecal fluorescein: Inject 0.5 mL of 1% fluorescein combined with 9.5 mL CSF, wait 30 minutes, and then examine nasal cavity with blue light endoscopy.
- Radionuclide cisternography (^{111}In-DPTA or ^{99m}Tc-DTPA) with intranasal pledgets to absorb CSF: Success for detection of intermittent leak is 25%-65%.
- MRI less sensitive but noninvasive and with no radioactivity.

Management
Posttraumatic

- Most traumatic CSF fistulas heal without intervention; if >7 days, usually need surgery.
- Acute trauma CSF leak, wait 2-3 weeks postinjury for edema resolution.
- Facial fracture reduction may allow resolution.

Post-ESS

- Intraoperative/surgical leaks should be repaired at time of primary surgery with free mucosal graft, with or without cartilage and/or bone. Graft may be harvested from septum or turbinates. Closure may be assisted by use of Fibrin glue.
- Small leaks detected postoperatively may resolve with bedrest and lumbar drain (150-240 mL/day); no bending, straining, or lifting; and use of laxatives.

Repair of Frontal Sinus Leak

Extracranial approach with osteoplastic flap
Technique

1. Perform coronal or brow incision. Use a plain film template to delineate bone cuts over the frontal sinus area (this limits inadvertent dural injury).
2. Create an inferiorly based osteoplastic flap.
3. Remove bone fragments and lining mucosa from the sinus if initial injury was secondary to trauma.
4. Use a drill with a diamond burr to remove mucosal remnants.
5. Identify the leak. If the tear is small, close the dura (suture or cautery).
6. Obliterate the frontal sinus and nasofrontal duct. A variety of substances have been used for frontal sinus obliteration, including abdominal fat (most common), lyophilized cartilage, cancellous bone, bio-activated glass, hydroxyapatite, pericranium, or glabellar muscle,
7. If a posterior table defect is detected and it is small, tuck the fascia between the edges and then obliterate the frontal sinus. If a large defect in the posterior defect is found, cranialize the sinus and obliterate the nasofrontal duct.

Results
- Failure rate of extracranial approach is 6%-30%.
- If unsuccessful, craniotomy is usually necessary.

Complications (7%-18%)
- Headache (suggesting recurrent disease).
- Mucocele as a result of incomplete mucosa ablation.
- Persistent hypesthesia in the supraorbital nerve distribution; seen more frequently with brow rather than coronal incision.
- Seroma or abscess at harvest site.
- Dural laceration.
- Nasal dorsum skin necrosis.
- Anosmia.
- Ptosis and frontalis muscle dysfunction.
- Neuralgia noted more often with brow incision.
- Scar or forehead abnormality (7%).

Extra-intracranial procedure
- Coronal incision; excision of anterior table, bilateral removal of posterior table, inspection of dura, closure of tear, and reinsertion of anterior plate with fixation.

Intracranial procedure
- Craniotomy with repair of posterior table or anterior skull base, typically with dural repair and large pericranial flap.
- Intranasal endoscopic repair as described previously useful for leaks emanating from ethmoid or sphenoid sinus, but not from frontal sinus.

Selected References from the Recent Literature

1. Bateman N, Mason J, Jones NS. Use of fluorescein for detecting cerebrospinal fluid rhinorrhoea: a safe technique for intrathecal injection. *Orl Journal of Oto-Rhino-Laryngology & Its Related Specialties* 2000;61:131-132.
2. Brodie HA. Prophylactic antibiotics for posttraumatic cerebrospinal fluid fistulae. A meta-analysis. *Archives of Otolaryngology—Head & Neck Surgery* 2000;123:749-752.
3. Castillo L, Jaklis A, Paquis P et al. Nasal endoscopic repair of cerebrospinal fluid rhinorrhea. *Rhinology* 2000;37:33-36.
4. Dodson EE, Gross CW, Swerdloff JL, Gustafson LM. Transnasal endoscopic repair of cerebrospinal fluid rhinorrhea and skull base defects: a review of twenty-nine cases. *Otolaryngology—Head & Neck Surgery* 2000;111:600-605.
5. Har-El G. What is "spontaneous" cerebrospinal fluid rhinorrhea? Classification of cerebrospinal fluid leaks [editorial]. [Review] [30 refs]. *Annals of Otology, Rhinology & Laryngology* 2000;108:323-326.
6. Hughes RG, Jones NS, Robertson IJ. The endoscopic treatment of cerebrospinal fluid rhinorrhoea: the Nottingham experience. *Journal of Laryngology & Otology* 2000;111:125-128.
7. Johnson DB, Brennan P, Toland J, O'Dwyer AJ. Magnetic resonance imaging in the evaluation of cerebrospinal fluid fistulae. *Clinical Radiology* 2000;51:837-841.
8. Kwartler JA, Schulder M, Baredes S, Chandrasekhar SS. Endoscopic closure of the eustachian tube for repair of cerebrospinal fluid leak. *American Journal of Otology* 2000;17:470-472.
9. Lanza DC, O'Brien DA, Kennedy DW. Endoscopic repair of cerebrospinal fluid fistulae and encephaloceles. *Laryngoscope* 2000;106:1119-1125.
10. Solomon P, Chen J, D'Costa M et al. Extracranial drainage of cerebrospinal fluid: a study of beta-transferrins in nasal and lymphatic tissues. *Laryngoscope* 2000;109:1313-1315.
11. Stone JA, Castillo M, Neelon B, Mukherji SK. Evaluation of CSF leaks: high-resolution CT compared with contrast-enhanced CT and radionuclide cisternography. *AJNR: American Journal of Neuroradiology* 2000;20:706-712.
12. Van D, Elmaleh M, Herman P et al. Transnasal endoscopic repair of congenital defects of the skull base in children. *Archives of Otolaryngology—Head & Neck Surgery* 2000;125:580-584.

ORBITAL DECOMPRESSION

Orbital decompression is indicated for the treatment of space-occupying lesions that compromise orbital function or cause visual loss.

Examples

Dysthyroid Orbitopathy or Graves' Disease
- Most common indication for orbital decompression.
- Between 30% and 70% of patients with hyperthyroidism develop orbital manifestations of the disease.
- Majority cosmetic.
- Between 2% and 5% develop significant sequela: optic neuropathy and exposure keratopathy.
- Risk factors for orbital complications: female gender, pretibial myxedema, and tobacco use.

Pathogenesis
- Autoimmune reaction against antigens shared by orbital fibroblasts and thyroid cells.
- Results in the infiltration of T lymphocytes and the deposition of mucopolysaccharides in orbital tissue.

Classification
Type I
- Female, symmetric proptosis, normal extraocular muscle function, and rarely, neuropathy or diplopia

Type II
- Asymmetric orbital involvement, restrictive diplopia, chemosis, acute orbital inflammation, and compressive neuropathy.

Outcome
- *Type I less likely to experience diplopia after decompression.*
- Type II responds better to steroids or XRT.

Clinical course
Acute phase
- The diseases lasts 6-18 months.
- Characterized by inflammation and congestion of the orbital tissues with resultant proptosis As the disease, originally cosmetic, progresses, corneal protection is inadequate and results in exposure keratitis and corneal ulcers.
- Enlargement of the extraocular muscles at the orbital apex may result in optic nerve compression and visual loss.

Chronic phase
- Develops up to 3 years after acute phase.

- Characterized by progressive enlargement and fibrosis of the extraocular muscles and increases in orbital fat.

Traumatic injuries
- With a significant blowout fracture, loss of support of the orbital tissues may occur with herniation of orbital tissue.
- Occasionally, muscle entrapment occurs.
- Orbital decompression and possibly reconstruction may be necessary to release the entrapped tissues and to prevent enophthalmos.
- Fractures of the orbit may also impinge on the optic nerve, compromising vision and requiring emergency intervention.

Orbital complications of sinusitis
- Include subperiosteal and orbital abscesses.
- Most frequently involve the medial wall of the orbit, where congenital or acquired defects exist in the bone.
- May be drained effectively endoscopically.

Sinus surgery
Most commonly results from injury to the anterior ethmoid artery just posterior to the nasofrontal recess, with retraction of the artery into the orbit and unrecognized, continued bleeding.

Patient Selection for Orbital Decompression

Graves' exophthalmopathy
Medical Therapy
- Majority of patients can be managed medically.
- First line: corticosteroids (often at high doses for prolonged periods of time).
- Irradiation (20 Gy) also effective.
- Surgery required when these therapies fail or corneal ulceration or visual loss imminent.
- Surgery increasingly done for cosmetic reasons.

Surgery
Surgical intervention is usually considered in the following order of procedures:
1. Orbital decompression.
2. Strabismus repair.
3. Eyelid adjustments.
4. Blepharoplasty.

Goals of Surgical Intervention
- Obtain maximal displacement of the eye posteriorly.
- Minimize displacement of the eye along other axes.
- Eliminate compression of the optic nerve.

Trauma
- Surgical intervention is indicated when displaced bone fragments impinge on the orbital tissues and

restrict orbital motility or compromise the optic nerve.

- Large blowout fractures, especially of the orbit floor, require repair to prevent posttraumatic enophthalmos.

Techniques

- A variety of techniques have been described for orbital decompression:
  - Krönlein: Removal of the lateral bony orbit.
  - Naffziger: Removal of orbital roof via a frontal craniotomy.
  - Sewall: Removal of the medial wall via ethmoidectomy.
  - Hirsch: Removal of orbital floor via Caldwell-Luc approach.
  - Walsh and Ogura: Combined removal of medial wall and orbital floor via a transantral procedure (combination of Hirsch and Sewall procedures). This is the most popular external approach for orbital decompression.

Decompression yields

- Single-wall decompression decreases proptosis by 0-4 mm.
- Medial and inferior walls decrease proptosis by 3-6 mm.
- Three-wall decompression decreases proptosis by 6-10 mm.
  Note: Yields are affected by degree of orbital stiffness, which is more likely to be increased in older patients with chronic disease.

Decompression of the medial and inferior walls
External transantral approach

- Described by Walsh and Ogura.
- Technique:
  - Caldwell-Luc approach to maxillary sinus.
  - Antrotomy medial to the infraorbital nerve is brought to the orbital rim to maximize exposure of the ethmoid cells.
  - Mucosa is stripped off roof and medial wall of the sinus.
  - Ethmoid cells are removed posterior to lacrimal crest and inferior to cribriform plate with curette and/or forceps.
  - Removal of maxillary sinus with osteotome or drill.
  - Removal of lamina papyracea, or fracture performed medially.
- Complications may include:
  - Infraorbital and lip anesthesia.
  - Asymmetric decompression of the two orbits.
  - Enophthalmos.
  - Medial ectropion.
  - Nasolacrimal duct obstruction (epiphora).
  - CSF rhinorrhea.
  - Oroantral fistula.
  - Chronic sinusitis.
  - Diplopia.
  - Blindness.

Endoscopic approach

CT scan posted in OR and reviewed.

1. Place the patient on the operating room table in the supine position, with the head elevated 15-30 degrees.
2. Decongest the nasal cavity with pledgets containing oxymetazoline, phenylephrine, or cocaine.
3. Inject the anterior edge of the middle turbinate, the lateral nasal wall, and the superior aspect of the inferior turbinate with a solution of 1% lidocaine and 1:100,000 epinephrine. Pack the nose for 10 minutes with 4% cocaine-soaked cotton pledgets.
4. Inspect the nose with a 4-mm, 0-degree ridged endoscope. Find the septum, turbinate, posterior choana, and adenoids. Holding the 0-degree telescope in the left hand and applying suction with the right hand, examine the nasal cavity. Identify the middle turbinate and then displace it medially using a Freer elevator. Delineate the uncinate process.
5. Perform an infundibulectomy by placing a sickle knife as close as possible to the superior attachment of the uncinate process. With a sawing action, move the knife firmly from the anterosuperior to the posteroinferior position, taking care not to violate the lamina papyracea. Extend the cut posteriorly in a line parallel to the lower borders of the middle turbinate. Displace the uncinate process toward the middle turbinate. Using a small Blakesley forceps, grasp the uncinate process at its superior attachment and twist medially while pushing posteroinferiorly (i.e., articulating the blade toward the orbit).
6. Perform an ethmoidectomy. Keeping the 0-degree telescope in the left hand, visualize the ethmoid bulla. Enter it by gentle, blunt dissection using a Blakesley forceps in the inferior medial aspect. The anterior ethmoidal artery is just anterosuperior to the bulla. Under direct visualization using the telescope, exenterate the ethmoidal cavity. Identify the basal lamella, which is the bony layer that defines the posterior extension of the anterior ethmoids and the insertion of the middle turbinate to the lateral nasal wall. Open the lamella in the inferomedial aspect with Blakesley forceps to enter the posterior ethmoids. Clean any diseased mucosa or polyps from the posterior ethmoids. The roof of the ethmoid sinus (e.g., fovea ethmoidalis) may be identified at this stage. Similarly, the lamina papyracea can be identified to expose the lateral wall of the ethmoid complex.
7. Perform a maxillary antrostomy. Introduce a 30-degree telescope medially and parallel to the inferior

border of the middle turbinate, with the instrument's beveled surface facing the lateral nasal wall. The maxillary sinus ostium can usually be visualized after the uncinate process has been removed. After identifying the ostium, cannulate it with a short, curved, suction, olive-tip cannula. Alternatively, if the ostium is not readily identified, gently insert a double-ended maxillary sinus ostium seeker inferoanteriorly, behind the uncinate process remnant and above the superior border of the inferior turbinate, under direct visualization with the same scope.

Enlarge the ostium posteriorly into the posterior fontanel using the Gruenwald cutting forceps. Perform anterior enlargement using sidebiting or backbiting cutting forceps. Enlarge the ostium eight to ten times its normal size. Take care to avoid injury of the sphenopalatine artery posteriorly and the nasal lacrimal duct or sac anteriorly.

8. Elevate the mucosa and remove it from the roof of the maxillary sinus to expose the bone over the infraorbital nerve bundle. Recall that the infraorbital nerve bundle may be dehiscent, so avoid direct manipulation of the nerve. Do not perform decompression lateral to the nerve because of the minimal additional decompression that is achieved and the risks of injury to the infraorbital nerve and hypoglobus.

9. With removal of bone, carefully palpate and fracture the bone of the lamina papyracea with the sharp end of a Cottle elevator. Take care to avoid lacerating the periorbita and subsequent herniation of orbital fat into the surgical field. Then carefully elevate and remove the fractured bone fragments using the Cottle elevator and Blakesley upbiting forceps. Continue removing the bone superiorly to within 2 mm of the fovea ethmoidalis, posteriorly to the anterior face of the sphenoid sinus, and laterally to within several millimeters of the infraorbital nerve. At the juncture of the inferior and medial orbital walls, preserve a buttress of bone anteriorly to avoid excessive inferior displacement of the globe and the development of hypoglobus.

10. Preform decompression. Pass a sickle knife intranasally and make a linear cut of the periorbita superiorly in a posterior-to-anterior direction. Then make approximately three to five linear incisions in a similar manner, proceeding from the superomedial to the inferolateral limits of the decompression. Take care to avoid excessive penetration of the sickle blade because the medial rectus muscle is often enlarged and at risk for injury. External pressure on the globe through the closed lids is helpful in breaking any fibrous bands and assessing the degree of orbital decompression.

Postoperative management
- Maximal orbital decompression may not be apparent immediately thus corneal lubricants may be necessary.
- Patients may experience increased diplopia and pain with extraocular movements.

Discharge instructions
- No bending, lifting, or straining is allowed, and coughing and sneezing is done with an open mouth.
- Pain medications with antiplatelet effects are avoided.
- Nasal saline is useful for loosening blood clots.

Follow-up
- Patients are seen at 1-week intervals for cleaning of the nasal cavity until adequate healing is noted.
- Mucosalization of the exposed orbital tissue occurs rapidly and is usually complete within 8 weeks.

Pitfalls and complications
Risks of orbital decompression include those of endoscopic sinus surgery (see previous section). Additional risks include:
- Infraorbital nerve hypesthesia/paresthesia. Rare in the absence of a Caldwell-Luc incision. Risk lessened by restricting the decompression to the orbital floor medial to the nerve bundle.
- Medial rectus muscle injury. Avoided by careful incision of the periorbita.
- Hypoglobus. Risk factors include decreased patient age (minimal orbital fibrosis and increased orbital fluidity), extent of bone removal, and incision of the periorbita.

Selected References from the Recent Literature

1. Goldberg RA, Weinberg DA, Shorr N, Wirta D. Maximal, three-wall, orbital decompression through a coronal approach. *Ophthalmic Surgery & Lasers* 2000;28:832-843.
2. Goldberg RA. The evolving paradigm of orbital decompression surgery [editorial]. [Review] [11 refs]. *Archives of Ophthalmology* 2000;116:95-96.
3. Goldberg RA, Steinsapir KD. Extracranial optic canal decompression: indications and technique. *Ophthalmic Plastic & Reconstructive Surgery* 2000;12:163-170.
4. Graham SM, Carter KD. Combined-approach orbital decompression for thyroid-related orbitopathy. *Clinical Otolaryngology & Allied Sciences* 2000;24:109-113.
5. Koay B, Bates G, Elston J. Endoscopic orbital decompression for dysthyroid eye disease. *Journal of Laryngology & Otology* 2000;111:946-949.

6. Lund VJ, Larkin G, Fells P, Adams G. Orbital decompression for thyroid eye disease: a comparison of external and endoscopic techniques. *Journal of Laryngology & Otology* 2000;111:1051-1055.

7. Luxenberger W, Stammberger H, Jebeles JA, Walch C. Endoscopic optic nerve decompression: the Graz experience. *Laryngoscope* 2000;108:873-882.

8. Sillers MJ, Cuilty-Siller C, Kuhn FA *et al.* Transconjunctival endoscopic orbital decompression. *Otolaryngology—Head & Neck Surgery* 2000;117:S137-S141

9. Ulualp SO, Massaro BM, Toohill RJ. Course of proptosis in patients with Graves' disease after endoscopic orbital decompression. *Laryngoscope* 2000;109:1217-1222.

10. Weetman AP, Wiersinga WM. Current management of thyroid-associated ophthalmopathy in Europe. Results of an international survey [see comments]. *Clinical Endocrinology* 2000;49:21-28.

11. West M, Stranc M. Long-term results of four-wall orbital decompression for Graves' ophthalmopathy. *British Journal of Plastic Surgery* 2000;50:507-516.

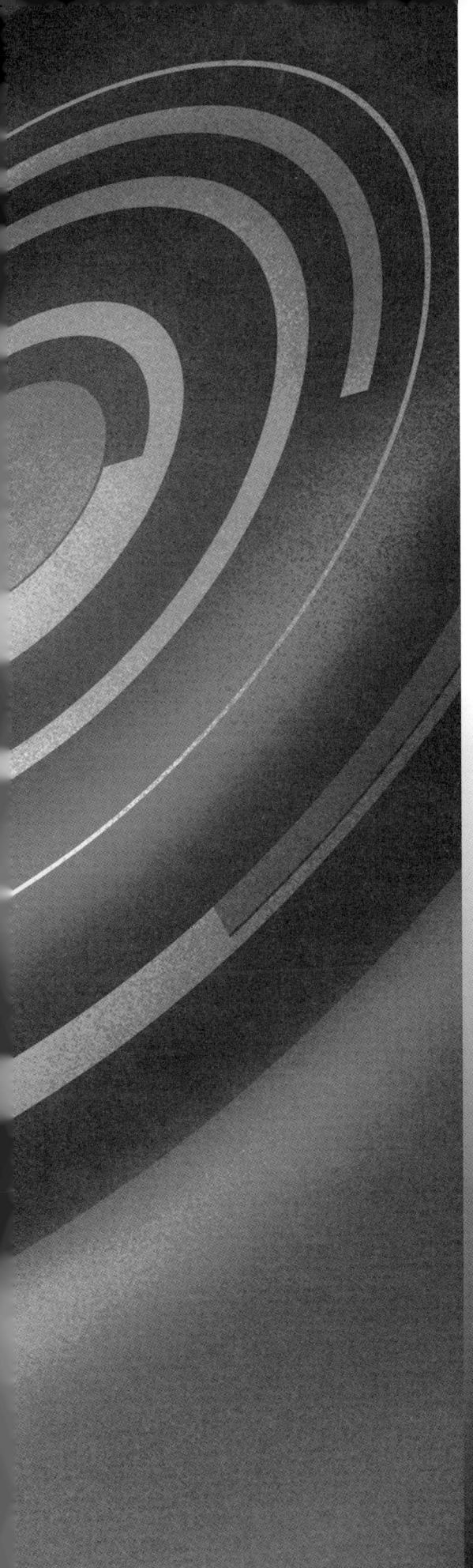

Disorders of the Oral Cavity and Oropharynx

COMMON BENIGN MUCOSAL LESIONS OF THE ORAL CAVITY

Vesicular or Ulcerative Lesions

Herpes simplex virus

- Primary infection most often presents as gingivostomatitis.
- Most frequently occurs in children between 1-3 years of age.
- Has 3-12 day incubation period.
- Initially presents with vesicles.
- Vesicle rupture results in yellowish, white superficial ulcer with red halo.
- Primary infection associated with fever, headache, gastrointestinal (GI) upset, enlarged nodes.
- Initial attack lasts 1-2 weeks.
- Histopathologic changes consist of ulcerative changes in mucosal surface and acute and chronic inflammatory infiltrates.
- Diagnosed by cultures or enzyme-linked immunoabsorbent assays (ELISA).
- Management is symptomatic, coupled with an antiherpetic agent (e.g., acyclovir [400 p.o. t.i.d]).

Recurrent aphthous stomatitis

- Commonly called "canker sore."
- Etiology unknown.
- Characterized by recurrent painful single or multiple necrotizing ulcers.
- Ulcerations of 5-30 days.
- Suspected predisposing factors: trauma, stress, hormonal changes.
- May be seen in systemic autoimmune diseases (e.g., Crohn's disease).
- Treatment: medical (e.g., amlexanox [Aphthasol] paste, anesthetic rinses, triamcinolone in Orabase paste, betamethasone diproprionate paste) or surgical (electrical or chemical cauterization).
- Thalidomide perhaps helpful in patients with human immunodeficiency virus (HIV)-related disease.

Syphilis

- Spirochete (Treponema pallidum)–mediated disease.
- Begins as solitary red, hard papule of up to several centimeters in diameter; superficially erodes to create shallow ulceration.
- Erodes to form a chancre with a red border and a dark red base; has 2-4–week incubation period.
- Detectable by silver impregnation, dark field microscopy, immunofluorescent techniques.
- Serologic test for syphilis (STS), inexpensive complement fixation test, unable to detect treponemal antigen, therefore many false positives produced.

- Florescent treponemal antigen (FTA): more specific and less false-positives.

Pemphigus vulgaris

- Characterized by systemic autoimmune disease of skin and mucosa.
- Average patient age = 55 years.
- Bullae within the oral cavity, which then rupture, leaving painful ulcers.
- Antibodies of patients directed against epithelium.
- Treated with systemic immunosuppressants

Benign mucous membrane pemphigoid (cicatricial pemphigoid)

- Bullae form, which then rupture and ulcerate.
- Average age is 66 years of age, female > male.
- May be autoimmune; immunoglobulin G (IgG) and C3 found in lesions.
- Ulcers may be asymptomatic.
- Lesions may also occur on conjunctiva.
- Treat with topical or systemic corticosteroids.

Hand, foot, and mouth disease

- Disease of children.
- Vesicular eruption on hands and feet and in oral cavity.
- Associated symptoms = fever, malaise, rhinitis, and diarrhea.
- Secondary to coxsackievirus infection (Group A).
- Symptomatic treatment.

Herpangina

- Disease of children.
- Papules and vesicles form on soft palate, tonsillar pillars, uvula.
- Vesicles rupture into ulcers.
- Associated symptoms include fever, headache, cervical lymphadenopathy.
- Caused by coxsackievirus or enteric cytopathic human orphan (ECHO) viruses.

Erythema multiforme

- Major form = Stevens-Johnson syndrome.
- Symptoms include bullae on the oral mucosa, pharynx, anogenital region, and conjunctiva; target-like lesions; and fever. Patient may have severe odynophagia impairing oral intake.
- Minor form is less likely to have oral involvement characterized by bullous lesions on skin, lips, and oral cavity. Fever may be present.
- Occurs in younger patients (10-30 years of age).
- Lesions of the skin and mucosa pass through the following stages:
1. Macular.
2. Bullous.
3. Sloughing.

4. Pseudomembranous.
5. Healing.

- Lesions appear to be provoked by a variety of exogenous exposures to infections (e.g., mycoplasma viruses) or by exposure to a variety of drugs (e.g., sulfonamides).
- Lesions are typically self-limited, resolving over 2-6 weeks.
- Supportive therapy may be required to allow patient to maintain oral intake.
- The use of systemic steroids is controversial because they may predispose some patients to fatal, secondary respiratory infections.

Reiter's syndrome

- Seronegative spondyloarthropathy.
- May be sexually transmitted; associated with infection by *Chlamydia trachomatis,* or associated with gastroenteritis, primarily caused by *Shigella, Salmonella, Yersinia,* or *Campylobacter,* as well as the *Chlamydia*-associated disease.
- The prevalence of the HLA-B27 tissue antigen 63%-96% in Reiter's syndrome.
- Clinical symptoms: arthritis, urethritis, cervicitis (in females), mucocutaneous vesicular/ulcerative lesions.
- Generally resolved over 3-4 months.
- In sexually transmitted form, treated with doxycycline.

Behcet's syndrome

- Inflammatory disease of unknown etiology.
- Associated with HLA-B51.
- Begins in third decade of life.
- Male > female.
- Characterized by painful ulcerative lesions of oral mucosa and genitalia.
- May involve central nervous system (CNS) (meningoencephalitis), eyes (uveitis), joints (arthritis).
- Treated with colchicine, systemic steroids, cyclosporine.

White Lesions

Candidiasis

- *Candida albicans.*
- Diagnosed clinically (lesions easily removed [pseudomembrane] and have erythematous base).
- Organism has nonbranching pseudohyphae.
- Stains used = Gram, periodic acid-Schiff (PAS), and silver.
- Treated with nystatin oral rinse, imidazole troches, oral fluconazole.

White sponge nevus

- Most frequently presents in childhood.
- Usually involves buccal mucosa.
- Autosomal dominant.
- Presents as large, raised, white corrugated patch.
- Pathology = increased thickness of epithelium with intracellular edema and nuclear pyknosis of stratum spinosum.
- No treatment necessary.

Nicotine stomatitis

- Seen in smokers.
- Whitened palate mucosa with multiple small papules evident; papules representative of inflamed obstructed orifices of the minor salivary glands.
- No treatment necessary.

Lichen planus

- Middle-age adults, female > male.
- Reticular = fine, interlacing striae on buccal mucosa; cannot be wiped off.
- Erosive = ulcerative lesion with surrounding keratosis on buccal mucosa, lateral tongue, gingiva.
- Pathology: hyperkeratosis, acanthosis, epithelial degeneration; T-cell infiltrate.
- Medication: reticular: no therapy; erosive: corticosteroids.
- May be associated with skin lesions: scaly, pruritic papules.

Leukoplakia

- White lesion.
- Cannot be scraped off.
- Male > female.
- 80% benign: hyperkeratosis, hyperparakeratosis, acanthosis.
- 20% premalignant or early malignant (e.g., dysplasia, carcinoma in situ [CIS]).
- More suspicious for malignancy when on lateral tongue, lower lip, floor of mouth.
- Treatment: removal of irritant, biopsy.

Hairy leukoplakia

- Shaggy, white lesion on tongue.
- Seen in patients affected with HIV.
- Not premalignant, no treatment necessary.

Red Lesions

Geographic tongue (benign migratory glossitis)

- Etiology unknown.
- Affects 1% of population.
- Waxing and waning of lesions.
- Central erythematous area of atrophic mucosa and absent papillae.
- Asymptomatic or mild tenderness.
- No treatment necessary.

Vascular lesions
- Isolated hemangiomas.
- Hemangiomas associated with Sturge-Weber syndrome (leptomeninges, skin, mucosa).
- Hereditary hemorrhagic telangiectasia (see epistaxis section).

Candidiasis
See similar section under white lesions.

Median rhomboid glossitis
- Central erythematous area of tongue with absent papillae.
- Etiology: embryologic defect (e.g., failure of lateral processes to grow medially) or *Candida* infection.
- Asymptomatic.
- Occasionally respond to antifungal agents.

Pernicious anemia
- Vitamin B_{12} deficiency may result in reddened, erythematous lesions on dorsal surface of tongue.

Erythroplakia
- Red patch on tongue.
- Premalignant or malignant change in up to 90%.

Burning tongue
- Female, postmenopausal.
- Rule out denture trauma, vitamin B_{12} deficiency, folate deficiency, diabetes mellitus, candidiasis, local trauma, psychological factors.
- May be idiopathic; treat with supportive care; hormone replacement therapy occasionally effective.

Other Lesions

Mucous retention cyst
- Results from rupture of minor salivary gland/duct with extravasation of mucous into surrounding tissues.
- Has epithelial lining (unlike mucocele).
- Presents as pale, nontender, cystic lesion filled with mucous.
- Treated with local excision.

Papilloma
- Most common benign lesion of oral cavity.
- Results from human papilloma virus infection.
- Found in palate > tongue > lips.
- Presents as exophytic, cauliflower-like, pink lesions.
- Histologic composition = fingerlike projections of a central vascular connective tissue core surrounded by stratified squamous epithelium.
- Treated with local cold knife or laser excision.

Selected References from the Recent Literature

1. Biron P, Sebban C, Gourmet R *et al*: Research controversies in management of oral mucositis. [Review] [19 refs]. *Supportive Care in Cancer* 2000;8:68-71.
2. Calabrese L, Fleischer AB: Thalidomide: current and potential clinical applications. [Review] [96 refs]. *American Journal of Medicine* 2000;108:487-495.
3. Eisen D, Essell J, Broun ER: Oral cavity complications of bone marrow transplantation. [Review] [47 refs]. *Seminars in Cutaneous Medicine & Surgery* 1997;16:265-272.
4. Epstein JB, Chow AW: Oral complications associated with immunosuppression and cancer therapies. [Review] [109 refs]. *Infectious Disease Clinics of North America* 1999;13:901-923.
5. Eversole LR: Immunopathogenesis of oral lichen planus and recurrent aphthous stomatitis. [Review] [134 refs]. *Seminars in Cutaneous Medicine & Surgery* 1997;16:284-294.
6. Feder HM, Jr.: Periodic fever, aphthous stomatitis, pharyngitis, adenitis: a clinical review of a new syndrome. [Review] [26 refs]. *Current Opinion in Pediatrics* 2000;12:253-256.
7. Ficarra G: Oral ulcers in HIV-infected patients: an update on epidemiology and diagnosis. [Review] [58 refs]. *Oral Diseases* 1997;3 Suppl 1:S183-S189
8. Karthaus M, Rosenthal C, Ganser A: Prophylaxis and treatment of chemo- and radiotherapy-induced oral mucositis—are there new strategies? [Review] [171 refs]. *Bone Marrow Transplantation* 1999;24:1095-1108.
9. MacPhail L: Topical and systemic therapy for recurrent aphthous stomatitis. [Review] [78 refs]. *Seminars in Cutaneous Medicine & Surgery* 1997;16:301-307.
10. MacPhail LA, Greenspan JS: Oral ulceration in HIV infection: investigation and pathogenesis. [Review] [39 refs]. *Oral Diseases* 1997;3 Suppl 1:S190-S193.
11. Meraw SJ, Mustapha IZ, Rogers RS: Cigarette smoking and oral lesions other than cancer. [Review] [52 refs]. *Clinics in Dermatology* 1998;16:625-631.
12. Peterson DE: Research advances in oral mucositis. [Review] [31 refs]. *Current Opinion in Oncology* 1999;11:261-266.
13. Popovsky JL, Camisa C: New and emerging therapies for diseases of the oral cavity. [Review] [86 refs]. *Dermatologic Clinics* 2000;18:113-125.
14. Porter SR, Scully C, Pedersen A: Recurrent aphthous stomatitis. [Review] [251 refs]. *Critical Reviews in Oral Biology & Medicine* 1998;9:306-321.
15. Reichart PA: Oral ulcerations in HIV infection. [Review] [30 refs]. *Oral Diseases* 1997;3 Suppl 1:S180-S182.
16. Reichart PA: Clinical management of selected oral fungal and viral infections during HIV-disease. [Review] [64 refs]. *International Dental Journal* 1999;49:251-259.
17. Rogers RS: Recurrent aphthous stomatitis: clinical characteristics and associated systemic disorders. [Review] [36 refs]. *Seminars in Cutaneous Medicine & Surgery* 1997;16:278-283.
18. Rosenthal C, Karthaus M, Ganser A: New strategies in the treatment and prophylaxis of chemo- and radiotherapy-induced oral mucositis. [Review] [159 refs]. *Antibiotics & Chemotherapy* 2000;50:115-132.
19. Roujeau JC: Treatment of severe drug eruptions. [Review] [33 refs]. *Journal of Dermatology* 1999;26:718-722.

20. Stanford TW, Rivera-Hidalgo F: Oral mucosal lesions caused by infective microorganisms. II. Fungi and parasites. [Review] [212 refs]. *Periodontology 2000* 1999;21: 125-144.

21. Stern RS: Improving the outcome of patients with toxic epidermal necrolysis and Stevens-Johnson syndrome [editorial; comment]. [Review] [16 refs]. *Archives of Dermatology* 2000;136:410-411.

22. Susser WS, Whitaker-Worth DL, Grant-Kels JM: Mucocutaneous reactions to chemotherapy [see comments]. [Review] [390 refs]. *Journal of the American Academy of Dermatology* 1999;40:367-398.

23. Trotti A: Toxicity in head and neck cancer: a review of trends and issues. [Review] [88 refs]. *International Journal of Radiation Oncology, Biology, Physics* 2000;47:1-12.

STOMATITIS AND PHARYNGITIS

Stomatitis

General considerations

- Inflammation of the oral mucosa, known as *stomatitis*, is usually symptomatic and is generally associated with mucosal erythema.
- Few cases present with pathognomonic physical signs, so a good history is the key to accurate diagnosis. Moreover, stomatitis and other oral lesions may be the presenting manifestations of serious systemic disease requiring comprehensive intervention.
- Treatment varies with etiology, but some basic principles are important:
  - Many cases will resolve with treatment of the underlying condition (e.g., nutritional deficiencies, ill-fitting dentures or prostheses).
  - Symptomatic treatment ensures both patient comfort and adequate nutritional intake. This may involve systemic analgesics, topical anesthetics, anti-inflammatory combinations (e.g., viscous lidocaine, various "magic mouthwashes"), and sialogogues.
  - The efficacy of topical medications in the oral cavity may be enhanced by combining them with specially designed delivery vehicles (e.g., Orabase, Zilactin-B).
  - Treatment is often more aggressive in immunocompromised patients.

Primary herpes simplex virus (HSV)

- Etiology: human herpesvirus type 1, occasionally type 2; spread by intimate contact.
- Presentation: more common in children, tends to be more severe in adults.
- Clinical symptoms: systemic illness (e.g., fever, headache, malaise, arthralgias, lymphadenopathy) and gingivitis featuring vesicles that rupture and ulcerate.
- Treatment: symptomatic.

Secondary HSV

- Etiology: After primary HSV infection, virus becomes latent, usually in trigeminal ganglia.
- Presentation: When reactivated (possibly by sunlight, stress, fatigue, etc.), a new ulcerating vesicular eruption appears, generally on the lips, hard palate, or fixed gingiva. Viral shedding occurs until the vesicles rupture.
- Treatment: Generally not necessary, but acyclovir is useful for prophylaxis.

Varicella

- Etiology: varicella zoster virus (VZV), spread by respiratory droplets.

- Presentation: incubates 2 weeks, causing systemic illness similar to HSV and a rash that progresses to a vesicular eruption, pustule formation, and crusting ulcers with an erythematous margin; in the oral cavity, lesions seen on the buccal mucosa, palate, pharynx.
- Treatment: symptomatic; vaccine now available.

Zoster

- Etiology: Like HSV, varicella leads to viral dormancy in cranial ganglia.
- Presentation: When reactivated, VZV leads to zoster (shingles), which manifests as a dermatomal rash, often associated with severe pain (postherpetic neuralgia) that may be worse and more protracted in the elderly.
- Treatment: Acyclovir, valacyclovir, or famciclovir decrease postherpetic neuralgia; topical capsaicin is effective.

Desquamative gingivitis

- This general term describes stomatitis with ulceration, diffuse erythematous desquamation, and, often, bulla formation. Severe forms of almost any stomatitis can become desquamative; these are the most common causes. Definitive diagnosis often requires biopsy.

Lichen planus

- Etiology: idiopathic lymphocytic destruction of basal cells; typically seen in women older than 40 years of age.
- Presentation: ulcerative buccal lesion with white interlacing Wickham's striae; can also cause atrophy, plaques, painful erosions; unclear if precancerous.
- Treatment: if asymptomatic, no treatment; if painful, topical or intralesional steroids; in severe cases, systemic agents (e.g., steroids, azathioprine, retinoids) useful.

Cicatricial pemphigoid (CP) and bullous pemphigoid (BP)

- Etiology: autoimmune destruction of the basement membrane that causes blisters, generally in elderly people. CP predominantly in females, BP in both sexes equally and milder than CP.
- Diagnosis: sometimes see Nikolsky's sign (rubbing of seemingly normal mucosa produces a vesicle or ulcer), but direct immunofluorescence required for definitive diagnosis.
- Treatment: topical steroids, occasionally systemic steroids or dapsone.

Pemphigus vulgaris
- Etiology: autoimmune destruction of intraepithelial components, causing blisters; more common in Ashkenazi Jews, but no sex predilection.
- Diagnosis: multiple painful blisters on buccal mucosa, hard palate, gingival; positive Nikolsky's sign; may be a sign of a visceral malignancy or a serious systemic autoimmune disease.
- Treatment: high-dose steroids, gold injections, plasmapheresis, cyclophosphamide.

Lupus erythematosus
- A generalized autoimmune disease, associated with multiorgan manifestations.

Discoid lupus (DLE)
- Etiology: usually women 20-40 years of age, rare visceral involvement; skin lesions in most, oral lesions in about 25%: erythematous plaques or erosions that lead to painful ulcers; sometimes characteristic white keratotic strands at edges of ulcers.
- Diagnosis: generally by history, in association with other DLE findings; positive direct immunofluorescence to basement membrane.
- Treatment: topical steroids, sunscreens.

Systemic lupus (SLE)
- Oral cavity involvement in 40% of patients; lesions similar to those in DLE.
- Diagnosis: positive antinuclear antibodies (ANA) test, positive direct immunofluorescence to basement membrane.
- Treatment: systemic treatment of disease, including salicylates, nonsteroidal antiinflammatory drugs (NSAIDs), steroids, cytotoxic agents

Erythema multiforme (EM)
- Possibly a hypersensitivity reaction, usually in young adults, causing explosive, symmetric erythematous lesions anywhere on the lips or oral mucosa; can be associated with severe pain, headache, and lymphadenopathy.
- Etiology: more than half of cases due to reactivated HSV-1, but can be caused by drugs, cancers, radiation or chemotherapy.
- Treatment: if mild, supportive care; in more severe cases, systemic steroids.
- Potential for EM to progress to Stevens-Johnson syndrome (high fever, malaise, ocular inflammation, and even blindness) and/or toxic epidermal necrolysis (generalized desquamation); usually the result of a drug reaction, the most common culprits being sulfonamides, barbiturates, phenytoin, allopurinol.

Candidiasis (fungal infection)
- Etiology: in immunocompetent patients, often due to poor oral hygiene or denture fitting problems.
- Diagnosis: presents as whitish plaques that can be scraped to reveal red, eroded mucosa; sometimes associated with angular chilitis; Gram stain or KOH stain often diagnostic, but rarely worthwhile.
- Treatment: topical (e.g., nystatin, clotrimazole) or systemic (e.g., ketoconazole); chlorhexidine rinses effective prophylactic agent.

Aphthous ulcers
- Etiology: idiopathic; seen in up to 25% of the population.
- Diagnosis: small (i.e., less than 1 cm) ulcers with a red border that last 7-10 days and leave no scar; occasionally larger and recurrent.
- Treatment: topical medications (e.g., triamcinolone in Orabase, Aphthasol); if large or frequent, occasional pulses of systemic steroids useful; thalidomide sometimes used in HIV-associated aphthous stomatitis.

Mucositis
- Etiology: local or systemic reaction to radiation therapy, chemotherapy, or bone marrow suppression.
- Diagnosis: diffuse erythema, pain, swelling, mucosal breakdown that can significantly interfere with adequate oral intake.
- Treatment: good oral hygiene, lip moisturization, topical anesthetics, systemic analgesics; of variety of prophylactic treatments proposed, none very effective in preventing mucositis.

Bacterial infections
- Etiology: usually odontogenic (strep, anaerobes).
- Diagnosis: erythema, pain, fever, lymphadenopathy.
- Treatment: penicillin, erythromycin, clindamycin, occasionally metronidazole.

Malnutrition
- Etiology: especially in alcoholics; usually B vitamins, but can also involve vitamin C, zinc, folic acid.
- Treatment: replacement of vitamins and minerals.

Special considerations in HIV/AIDS patients
- Most stomatitis presents and responds similarly in immunocompromised patients. Nonetheless, a few differences are worth noting:
  - Candidiasis: may require permanent prophylaxis.
  - Cryptococcus: ulcers, nodules, swellings on palate; treat with amphotericin B and then fluconazole.
  - Histoplasmosis: ulcers, nodules, vegetations; treat with amphotericin B or itraconazole.
  - HSV and VZV: can be more severe; treat with acyclovir or foscarnet.
  - Oral hairy leukoplakia: a white thickening, usually on the lateral tongue; associated with Epstein-Barr virus (EBV); generally asymptomatic.

- Kaposi's sarcoma: dark macules or nodules, diagnosed by biopsy and associated with a herpesvirus; treated with x-ray therapy (XRT), intralesional chemotherapy, or interferon or surgical excision.
- Gingivitis and periodontitis: more painful and persistent, wider spectrum of flora; can progress to necrotizing stomatitis with frank osteitis and fistulization, requiring aggressive surgery.
- Non-Hodgkin's lymphoma: often EBV-associated B-cell and aggressive; may present with masses in the oral cavity.

Pharyngitis

General considerations

- Any inflammation of the nasopharynx, oropharynx, or hypopharynx is known as *pharyngitis*. Infectious pharyngitis is extremely common and in most cases is diagnosed clinically and treated supportively.
- A variety of conditions can mimic simple self-limiting pharyngitis, and a thorough head and neck examination and selected pathologic studies may be required for appropriate management. Furthermore, it should be remembered that certain pharyngitides (e.g., epiglottitis) or similar conditions (e.g., the sore throat accompanying an expanding tumor) can herald airway obstruction, and they must be treated as aggressively as any other airway emergency.

Bacterial pharyngitis

- The normal flora of the pharynx consists mostly of gram-positive aerobes and various anaerobes, many of which can be implicated singly or multiply in pharyngitis.

Streptococcal

- Usually group A (beta-hemolytic), streptococcal, or "strep throat" as it is commonly known, presents with fever, sore throat, and odynophagia.
- On examination the pharynx is erythematous, and an exudate is often obvious.
- Cervical lymphadenopathy is common.
- Both rapid antigen and more accurate culture tests are available for diagnosis.
- Treatment of choice is penicillin.
- Streptococcal infections can lead to scarlet fever (which includes a generalized rash and strawberry tongue), rheumatic fever (with rheumatic heart disease many years later), and acute poststreptococcal glomerulonephritis.

Staphylococcus

- Clinically similar to strep throat (without the sequelae), staphylococcus infection is generally treated with a cephalosporin.

Diphtheria

- Although rare in developed countries due to vaccination, *Corynebacterium diphtheriae* infects the pharynx and produces an exotoxin that leads to the formation of grayish black necrotic pseudomembranes that can cause airway obstruction.
- The toxin can occasionally access the bloodstream, causing circulatory shock and requiring aggressive support and antitoxin administration.
- Treatment consists of penicillin or erythromycin.

Whooping cough

- Caused by *Bordetella pertussis*, whooping cough is also now rare in developed nations.
- The disease presents with upper respiratory infection symptoms and a low-grade fever and progresses to characteristic paroxysmal coughing fits; a mucopurulent exudate in the pharynx is seen.
- Treatment is supportive because the disease is unaffected by antibiotics when in the whooping stage.

Acute epiglottitis

- Although on the decrease due to vaccination against *Haemophilus influenzae*, epiglottitis is still seen occasionally in its typical 2-5 years-of-age group.
- After presenting with sore throat, fever, and dysphagia, symptoms can rapidly progress to airway obstruction.
- Treatment is with a second-generation cephalosporin.
- Protection of the airway is paramount. Children are typically intubated. Adult may be observed in a monitored unit.

Gonorrhea

- *Neisseria gonorrhoeae,* which is spread by sexual contact, can cause pharyngitis.
- Although generally asymptomatic, patients can experience sore throat, tonsillar hypertrophy, and cervical lymphadenopathy.
- Detection of the gram-negative diplococci is difficult, generally requiring special cultures that guide appropriate antibiotic therapy.

Other bacterial infections

- Many organisms can cause infectious pharyngitis, often in concert with their more typical manifestations.
- Examples include Salmonella, *Yersinia, Moraxella, Mycoplasma, Mycobacteria,* and *Rickettsial* organisms.

Syphilis

- *Treponema pallidum* infection can affect the head and neck in any of its three stages.

Primary stage

- Infected patients have a painless, ulcerated chancre, which can be anywhere on the site of entry, including the soft palate, tonsils, or tongue.
- The chancre is usually accompanied by localized, painless lymphadenopathy.
- Treatment for primary syphilis is penicillin.

Secondary stage

- Patients develop mucous patches, silvery painless erosion with raised red edges.
- Patients may complain of a sore throat at this time.

Tertiary stage

- Tertiary syphilis, which occurs years later, produces gummas, firm tumorlike masses all over the body, including the oropharynx.
- They can be mistaken for malignancies, and histologic diagnosis is essential.

Viral infections

- Viruses (including adenoviruses, parainfluenza, rhinoviruses, ECHO, and coxsackievirus) are the usual cause of mild, self-limiting pharyngitis.
- Patients often have mild pharyngeal erythema, cough, rhinorrhea, myalgias, headache, and fever.
- Although it is often hard to distinguish viral from bacterial pharyngitis, a normal white blood cell count and lack of exudate on examination favor a viral etiology.
- In immunocompromised patients a culture may be helpful to guide possible treatment, but in most patients a culture is unnecessary.
- Treatment is supportive.

Measles

- Infection with measles virus causes fever, conjunctivitis, coryza, rash, and typical spotty lesions on the buccal mucosa (Koplik's spots).
- Giant cell formation in lymphoid tissue causes tonsillar hypertrophy.
- Treatment is supportive.

Herpes

- Although it generally causes gingivostomatitis, HSV-1 can present with exudative pharyngitis.

Infectious mononucleosis

- Caused by EBV or, less commonly, cytomegalovirus, mononucleosis is a systemic infection that typically causes fever, malaise, membranous pharyngitis, lymphadenopathy, and hepatosplenomegaly in young adults.
- Diagnosis is by serologic testing, and care is supportive.

Fungal infections

- A variety of fungi, including cryptococcus, histoplasma, and rhinosporidia, can cause pharyngitis, but the most common fungus implicated is *Candida albicans*.
- Usually seen with oral cavity involvement, candidiasis presents with white, sometimes cheesy, plaques.
- Depending on whether or not other organs are involved, either local or systemic antifungal therapy is the treatment of choice.

Idiopathic pharyngitis

- Sore throat is a common complaint, and an obvious etiology is often not found.
- Some other causes of pharyngitis include:
  - Postnasal drip.
  - Gastroesophageal reflux.
  - Tobacco.
  - Alcohol.
  - Spicy, hot, scratchy foods.
  - Medications: mouthwashes.

Selected References from the Recent Literature

1. Gooch WM: Potential infectious disease complications of upper respiratory tract infections. [Review] [26 refs]. *Pediatric Infectious Disease Journal* 1998;17:S79-S82.
2. Olivier C: Rheumatic fever—is it still a problem?. [Review] [53 refs]. *Journal of Antimicrobial Chemotherapy* 2000;45 Suppl:13-21.
3. Rogers RS: Recurrent aphthous stomatitis: clinical characteristics and associated systemic disorders. [Review] [36 refs]. *Seminars in Cutaneous Medicine & Surgery* 1997;16:278-283.
4. Scaglione F, Demartini G, Arcidiacono MM et al: Optimum treatment of streptococcal pharyngitis. [Review] [106 refs]. *Drugs* 1997;53:86-97.
5. Smith SA: Respiratory failure as a complication of pharyngitis: Lemierre's syndrome. [Review] [15 refs]. *Pediatric Emergency Care* 1999;15:402-403.
6. Tsevat J, Kotagal UR: Management of sore throats in children: a cost-effectiveness analysis [see comments]. [Review] [73 refs]. *Archives of Pediatrics & Adolescent Medicine* 1999;153:681-688.
7. Williams A, Nagy M, Wingate J et al: Lemierre syndrome: a complication of acute pharyngitis. [Review] [5 refs]. *International Journal of Pediatric Otorhinolaryngology* 1998;45: 51-57.

SWALLOWING DISORDERS AND THEIR TREATMENT

Normal Deglutition

1. *Oral preparatory phase:* Food is masticated and mixed with saliva (need mobile tongue and competent palatoglossal sphincter to prevent premature bolus loss).
2. *Oral propulsive phase:* Palatoglossal sphincter opens, tongue base descends and uvula elevates, and tongue pumps bolus into oropharynx.
3. *Pharyngeal phase (takes less than 1 second):* Soft palate elevates, tongue thrusts, larynx elevated (to obstruct the airway) and descends, upper esophageal sphincter (UES) relaxes, and the bolus passes aided by pharyngeal constrictor peristalsis.
   - UES
     - Junction between hypopharynx and esophagus; closed at rest.
     - Opening related to cricopharyngeal relaxation and laryngeal elevation.
     - Length of 4-6 cm; contributions mainly from cricoid lamina, with contributions from the thyropharyngeus and cricopharyngeus.
4. *Esophageal phase:* Bolus is pushed through the esophagus by peristalsis.

Airway Protection

- Fully protected only in pharyngeal phase.
- Sequential order of closure (vocal cords, false vocal cords, contact of cuneiform cartilages against epiglottis, epiglottic retroversion).

Dysphagia

Etiology

- Stricture (e.g., cancer, Zenker's diverticulum, esophageal strictures).
- Function (e.g., neurologic disease, neuromuscular disease, gastroesophageal reflux disease [GERD], cricopharyngeal spasm, psychogenic, drugs, radiotherapy, after head and neck surgery).

Pathophysiology

- Inefficient transit (normally takes 2 seconds from mouth to esophagus) secondary to:
  - Lingual weakness, pharyngeal palsy, failure of laryngeal elevation.
  - Tumor, Zenker's diverticulum, UES obstruction.

Aspiration (Passage of Material Below the Level of the Vocal Cords)

1. Prandial aspiration (aspiration of food during swallowing)
   - Most of the time the cord closure is normal, but sequential timing of closure is abnormal (food is aspirated either before or after glottic closure).
   - Use modified Barium swallow or swallowing nasopharyngolaryngoscopy (e.g., endoscopic evaluation of swallowing [EES]) to diagnose.
   - Successful treatment includes cessation of feeding and/or swallowing therapy.
   - Aspiration **before pharyngeal phase** is most commonly neurologic in nature and responds to thickened diets, neck flexion during swallowing, and other conservative measures. Surgical management includes horizontal epiglottoplasty, tongue base flaps, and laryngeal suspension.
   - Aspiration **during the pharyngeal phase** is the least common, usually due to vocal paresis, palsy, or incoordination, and responds to vocal cord adduction exercises. Surgical management includes vocal cord augmentation.
   - Aspiration **after the pharyngeal phase** is usually due to inhalation of uncleared residue at the laryngeal inlet and responds to thinning of the diet, alternating of liquids, and other physical techniques. Surgical management includes translaryngeal resection of the cricoid lamina, cricopharyngeal myotomy, and laryngeal elevation.
2. Salivary aspiration
   - Small amounts may occur in normal sleep.
3. Reflux aspiration
   - Tissue is destroyed by acid.

Gastroesophageal Reflux Disease (Laryngopharyngeal Reflux)

- Symptoms include heartburn and acid regurgitation, chronic sore throat, globus sensation, chronic cough, throat clearing, otalgia, and hoarseness.
- Small amount of reflux is normal after meals; however, pathologic reflux occurs after meals and when lying in bed. Low pH causes inflammation, which leads to the complications of reflux.

Clinical Assessment of Swallowing Function

History

- Diet, feeding method, duration of meals.
- Recent weight loss.

- Coughing during feeding.
- Symptoms of reflux.
- Throat clearing and chronic cough.
- History of neurologic disorder.
- History of medical illness that may impair swallowing.
- History of surgery that may disrupt upper airway or swallowing reflexes (e.g., cancer of the upper airway, thoracotomy, thyroid surgery).
- Previous pneumonia.
- Medications (antihistamines and antidepressants cause dryness; antipsychotics can impair movement), smoking, alcohol.

Examination

- Examine structure and function (cranial nerve exam, vocal cord mobility, evidence of reflux, glottic closure).
- Patients may have aspiration in the face of normal examination due to impairment of coordination and timing of swallowing.

Swallowing nasolaryngoscopy

- Directly observe foods of different consistency (e.g., solid, paste, and liquid) for aspiration into in the airway or in the subglottis.
- In a normal person the view will be obscured by normal pharyngeal closure during the pharyngeal phase.
- This technique can be used with patients as a visual feedback mechanism in a rehabilitation setting.

Modified barium swallow (MBS)

- First, look at the lateral view for aspiration (barium below the vocal cords) with small volumes, then increase volume and try different consistencies.
- Penetration: assess for leakage into the larynx into the level of the vocal folds.
- Aspiration: document relation to pharyngeal phase and severity. Assess for silent aspiration and ability to deal with different food consistencies
- Swallowing efficiency: measure time taken to swallow the bolus.

Manometry

- Used in the evaluation of esophageal motility.
- Must be assessed in conjunction with MBS.
- Most common diagnoses: motor disorders secondary to GERD and primary neurogenic disorders secondary to diabetes mellitus, aging, alcohol, amyotrophic lateral sclerosis, multiple sclerosis, Parkinson's disease.
- More rare diagnoses: chalasia, Nutcracker esophagus, diffuse esophageal spasm.

24-hour pH monitoring

- Gold standard for evaluation of GERD.
- Used in patients who do not have signs of reflux based on results from other testing modalities.

Treatment of Dysphagia

1. Evaluate for the safety of oral feeding and severity of aspiration. Silent aspiration is present in 40% of those with dysphagia.
2. Assess the adequacy of oral intake.
3. Institute nonoral feeding (e.g., nasogastric tube [NGT] or feeding gastrostomy) if oral feeding is unsafe.
- Risks of NGT feeding include GERD, pharyngeal swallowing impairment, tracheal misplacement, aspiration pneumonia, and laryngeal edema.
4. Institute conservative swallowing therapy (e.g., change in diet or posture).
5. Efficacy can be assessed by MBS or endoscopic evaluation of swallowing.
6. Patients who do not respond to conservative management are candidates for conservative surgery or gastrostomy/jejunostomy.

Treatment of GERD

Initial therapy

- Proton pump inhibitors, H_2 blockers, agents that increase esophageal motility (e.g., metoclopramide).
- Weight loss.
- Avoidance of smoking.
- Reverse Trendelenburg position of bed at night.
- Small meals before bed but avoid coffee, chocolate, tea, alcohol, fatty and spicy foods.

Failure of maximal medical management

- Fundoplication.

Treatment of Salivary Aspiration

1. Reduce salivary production (atropine, hyoscine).
2. Attempt to suction through a mini-tracheostomy.
3. Cease oral feeding.
4. Evaluate mechanism of salivary aspiration and treat appropriately (cricopharyngeal myotomy, translaryngeal cricoid resection, or laryngeal elevation).

Surgery

Alternate nutrition

- Gastrostomy.
- Jejunostomy.
- Cervical esophagostomy.

Conservative surgery (preserve speech and swallowing function)

- Cricopharyngeal myotomy: obstruction due to cricopharyngeal bar (5%-15% of population), leading to residue in the pharynx.
- Vocal augmentation: pharyngeal phase only time vocal cords close.
- Horizontal epiglottoplasty: keeps the epiglottis in the horizontal position.
- Translaryngeal cricoid resection: opens UES to prevent residue buildup.
- Laryngeal suspension.

Radical surgery (disconnect swallowing passages from the airway, does not preserve glottic function)

- Tracheostomy (for pulmonary toilet): ideal for short-term therapy in acute illness; can impair swallowing; patients aphonic; scarring can hurt long-term recovery
- Laryngeal stent: short-term for those with tracheostomy; used to cork airway off above trachea.
- Laryngeal diversion: airway disconnected from the upper trachea, bringing lower trachea out through skin as a permanent stoma and diverting upper trachea into the esophagus.
- Laryngeal closure: closes airway at glottic or supraglottic levels (sometimes using an epiglottic flap, all of which requires a permanent tracheostomy).
- Laryngectomy: irreversible (used in end-stage disease or progressive illness in patient who is aphonic).

Selected References from the Recent Literature

1. Cook IJ: Diagnosis and management of cricopharyngeal achalasia and other upper esophageal sphincter opening disorders. [Review] [33 refs]. *Current Gastroenterology Reports* 2000;2:191-195.
2. Davies S: Dysphagia in acute strokes [see comments]. [Review] [20 refs]. *Nursing Standard* 1999;13:49-54.
3. Spechler SJ: AGA technical review on treatment of patients with dysphagia caused by benign disorders of the distal esophagus [see comments]. [Review] [210 refs]. *Gastroenterology* 1999;117:233-254.
4. Brais B, Rouleau GA, Bouchard JP et al: Oculopharyngeal muscular dystrophy. [Review] [84 refs]. *Seminars in Neurology* 1999;19:59-66.
5. Kelly JH: Management of upper esophageal sphincter disorders: indications and complications of myotomy. [Review] [24 refs]. *American Journal of Medicine* 2000;108 Suppl 4a:43S-46S.
6. Walker SJ, Byrne JP, Birbeck N: What's new in the pathology, pathophysiology and management of benign esophageal disorders? [Review] [500 refs]. *Diseases of the Esophagus* 1999;12:219-237.

7. Mason RJ, Bremner CG: Myotomy for pharyngeal swallowing disorders. [Review] [145 refs]. *Advances in Surgery* 1999;33:375-411.
8. Gleeson DC: Oropharyngeal swallowing and aging: a review. [Review] [98 refs]. *Journal of Communication Disorders* 1999;32:373-395.
9. Miller RM, Chang MW: Advances in the management of dysphagia caused by stroke. [Review] [78 refs]. *Physical Medicine & Rehabilitation Clinics of North America* 1999;10:925-941.
10. Langmore SE: Issues in the management of dysphagia. [Review] [35 refs]. *Folia Phoniatrica et Logopedica* 1999;51:220-230.
11. Shin T, Tsuda K, Takagi S: Surgical treatment for dysphagia of neuromuscular origin. [Review] [16 refs]. *Folia Phoniatrica et Logopedica* 1999;51:213-219.
12. Logemann JA: Behavioral management for oropharyngeal dysphagia. [Review] [56 refs]. *Folia Phoniatrica et Logopedica* 1999;51:199-212.
13. Schroter-Morasch H, Bartolome G, Troppmann N et al: Values and limitations of pharyngolaryngoscopy (transnasal, transoral) in patients with dysphagia. [Review] [43 refs]. *Folia Phoniatrica et Logopedica* 1999;51:172-182.
14. Fujiu-Kurachi M: Food measures and other critical diagnostic measures. [Review] [66 refs]. *Folia Phoniatrica et Logopedica* 1999;51:147-157.
15. Broniatowski M, Sonies BC, Rubin JS et al: Current evaluation and treatment of patients with swallowing disorders. [Review] [35 refs]. *Otolaryngology—Head & Neck Surgery* 1999;120:464-473.
16. Domenech E, Kelly J: Swallowing disorders. [Review] [90 refs]. *Medical Clinics of North America* 1999;83:97-113.
17. Cook IJ, Kahrilas PJ: AGA technical review on management of oropharyngeal dysphagia. [Review] [197 refs]. *Gastroenterology* 1999;116:455-478.
18. McHorney CA, Rosenbek JC: Functional outcome assessment of adults with oropharyngeal dysphagia. [Review] [69 refs]. *Seminars in Speech & Language* 1998; 19:235-246.
19. DiMarino AJJ, Allen ML, Lynn RB et al: Clinical value of esophageal motility testing [see comments]. [Review] [128 refs]. *Digestive Diseases* 1998;16:198-204.
20. Schechter GL: Systemic causes of dysphagia in adults. [Review] [43 refs]. *Otolaryngologic Clinics of North America* 1998;31:525-535.
21. Derkay CS, Schechter GL: Anatomy and physiology of pediatric swallowing disorders. [Review] [14 refs]. *Otolaryngologic Clinics of North America* 1998;31:397-404.
22. Kosko JR, Moser JD, Erhart N et al: Differential diagnosis of dysphagia in children. [Review] [43 refs]. *Otolaryngologic Clinics of North America* 1998;31:435-451.
23. Arvedson JC: Management of pediatric dysphagia. [Review] [75 refs]. *Otolaryngologic Clinics of North America* 1998;31:453-476.
24. Plant RL: Anatomy and physiology of swallowing in adults and geriatrics. [Review] [24 refs]. *Otolaryngologic Clinics of North America* 1998;31:477-488.
25. Bastian RW: Contemporary diagnosis of the dysphagic patient. [Review] [27 refs]. *Otolaryngologic Clinics of North America* 1998;31:489-506.

26. Dray TG, Hillel AD, Miller RM: Dysphagia caused by neurologic deficits. [Review] [60 refs]. *Otolaryngologic Clinics of North America* 1998;31:507-524.

27. Wisdom G, Blitzer A: Surgical therapy for swallowing disorders. [Review] [83 refs]. *Otolaryngologic Clinics of North America* 1998;31:537-560.

28. Poertner LC, Coleman RF: Swallowing therapy in adults. [Review] [31 refs]. *Otolaryngologic Clinics of North America* 1998;31:561-579.

29. Klinkenberg-Knol EC: Otolaryngologic manifestations of gastro-oesophageal reflux disease. [Review] [45 refs]. *Scandinavian Journal of Gastroenterology–Supplement* 1998;225: 24-28.

ODONTOGENIC CYSTS AND TUMORS

Odontogenic Cysts

Arise from enamel organ or follicle (follicular cysts): potential of becoming ameloblastomas
Primordial cyst

- Arises from tooth germ and forms a cyst (associated with missing tooth); mandible > maxilla.
- Usually arises in second to third decade of life.
- Painless; may cause migration of erupted teeth or enlargement of jawbone.
- Treatment: local excision and curettage.

Dentigerous cyst

- Most common of all follicular cysts.
- Male > female.
- Arise in the second to third decade of life.
- Mandible > maxilla; mostly in molar area.
- Arises in the from enamel organ after partial completion of crown.
- Children: eruption cysts (often rupture on eruption of tooth into oral cavity) rarely malignant transformation to squamous cell carcinoma.

Multilocular cyst (<1% of all follicular cysts)

- Not associated with developed teeth; found often in mandibular molar area.
- Lined with stratified squamous epithelium.
- Associated with basal cell nevus syndrome.
  - Multilocular cysts.
  - Multiple basal cell carcinoma.
  - Sebaceous cysts of skin.
  - Skeletal deformities (frontal bossing, splayed ribs, fusion of vertebrae).

Arise from epithelial rests of Malassez
Radicular cyst

- Secondary to inflammation; proliferation of epithelial rests.
- Asymptomatic with no gross deformity, occasionally sensitive to percussion.
- Rare association with fistula.
- Maxilla > mandible, associated tooth is nonvital.
- Treatment: extraction of tooth, root canal filling, curettage.

Residual cyst

- Cyst remaining after tooth associated with a radicular cyst has been extracted.
- Treatment: surgical enucleation.

Arise from enamel organ or rests of malassez
Odontogenic keratocyst

- Rare keratin-producing cysts found in basal cell nevus syndrome.
- Mandible > maxilla.

Calcifying odontogenic cyst

- Patients often less than 40 years of age.
- Benign, often cystic.
- Treatment: local conservative removal.

Odontogenic Tumors

Epithelial tumors

- Ameloblastoma tumor:
  - Most aggressive of odontogenic tumors of the jaw, but slow growing.
  - Arises from dental lamina or derivative (e.g., enamel organ, epithelial rests, follicular cysts).
  - Occurrence at 20-50 years of age, mean 39 years of age.
  - 80% mandible, 20% maxilla; 80% molar.
  - Painless; may appear enlarged with displacement/malocclusion of regional teeth.
  - Treatment: surgical resection with mandibular reconstruction.
  - May be aspirated during surgery, giving rise to a secondary pulmonary focus.
  - Recurrence common due to incomplete removal.
  - Rarely becomes malignant with metastasis to regional nodes or lungs.
- Acanthomatous ameloblastoma tumor.
- Odontogenic adenomatoid tumor (adenoameloblastoma).
- Neuroectodermal tumor of infancy (melanoameloblastoma).

Mesenchymal tumors

- Cementoma:
  - 70% in African-Americans, 10× female > male.
  - Periapical lesion found most often in mandible incisors.
  - Extremely slow, limited growth; asymptomatic.
  - Requires no treatment.
- Benign cementoblastoma (true cementoma) tumor.
- Cementifying fibroma tumor.
- Odontogenic myxoma tumor.
- Odontogenic fibroma tumor.
  - Most common tumor of jaw (limited, slow growth).
  - Mandible > maxilla; second decade of life.
  - Asymptomatic or slight enlargement of jaw with impacted tooth.
  - Often misdiagnosed: radiographic appearance of dentigerous cyst.

- ◻ Solid, not cystic.
  - ◻ Treatment: curettage.
- Dentinoma tumor.

Mixed tumors (epithelial and mesenchymal)
- Ameloblastic fibroma tumor.
- Granular cell ameloblastic fibroma tumor.
- Ameloblastic fibroodontoma tumor.
- Ameloblastic odontoma (odontoameloblastoma) tumor.
- Odontoma (compound, complex, cystic) tumor:
  - ◻ Compound; maxilla > mandible; second decade of life
  - ◻ Complex; posterior upper/lower jaw; male > female.
  - ◻ Slow growing; often asymptomatic or presents with impacted teeth.
  - ◻ Rare deformity of normal jaw contour.
  - ◻ Treatment: local removal (easily enucleated, will not recur).

Rare odontogenic tumors
- Granular cell ameloblastoma tumor.
- Calcifying epithelial odontogenic tumor.
- Ameloblastic fibrosarcoma tumor.
- Squamous odontogenic tumor.
- Extraosseous odontogenic tumor.

Selected References from the Recent Literature

1. Bataineh AB: Effect of preservation of the inferior and posterior borders on recurrence of ameloblastomas of the mandible. [Review] [54 refs]. *Oral Surgery, Oral Medicine, Oral Pathology, Oral Radiology, & Endodontics* 2000;90: 155-163.
2. Chow HT, Teh LY: Sensory impairment after resection of the mandible: a case report of 10 cases. *Journal of Oral & Maxillofacial Surgery* 2000;58:629-635.
3. Eversole LR: Malignant epithelial odontogenic tumors. [Review] [79 refs]. *Seminars in Diagnostic Pathology* 1999;16:317-324.
4. Hao SP, Chen HC, Chang YM *et al:* A combined approach to benign but advanced mandibular tumor. *Auris, Nasus, Larynx* 1998;25:285-288.
5. Li KK, Fabian RL, Goodman ML: Malignant fibrous histiocytoma after radiation for ameloblastoma of the maxilla. [Review] [19 refs]. *Journal of Oral & Maxillofacial Surgery* 1997;55:85-88.
6. Li TJ, Wu YT, Yu SF *et al:* Unicystic ameloblastoma: a clinicopathologic study of 33 Chinese patients. *American Journal of Surgical Pathology* 2000;24:1385-1392.
7. Manor Y, Merdinger O, Katz J *et al:* Unusual peripheral odontogenic tumors in the differential diagnosis of gingival swellings. [Review] [28 refs]. *Journal of Clinical Periodontology* 1999;26:806-809.
8. Mathew S, Rappaport K, Ali SZ *et al:* Ameloblastoma. Cytologic findings and literature review. [Review] [15 refs]. *Acta Cytologica* 1997;41:955-960.
9. Melrose RJ: Benign epithelial odontogenic tumors. [Review] [36 refs]. *Seminars in Diagnostic Pathology* 1999;16:271-287.
10. Oji C: Late presentation of orofacial tumours. *Journal of Cranio-Maxillo-Facial Surgery* 1999;27:94-99.
11. Okada H, Davies JE, Yamamoto H: Malignant ameloblastoma: a case study and review. *Journal of Oral & Maxillofacial Surgery* 1999;57:725-730.
12. Olaitan AA, Adekeye EO: Unicystic ameloblastoma of the mandible: a long-term follow-up. *Journal of Oral & Maxillofacial Surgery* 1997;55:345-348.
13. Olaitan AA, Arole G, Adekeye EO: Recurrent ameloblastoma of the jaws. A follow-up study. *International Journal of Oral & Maxillofacial Surgery* 1998;27:456-460.
14. Orringer JS, Shaw WW, Borud LJ *et al:* Total mandibular and lower lip reconstruction with a prefabricated osteocutaneous free flap. *Plastic & Reconstructive Surgery* 1999;104:793-797.
15. Sampson DE, Pogrel MA: Management of mandibular ameloblastoma: the clinical basis for a treatment algorithm. *Journal of Oral & Maxillofacial Surgery* 1999;57:1074-1077.
16. Sand L, Jalouli J, Larsson PA *et al:* Presence of human papilloma viruses in intraosseous ameloblastoma. *Journal of Oral & Maxillofacial Surgery* 2000;58:1129-1134.
17. Schafer DR, Thompson LD, Smith BC *et al:* Primary ameloblastoma of the sinonasal tract: a clinicopathologic study of 24 cases. *Cancer* 1998;82:667-674.
18. Schmidt R, Moses RL, Loggi D *et al:* Unusual otolaryngic presentations of ameloblastoma. *Otolaryngology—Head & Neck Surgery* 1999;121:285-289.
19. Tomich CE: Benign mixed odontogenic tumors. [Review] [14 refs]. *Seminars in Diagnostic Pathology* 1999;16:308-316.
20. Yamamoto H, Inui M, Mori A *et al:* Clear cell odontogenic carcinoma: a case report and literature review of odontogenic tumors with clear cells. [Review] [19 refs]. *Oral Surgery, Oral Medicine, Oral Pathology, Oral Radiology, & Endodontics* 1998; 86:86-89.

SALIVARY GLAND INFECTIONS

Acute Suppurative Sialadenitis

- Infection of salivary gland parenchyma caused by retrograde bacterial migration from oral cavity.
- Parotid gland most frequently involved.
- Secondary to reduction of salivary flow resulting from dehydration, anticholinergics, diuretics.
- Poor oral hygiene.
- May also occur secondary to stone formation, particularly in submandibular gland.

Microbiology
- Elderly or debilitated: penicillin-resistant *Staphylococcus aureus*.
- Community acquired: *Staphylococcus pyogens, Streptococcus viridans, Streptococcus pneumoniae, Haemobartonella influenza*.

Clinical symptoms
- Local: rapid onset of pain, swelling, induration of involved gland.
- Systemic: fever, chills, malaise, leukocytosis with neutrophilia.

Treatment
- Parenteral antibiotics β-lactamase–resistant penicillin or cephalosporin.
- Fluid and electrolyte replacement.
- Oral hygiene, sialogogues, analgesics, local heat application.
- External or bimanual massage.
- Intraoral stone extraction.
- If conservative measures fail, surgical drainage or excision of gland.

Recurrent Suppurative Parotitis of Childhood

- Infrequently occurs in otherwise healthy children.
- Males > females.

Microbiology
- *Str. viridans*.

Clinical symptoms
- Recurrent episodes of glandular swelling, generalized malaise, pain frequently following meals.

Treatment
- Antibiotics administered.
- Most symptoms abate with adolescence.

Chronic Sialadenitis

- Predisposing factors: ductal stricture, ductal dilation, intraductal calculus, mucous plug, depressed glandular secretion, immunodeficiency, autoimmune disorder.
- Parotid gland most commonly affected; submandibular gland also commonly affected.
- Asymptomatic intervals range from weeks to several months.

Microbiology
- *S. aureus*.

Clinical symptoms
- Recurring painful episodes of swelling with thickening and diminution of saliva.

Treatment
- Antibiotics.
- Correction of anatomically predisposing factors.
- Disruption of neuronal innervation of gland, salivary duct ligation, salivary gland excision.

Viral Infections

Microbiology
- Mumps: paramyxovirus.
- Primarily in children.

Clinical symptoms
- Bilateral parotid gland swelling; rarely submandibular gland swelling.
- Pain exacerbated by eating.
- Low-grade fever, arthralgia, malaise, headache.

Treatment
- Hydration and rest.
- Dietary modifications to minimize glandular secretory activity.

HIV-Associated Salivary Gland Disease (HIV-SGD)

- Described among HIV-seropositive and high-risk HIV-seronegative patients.
- Parotid gland most frequently affected.

Clinical symptoms
- Gradual nontender enlargement of one or more salivary glands with xerostomia, dry eyes, arthralgia.

Pathology
- Multiple cysts of parotid gland; can be diagnosed on ultrasound, computed tomography (CT) scan or magnetic resonance imaging (MRI).

Treatment

- Reassurance.
- Cyst aspiration and injection of doxycycline to sclerose cysts.
- Parotidectomy (rarely indicated).

Granulomatous Salivary Gland Infections

Mycobaterial disease

- Enlargement (mimicking slow-growing neoplasm).
- *Mycobacterium tuberculosis.*
  - Most common in parotid.
  - Constitutional signs: fever, night sweats, weight loss; facial nerve involvement rare.
  - Diagnosis: biopsy and culture.
  - Treatment: antituberculosis therapy.

Nontuberculous mycobacterium

- Most common in children 16-36 months of age.
- *Mycobacterium kansasii, Mycobacterium scrofulaceum,* and *Mycobacterium avium-intracellulare.*
- Involvement most often of periparotid and submandibular lymph nodes.
- Sinus tracts sometimes form and drain to skin.
- Diagnosis: biopsy and culture.
- Treatment: response of these infections to antituberculosis medications generally not good; local surgical control of draining fistulas, skin, and soft tissue necrosis sometimes necessary; treatment of lesions often unnecessary.

SALIVARY GLAND TRAUMA

Etiology

- Nearly all injuries to the salivary glands are caused by penetrating trauma (e.g., stab wounds and gunshot wounds).
- Blunt trauma can occasionally result in contusions, edema, or hemorrhage.

Clinical manifestations

- Location of wound consistent with salivary gland trauma.
- With parotid, may often see duct in the wound.
- Pooling of secretions in wound.
- Pass probe through duct to assess whether is intact.

Management

- Possible to manage lacerations to the parenchyma conservatively: close parenchyma and capsule with interrupted sutures.
- Explore wound posterior to anterior border of the masseter muscle for likely ductal injury.
- Close ducts with end-to-end anastomosis over a catheter; catheter left in place for at least 2 weeks.
- Excise gland when repair is not possible.

Complications

- Treatment of salivary cutaneous fistula: repeated aspirations and pressure dressing.
- Duct obstruction possible if persistence of fistula past 2 weeks.
- Contusions.
- Edema.
- Hemorrhage.
- Facial nerve paralysis: seen in parotid gland trauma:
  - Facial nerve exploration is indicated in cases of complete paralysis.
  - Lacerated nerve branches are repaired by either anastomosis or interposition graft.
  - Isolated marginal branch injury in submandibular trauma should not be explored.

Selected References from the Recent Literature

1. Bova R, Walker P: Neonatal submandibular sialadenitis progressing to submandibular gland abscess. *International Journal of Pediatric Otorhinolaryngology* 2000;53:73-75.
2. Smith AD, Elahi MM, Kawamoto HKJ *et al*: Excision of the submandibular gland by an intraoral approach. *Plastic & Reconstructive Surgery* 2000;105:2092-2095.
3. Fowler CB, Brannon RB: Subacute necrotizing sialadenitis: report of 7 cases and a review of the literature. [Review] [7 refs]. *Oral Surgery, Oral Medicine, Oral Pathology, Oral Radiology, & Endodontics* 2000;89:600-609.
4. Hogg RP, Ayshford C, Watkinson JC: Parotid duct carcinoma arising in bilateral chronic sialadenitis. [Review] [4 refs]. *Journal of Laryngology & Otology* 1999;113:686-688.
5. Sumi M, Izumi M, Yonetsu K et al: The MR imaging assessment of submandibular gland sialoadenitis secondary to sialolithiasis: correlation with CT and histopathologic findings. *American Journal of Neuroradiology* 1999;20:1737-1743.
6. Rice DH: Noninflammatory, non-neoplastic disorders of the salivary glands. [Review] [6 refs]. *Otolaryngologic Clinics of North America* 1999;32:835-843.
7. McQuone SJ: Acute viral and bacterial infections of the salivary glands. [Review] [65 refs]. *Otolaryngologic Clinics of North America* 1999;32:793-811.
8. Bodner L: Parotid sialolithiasis. [Review] [15 refs]. *Journal of Laryngology & Otology* 1999;113:266-267.
9. Haga HJ, Hulten B, Bolstad AI *et al*: Reliability and sensitivity of diagnostic tests for primary Sjogren's syndrome. *Journal of Rheumatology* 1999;26:604-608.
10. Harris NL: Lymphoid proliferations of the salivary glands. *American Journal of Clinical Pathology* 1999;111:S94-103.
11. Goh YH, Sethi DS: Submandibular gland excision: a five-year review. *Journal of Laryngology & Otology* 1998;112:269-273.
12. Harrison JD, Epivatianos A, Bhatia SN: Role of microliths in the aetiology of chronic submandibular sialadenitis: a clinicopathological investigation of 154 cases. *Histopathology* 1997;31:237-251.

13. Seifert G: Aetiological and histological classification of sialadenitis [editorial]. [Review] [113 refs]. *Pathologica* 1997;89:7-17.

14. Kim RH, Strimling AM, Grosch T et al: Nonoperative removal of sialoliths and sialodochoplasty of salivary duct strictures. *Archives of Otolaryngology—Head & Neck Surgery* 1996;122:974-976.

15. Ottaviani F, Capaccio P, Campi M *et al:* Extracorporeal electromagnetic shock-wave lithotripsy for salivary gland stones. *Laryngoscope* 1996;106:761-764.

16. Bodner L, Fliss DM: Parotid and submandibular calculi in children. *International Journal of Pediatric Otorhinolaryngology* 1995;31:35-42.

SLEEP APNEA

Definitions

- Apnea: cessation of airflow for longer than 10 seconds; complete airway closure.
- Hypopnea: 50% decrease in airflow or >4% reduction in oxygen saturation or an electroencephalogram (EEG) arousal due to partial airway closure.
- Upper airway resistance syndrome (UARS): increased ventilatory effort, crescendo snoring, arousal and sleep fragmentation without apneas, hypopneas, or oxygen desaturation; will have excessive daytime sleepiness.
- Obstructive breathing disorders on a continuum:
  - Snoring with sleep disturbance.
  - UARS.
  - OSAS (obstructive sleep apnea syndrome).
- Apnea index (AI): number of apnea events per hour of sleep; historically <5 events per hour normal, usually AI >20 for clinically symptomatic patients.
- Respiratory distress index (RDI): more valid measure to define presence of sleep apnea; number of apneas and hypopneas per minute:
  - <5 = normal.
  - <20 = mild apnea.
  - 20-40 = moderate apnea.
  - >40 = severe apnea.
- Obstructive sleep apnea: most common, resulting in obstruction of the upper airway with ventilatory effort.
- Central sleep apnea: due to absent ventilatory effort (rare).
- Mixed sleep apnea: initial central apnea followed by obstructive apnea and arousal; improvement with treatment of obstruction and considered obstructive sleep apnea syndrome (OSAS).

Incidence and etiology

- Between 4% and 9% of males and 2%-4% of females older than 30 years of age.
- Male:female = 2:1.
- Habitual snorers have 34%-60% incidence of OSA.
- Obese patients most commonly affected; obesity (>120% of ideal body weight) major risk factor.
- Associated conditions include hypothyroidism, acromegaly, Down syndrome, Treacher Collin's-Franceschetti syndrome, achondroplasia.
- Alcohol, sedatives, hypnotics.

Pathophysiology

- Upper airway obstruction occurs at one or more levels of the pharynx.
- Collapsing forces of the airway (e.g., structural characteristics promoting collapse, negative inspiratory forces) are greater than the dilating forces (e.g., structural characteristics promoting patency, neuromuscular tone).
- Dilating muscles of pharynx include genioglossus, geniohyoid, medial pterygoid, tensor veli palatini, and sternohyoid. There is a sleep-related loss of neuromuscular tone of the pharynx.
- Structural abnormalities predisposing to obstruction include:
  - Thick, long soft palate.
  - Large uvula.
  - Redundant pharyngeal mucosal folds.
  - Prominent lingual tonsils.
  - Macroglossia.
  - Low hyoid bone.
  - Nasal obstruction.
  - Retrusive mandible.
  - Increased neck girth.
- Collapse may be at multiple sites.
  - Nineteen percent of OSAS patients have only palate collapse.
  - Between 50% and 80% of patients have collapse at the palatal level and other sites.
  - Three sites of obstruction:
    - Type I: oropharyngeal (upper pharyngeal).
    - Type II: orohypopharyngeal (combined upper and lower pharyngeal).
    - Type III: hypopharyngeal (lower pharyngeal).

Clinical Manifestations

- Loud snoring, witnessed apneas, gasping/choking while asleep, enuresis (children), nocturnal awakening, daytime somnolence, personality change, moodiness, depression, decreased mental acuity, automobile or work-related accidents, decreased libido, cardiovascular morbidity.
- Obesity, increased neck size (>17 inches males, >16 inches females); hypertension in 50% of patients with OSAS.
- Oropharynx: elongated, thickened soft palate, narrow width and depth of oropharynx, large uvula, wide posterior pillar, redundant lateral mucosal folds.
- Lower oropharynx/hypopharynx: Prominent lingual tonsils, large tongue, redundant epiglottis or arytenoid mucosa with collapse on inspiration, retrodisplaced epiglottis.
- Other manifestations: nasal obstruction, retrusive mandible or maxilla with or without Type II or III occlusion, inferiorly positioned laryngohyoid complex.
- Mueller maneuver:
  - Patient attempts an inspiration with mouth closed and nostrils occluded during fiberoptic endoscopy.
  - Collapse of the airway is speculated to reflect collapse during sleep.
  - Maneuver has a 60% false-negative and false-positive rate.

Investigations
Sleep physiology
Stages

- Non-rapid eye movements (REM): quiet or slow-wave sleep, divided into Stage I (lightest) through Stage IV (delta sleep = deepest):
  - Stage I (10%-20% of normal sleep): transition form from wakefulness to sleep, increased in OSAS.
  - Stage II (30%-40% of sleep time): "true sleep," consolidated periods of sleep without spontaneous arousals.
  - Stages III and IV (<10% of sleep time): deeper sleep, reduced in OSAS.
- REM
  - Approximately every 90 minutes.
  - High levels of brain wakefulness.
  - Muscle atonia.
  - Characteristic EEG and bursts of rapid eye movements.
  - Airway collapse may worsen due to decreased skeletal muscle tone.

Terms

- Sleep latency: time to onset of sleep, 10-15 minutes in normal, shortened in OSAS.
- REM latency: time to onset of REM; shortened in OSAS, narcolepsy, and depressive disorders.
- Arousal: transient awakening, often the result of apnea, periodic leg movement, noise.

Polysomnography

- Gold standard for the diagnosis of OSAS; defines its severity.
- Includes the determination of the stages of sleep via EEG, electrooculograph (EOG), submental electromyogram (EMG) and identification of the types of apneic events with pulse oximetry, cardiac monitoring, monitoring of thoracic breathing movements.

Submental EMG

- Records static and phasic muscle tone.
- Increased activity during arousals.

Electrooculogram (EOM)

- Records blinks, rapid eye movements, slow movements.
- Distinguishes wakefulness and REM versus non-REM sleep.

EEG

- Records brainwaves necessary to define sleep levels.
- Expected changes with OSAS include:
  - Increased light sleep.
  - Decreased slow-wave sleep (Stages III and IV).
  - Decreased REM sleep.
  - Multiple arousals coinciding with the apneas.
  - 56% of obstructive apneas during REM sleep.
  - 3% of obstructive apneas during Stage I.
  - 33% of obstructive apneas during Stage II.
  - 7% of obstructive apneas during slow-wave sleep.

Respiratory tests performed in polysomnography

- Respiratory airflow: nasal airflow and oral airflow.
  - Measured using a thermistor: measures small increases and decrease in ambient temperature corresponding to inhalation and exhalation.
  - Can determine decreased, absent, normal airflow.
- Respiratory effort.
- Abdominal and chest belts worn; attached to strain gauges and used to measure chest wall movement and abdominal wall movement.
  - Presence of respiratory effort during an apneic episode typical for obstructive apnea.
  - Absence of respiratory effort leading to apnea = central apnea.
  - Chest and abdominal movements usually synchronized.
  - Paradoxical movements typical in some sleep disordered breathing patterns.
- Oxygen saturation (SaO_2)
  - Usually a 10-12–second delay before desaturation is detected if measured at the finger.
  - Measurement of the degree of desaturation coinciding with apneas and hypopneas.
  - Greater than 3% reduction in SaO_2 considered abnormal.

Electrocardiogram (ECG)

- Abnormalities of rate and rhythm may correspond to apneas.
- Tachycardia-bradycardia episodes are common with apneas.
- Life-threatening dysrhythmias may occur with apneas.
- 25% of patients with OSAS have ischemic heart disease.
- 40% of patients with cardiovascular accident (CVA) or myocardial infarction (MI) have OSA.

Tibialis (EMG)

- Periodic limb movements may be associated with apneas and can result in frequent arousals secondary to sleep fragmentation.

Body position

- Obstructive episodes tend to be worse in the supine position (versus lateral decubitus).
- Monitored by the sleep attendant or a position sensor.

Habitual, loud, irregular snoring

- Prominent feature of OSAS and may be included in polysomnography.

Split night polysomnography
- Polysomnogram plus continuous positive airway pressure (CPAP) titration.

Esophageal manometry
- Still in clinical trials.

Objective evaluations of sleepiness
- Epworth sleepiness scale:
  - Eight questions.
  - Measures the likelihood of falling asleep.
- Multiple sleep latency test (MSLT).
  - Five scheduled naps performed and latency to Stage I sleep measured.
  - Indicated when narcolepsy is considered as a diagnosis or when daytime sleepiness needs to be evaluated objectively.

Radiography
Cephalometrics (standard measurements of airway based on lateral skull films)
- SNA: angle from sphenoid to nasion to supradentale (normal = 83° +/− 2°).
- SNB: angle from sphenoid to nasion to infradentale (normal = 80° +/− 2°).
- Used primarily by oral surgeons to evaluate tongue base obstruction.

MRI, CT, cine CT, and airway fluoroscopy
- Also obtained at some centers.

Complications
- Cardiovascular disease (cardiac hypertension [HTN], pulmonary HTN, cardiac arrhythmias).
- Chronic obstructive pulmonary disease (COPD).
- Motor vehicle accidents: risk increased up to seven times that of the general population.
- Increased mortality.
  - Related to vascular disease.
  - AI >20 associated with increased mortality.
  - Risk eliminated with successful treatment.

Treatment
General measures
- Weight loss.
- Discontinue alcohol, sedatives, hypnotics.

Medications (less effective)
- Acetazolamide: increases respiratory drive; useful in central but not obstructive sleep apnea.
- Methylprogesterone: decreases $PaCO_2$ in hypoventilation syndromes; no role in OSAS.
- Protriptyline: decreases REM sleep where most apnea occur; rarely used.

- Oxygen therapy: rarely used since it does not decrease apneas and, due to increased oxygenation, decreases arousal threshold.

Positional therapy
- For patients who only have apnea in supine position.
- Use devices (e.g., tennis balls sewn to back of shirt) to prevent supine positioning.

Continuous positive airway pressure
- Provides pneumatic splint to airway; increases airway caliber.
- Optimal CPAP determined during sleep study; ranges from 5-20 cm H_2O.
- Can be applied via nasal mask or nasal pillows; tight seal required.
- Mask slip may require chin strap.
- Compliance major issue; general compliance rate for effective treatment approximately 60%.

Minor side effects
- Nocturnal arousals.
- Rhinitis, nasal irritation, and nasal mucosa dryness.
- Mask and mouth leaks.
- Facial skin discomfort.
- Difficulty in exhaling.
- Claustrophobia.
- Chest and back pain.

Bilevel CPAP (BiPAP)
- Allows independent regulation of inspiratory and expiratory phase pressures.
- Not yet shown to be more efficacious or better tolerated than CPAP.
- BiPAP currently reserved for patients intolerant of CPAP, especially if patient intolerant due to difficulty in exhalation or chest pain.

Auto-CPAP
- Adjusts CPAP levels throughout night based on detection of apnea, snoring, or inspiratory flow limitation.
- Attractive because it accommodates for levels of sleep, degree of sedation, change in sleep position.
- Reduces pressure-related side effects and reduces risk of inadequate CPAP.

Intraoral devices
- Mandibular advancement: best studied; tongue retaining devices.
- Advance to 50%-75% of maximal forward protrusion of jaw.
- Lessen but do not abolish sleep apnea.

- Useful in patients with mild to moderate sleep apnea, particularly with retrognathia or micrognathia.

Surgery

Indications
- Failed or noncompliant with medical therapy.

Work-up
- Determine level of obstruction: by physical exam, may need adjunctive cephalometrics or MRI.
  - Type I: oropharyngeal.
  - Type II: oropharyngeal and hypopharyngeal.
  - Type III: hypopharyngeal.

Laser-assisted uvulopalatoplasty (LAUP)
- Developed in the late 1980s, this procedure was first used in the United States in 1993 for snoring without apnea.
- LAUP addresses only the redundant tissue of the pharynx, as opposed to the uvulopalatopharyngoplasty (UPPP), which addresses the lateral pharyngeal walls and the tonsils.
- This procedure is designed to correct breathing abnormalities by reducing the amount of tissue in the velum and uvula and reducing soft tissue vibration at the soft palate.
- LAUP often requires multiple procedures, as opposed to other methods with electrocautery or a cold-knife.

Indications
- LAUP may be offered to patients with mild sleep apnea or snoring.
  - RDI <20.
  - Oxygen saturation not less than 85%.

Contraindications
- Patients with a hyperactive gag reflex.
- Mandibular retrognathia with relative macroglossia.
- Velopharyngeal insufficiency.
- Bleeding disorders or receiving anticoagulation.
- Submucous cleft palate.

Technique
- This procedure is performed in the office using the standard CO_2 laser precautions, with special pieces designed to protect the posterior pharyngeal wall.
- The patient is placed in a semi-Fowler position and instructed to relax the tongue. The patient is then usually instructed to inhale and hold their breath, which stops movement in the mouth, and allows for exhalation at the end of the burst to clear the plume. Anesthesia consists of 10% lidocaine spray applied to the palate and the base of tongue. Both sides of the soft palate and occasionally the base of the uvula are then infiltrated with local anesthesia (+/− corticosteroids).
- The laser power is usually set at 15-20 watts in a continuous mode, and vertical transpalatal incisions are made bilaterally lateral to the base of the uvula, followed by a partial vaporization of the uvula itself. Incisions are usually no more than 1 cm (longer incisions have been shown to bleed more frequently at the apex), and optimally are at a 5° angle from the vertical-oriented superolaterally. The beam is used in focus mode for cutting and defocused mode for ablation and coagulation. Patients then wash out their mouths with cold water to cool the operative site.
- Patients are usually sent home on antibiotics, with pain elixirs, and are often given perioperative steroids as well as oral rinses (peroxide based) to reduce eschar formation. Multiple procedures spaced 4-6 weeks apart are required to reshape the palate to overcome a patient's symptoms of snoring. The endpoint is determined by the satisfaction of the patient, alleviation of snoring, or if the patient cannot make a snorting sound mimicking snoring (suggests another etiology).

Complications
- Minor bleeding (1%-3%), mostly within 48 hours of the procedure (silver nitrate usually controls this bleeding).
- Oral candidiasis, usually responsive to antifungals.
- Temporary velopharyngeal insufficiency (VPI), usually resolving within 2 weeks of the procedure.
- Temporary change in taste.
- No cases of permanent VPI, nasopharyngeal stenosis, airway compromise, death reported.
- Vasovagal reactions during anesthesia reported.

Therapeutic success
- More effective for snoring than sleep apnea.
- Generally, a 50% reduction in the postoperative RDI achievable in 50%-60% of selected patients.

Advancement genioplasty with hyoid suspension
Indications
- Obstructive sleep apnea (OSA) with clinical suspicion for contribution of the base of tongue to airway collapse.
- Candidates: traditionally, patients who have more severe forms of OSA (RDI >50) or have failed other surgical procedures. In particular, patients with retrognathic or micrognathic phenotypes better candidates for procedure.

Contraindications
- Mild OSA or OSA treated with compliant use of CPAP.

- Lack of tongue base contribution to airway obstruction or lack of micrognathia/retrognathia.

Technique
- The most popular method is advancement genioplasty combined with hyoid suspension.
- In this procedure, the genial tubercle of the mandible, which attaches to the genioglossus muscle, is advanced anteriorly. Inferior sagittal osteotomy (ISO) is the most common method employed, in which a rectangular portion of the midline mandible is resected below the apices of the anterior teeth, rotated 90°, and secured in its new position.
- This advances the genioglossus musculature and the tongue base by a dimension equal to the thickness of the mandible. The hyoid bone is then freed from its inferior muscular attachments and suspended from the mandible (thereby anteriorly displacing the hyoid and tongue base) with permanent sutures or wires. This results is an enlarged airway at the base of tongue.

Complications
- Airway loss (perioperative sedatives, failed intubation, postoperative swelling).
- Bleeding (lingual artery).
- Temporary anesthesia to lower anterior teeth.
- Poor postoperative pain management.
- Loss of taste and tongue numbness (injury to lingual nerve).
- Wound breakdown and infection (due to excessive tension and unsterile surgical environment).
- Postoperative relaxation in tissues resulting in a partial loss of clinical benefit.

Base of tongue somnoplasty
Indications
- OSA with clinical suspicion for contribution of the base of tongue to airway collapse.
- Done in conjunction with more traditional forms of surgical therapy (e.g., UPPP) to address the tongue base.
- Also used independently to address many areas that contribute to OSA, including nasal turbinates, soft palate, base of tongue, tonsils, and pharyngeal walls.

Contraindications
- Mild OSA or OSA treated with compliant use of CPAP.
- Lack of tongue base contribution to airway obstruction.

Technique
- With the patient under local anesthesia, an insulated needle is placed in the areas with the most bulk (typically between the foramen caecum and the vallecula). Radiofrequency energy (Rfe) is then delivered submucosally to the base of tongue.
- Somnoplasty creates limited zones of coagulation beneath the tissue surface. As lesions resorb, they stiffen and reduce the tissue volume in the base of tongue.
- Typically, separate (5-6) Rfe treatments (approximately 1543 J for 9 minutes at 80°C) are delivered at 4-week intervals.

Complications
- Wound breakdown and infection (suppurative infections requiring incision and drainage [I & D] have been reported at a frequency of 1.4%).
- Airway loss (postoperative swelling and airway anesthesia).
- Bleeding (lingual artery).
- Nerve injury (lingual and hypoglossal).

Maxillomandibular advancement osteotomy for OSA
Description
- Skeletal advancement (of the maxilla and/or mandible) that results in the attached soft tissues being displaced, allowing less collapse during OSA events.
- Maxillomandibular advancement osteotomy one of three common maxillofacial procedures used in OSAS:
  □ Mandibular advancement with genioglossus advancement.
  □ Hyoid myotomy and suspension.
  □ Maxillomandibular osteotomy and advancement.

Indications
- Commonly performed after other more conservative procedures have failed.
- In patients who have severe OSAS and obvious maxillo-mandibular deficiency, maxillofacial surgery an option in combination with soft tissue procedures as the initial treatment.
- Alternative to permanent tracheostomy in those patients who have failed more conservative surgical alternatives.

Contraindications
- Poor cardiopulmonary status.
- Failure to attempt other surgical therapies in cases without obvious maxillofacial abnormalities.

Technique
- Bilateral maxillary and mandibular osteotomies performed and anterior segments advanced as far anteriorly as possible.

- Osteotomies are performed on the mandibular ramus below and in a LeFort I fashion on the maxilla.
- A variety of stabilizing devices used, with plates gaining the most favor recently.
- Limitations: ability to stabilize maxillofacial segments after osteotomies and aesthetic facial changes associated with procedure.

Therapeutic success

- In selected patients, procedure highly effective (>95% of cases report a significant reduction in RDI) within 1 year of procedure.
- Transient anesthesia of face and cardiac arrhythmias reported as complications associated with procedure.

Other Sleep Disorders

- Sleep deprivation: Average adult up to 8 hours of sleep per night; children more.
- Insomnia: Inadequate or poor quality sleep.
- Narcolepsy: sleep attacks, cataplexy, sleep paralysis (REM skeletal muscle paralysis persisting into wakefulness), hypnagogic hallucinations (vivid dreams intruding into wakefulness).
- Periodic leg movements: rapid repetitive myoclonic movements during sleep.
- Obesity-hypoventilation syndrome (Pickwickian syndrome)
  - Usually coexists with OSA.
  - Obesity (usually morbid).
  - Chronic hypoventilation.
  - $PaCO_2$ >45.

Selected References from the Recent Literature

1. Alwani A, Rubinstein I: The nose and obstructive sleep apnea. [Review] [12 refs]. *Current Opinion in Pulmonary Medicine* 1998;4:361-362.
2. Anonymous: Sleep-related breathing disorders in adults: recommendations for syndrome definition and measurement techniques in clinical research. The Report of an American Academy of Sleep Medicine Task Force [see comments]. [Review] [122 refs]. *Sleep* 1999;22:667-689.
3. Anstead M, Phillips B: The spectrum of sleep-disordered breathing. [Review] [58 refs]. *Respiratory Care Clinics of North America* 1901;5:363-377.
4. Anstead M, Phillips B, Buch K: Tolerance and intolerance to continuous positive airway pressure. [Review] [26 refs]. *Current Opinion in Pulmonary Medicine* 1998;4:351-354.
5. Ayas NT, Epstein LJ: Oral appliances in the treatment of obstructive sleep apnea and snoring. [Review] [36 refs]. *Current Opinion in Pulmonary Medicine* 1998;4:355-360.
6. Badr MS: Pathogenesis of obstructive sleep apnea. [Review] [37 refs]. *Progress in Cardiovascular Diseases* 1999;41:323-330.
7. Bower CM, Gungor A: Pediatric obstructive sleep apnea syndrome. [Review] [103 refs]. *Otolaryngologic Clinics of North America* 2000;33:49-75.
8. Bridgman SA, Dunn KM: Surgery for obstructive sleep apnea. [Review] [203 refs]. *Cochrane Database of Systematic Reviews* [computer file] 2000;CD001004
9. Chin K, Ohi M: Obesity and obstructive sleep apnea syndrome. [Review] [20 refs]. *Internal Medicine* 1999;38:200-202.
10. Coleman J: Sleep studies. Current techniques and future trends. [Review] [25 refs]. *Otolaryngologic Clinics of North America* 1999;32:195-210.
11. Coleman J: Disordered breathing during sleep in newborns, infants, and children: symptoms, diagnosis, and treatment. [Review] [23 refs]. *Otolaryngologic Clinics of North America* 1999;32:211-222.
12. Coleman J: Complications of snoring, upper airway resistance syndrome, and obstructive sleep apnea syndrome in adults. [Review] [39 refs]. *Otolaryngologic Clinics of North America* 1999;32:223-234.
13. Coleman J: Oral and maxillofacial surgery for the management of obstructive sleep apnea syndrome. [Review] [11 refs]. *Otolaryngologic Clinics of North America* 1999;32:235-241.
14. Coleman J, Rathfoot C: Oropharyngeal surgery in the management of upper airway obstruction during sleep. [Review] [33 refs]. *Otolaryngologic Clinics of North America* 1999;32:263-276.
15. Coleman J, Bick PA: Suspension sutures for the treatment of obstructive sleep apnea and snoring. [Review] [8 refs]. *Otolaryngologic Clinics of North America* 1999;32:277-285.
16. Day R, Gerhardstein R, Lumley A *et al*: The behavioral morbidity of obstructive sleep apnea. [Review] [80 refs]. *Progress in Cardiovascular Diseases* 1999;41:341-354.
17. Fogel RB, White DP: Obstructive sleep apnea. [Review] [152 refs]. *Advances in Internal Medicine* 2000;45:351-389.
18. George CF: Diagnostic techniques in obstructive sleep apnea. [Review] [78 refs]. *Progress in Cardiovascular Diseases* 1999;41:355-366.
19. Henderson JH, Strollo PJ, Jr.: Medical management of obstructive sleep apnea. [Review] [109 refs]. *Progress in Cardiovascular Diseases* 1999;41:377-386.
20. Hudgel DW, Auckley DH: Treatment of obstructive sleep apnea. [Review] [75 refs]. *Respiratory Care Clinics of North America* 1999;5:379-394.
21. Jones TM, Swift AC: Snoring: recent developments. [Review] [71 refs]. *Hospital Medicine (London)* 2000;61:330-335.
22. Littner M: Polysomnography in the diagnosis of the obstructive sleep apnea-hypopnea syndrome: where do we draw the line? [editorial; comment]. [Review] [12 refs]. *Chest* 2000;118:286-288.
23. Marais J, Armstrong MW: Effect of laser uvulopalatoplasty on middle ear function. [Review] [11 refs]. *Laryngoscope* 1999;109:1947-1949.
24. Marcus CL: Sleep-disordered breathing in children. [Review] [43 refs]. *Current Opinion in Pediatrics* 2000;12:208-212.
25. Marcus CL: Pathophysiology of childhood obstructive sleep apnea: current concepts. [Review] [72 refs]. *Respiration Physiology* 2000;119:143-154.
26. Messner AH, Pelayo R: Pediatric sleep-related breathing disorders. [Review] [90 refs]. *American Journal of Otolaryngology* 2000;21:98-107.

27. Mirza N, Lanza DC: The nasal airway and obstructed breathing during sleep. [Review] [61 refs]. *Otolaryngologic Clinics of North America* 1999;32:243-262.

28. Roux F, D'Ambrosio C, Mohsenin V: Sleep-related breathing disorders and cardiovascular disease. [Review] [90 refs]. *American Journal of Medicine* 2000;108:396-402.

29. Sher AE: Surgical management of obstructive sleep apnea. [Review] [47 refs]. *Progress in Cardiovascular Diseases* 1999;41:387-396.

30. Simonds AK: New developments in the treatment of obstructive sleep apnoea. [Review] [32 refs]. *Thorax* 2000;55 Suppl 1:S45-S50.

31. Skomro RP, Kryger MH: Clinical presentations of obstructive sleep apnea syndrome. [Review] [76 refs]. *Progress in Cardiovascular Diseases* 1999;41:331-340.

32. Weiss JW, Launois SH, Anand A *et al:* Cardiovascular morbidity in obstructive sleep apnea. [Review] [68 refs]. *Progress in Cardiovascular Diseases* 1999;41:367-376.

33. Woodson BT: Surgical approaches to obstructive sleep apnea. [Review] [96 refs]. *Current Opinion in Pulmonary Medicine* 1998;4:344-350.

34. Wright J, White J: Continuous positive airways pressure for obstructive sleep apnoea. [Review] [7 refs]. *Cochrane Database of Systematic Reviews* [computer file] 2000; CD001106.

TONSILLECTOMY AND ADENOIDECTOMY

Indications

Chronic tonsillitis

- Seven or more episodes in the preceding year.
- Five or more episodes in each of the 2 preceding years.
- Three or more episodes in each of the 3 preceding years.
- Each episode had one or more of:
  - Oral temperature >38.3° C.
  - Cervical lymphadenopathy >2 cm, or tender nodes.
  - Tonsillar exudates.
  - Positive throat culture for group A β-hemolytic strep.
- Obstructive sleep apnea, particularly in children.
- Cor pulmonale (secondary to OSA).
- Peritonsillar abscess (controversial: single episode of abscess does not mandate performance of tonsillectomy).
- Suspected malignancy.

Contraindications

- Bleeding diathesis.
- Cleft palate (absolute contraindication for adenoidectomy).
- Active infection (relative contraindication).

Complications

- Death (1 in 20,000).
- Primary hemorrhage (0.5-2.2 per 100).
  - Management.
    - Control hemodynamic status (fluids, blood transfusion).
    - Pressure.
    - Cautery.
    - Hemostatic agents (e.g., Surgicel, Avitene, Gelfoam).
    - Suture ligation of superior or inferior poles (inferior pole ligation carries higher risk due to closer proximity to internal carotid artery).
    - Ligation of external carotid artery.
    - Angiogram and embolization.
    - If internal carotid artery is violated, usually due to a tortuous course that brings it close to the tonsillar bed, control bleed with pack. Diagnosis is confirmed with angiogram. Balloon occlusion test may be performed at that time. If angiogram confirms ICA trauma, the patient is returned to the operating room for immediate attempt at intraoperative vascular repair. ICA ligation is a last resort treatment.
- Late hemorrhage (0.1-3 per 100); manage as per above.
- Airway obstruction secondary to:
  - Grossly enlarged tonsils obstructing airway at intubation.
  - Aspiration of:
    - Blood.
    - Tonsillar tissue.
  - Postoperative airway edema (rare).
- Aspiration pneumonia.
- Severe odynophagia leading to dehydration.
- Factors that have been proposed to decrease postoperative pain include:
  - Intraoperative and postoperative corticosteroids.
  - Intraoperative and postoperative antibiotics.
  - Infiltration of tonsillar bed with local anesthetic.
  - Minimization of use of electrocautery.
- Otalgia.
- Uvular hypertrophy.
- Palatopharyngeal insufficiency (velopharyngeal insufficiency).
  - Predisposing factors include:
    - Submucous cleft.
    - Neurologic disorders.
    - Preoperative hypernasality.
    - History of nasal regurgitation.
    - Family history of cleft or velopharyngeal insufficiency (VPI).
  - Treatment includes:
    - Observation; majority recover within first 3 weeks to 3 months.
    - Speech therapy; indicated in persistent cases.
    - Pharyngoplasty; indicated with speech therapy failure, generally considered 1 year posttonsillectomy/adenoidectomy.
- Nasopharyngeal stenosis.
- Refractory torticollis.
  - Hyperextension injury.
  - Must rule out atlantoaxial dislocation.
- Lymphoid tissue regrowth.
- Facial edema.
- Dental trauma (most common = maxillary incisors).
- Temporal joint disorder dislocation (treat with immediate intraoperative relocation).

Selected References from the Recent Literature

1. Allen GC, Armfield DR, Bontempo FA *et al:* Adenotonsillectomy in children with von Willebrand disease. *Archives of Otolaryngology—Head & Neck Surgery* 1999;125:547-551.
2. Deutsch ES: Tonsillectomy and adenoidectomy. Changing indications. [Review] [102 refs]. *Pediatric Clinics of North America* 1996;43:1319-1338.
3. Herzon FS, Nicklaus P: Pediatric peritonsillar abscess: management guidelines. [Review] [45 refs]. *Current Problems in Pediatrics* 1996;26:270-278.
4. Husband AD, Davis A: Pain after tonsillectomy. [Review] [44 refs]. *Clinical Otolaryngology & Allied Sciences* 1996;21:99-101.

5. Kieff DA, Bhattacharyya N, Siegel NS *et al:* Selection of antibiotics after incision and drainage of peritonsillar abscesses. *Otolaryngology—Head & Neck Surgery* 1999;120: 57-61.

6. Mui S, Rasgon BM, Hilsinger RL, Jr.: Efficacy of tonsillectomy for recurrent throat infection in adults. *Laryngoscope* 1998;108:1325-1328.

7. Murthy P, Laing MR: Dissection tonsillectomy: pattern of post-operative pain, medication and resumption of normal activity. *Journal of Laryngology & Otology* 1998;112: 41-44.

8. Nunez DA, Provan J, Crawford M: Postoperative tonsillectomy pain in pediatric patients: electrocautery (hot) vs cold dissection and snare tonsillectomy—a randomized trial. *Archives of Otolaryngology—Head & Neck Surgery* 2000;126: 837-841.

9. Randall DA, Hoffer ME: Complications of tonsillectomy and adenoidectomy. [Review] [93 refs]. *Otolaryngology—Head & Neck Surgery* 1998;118:61-68.

10. Stewart MG: Pediatric outcomes research: development of an outcomes instrument for tonsil and adenoid disease. *Laryngoscope* 2000;110:12-15.

11. Woolford TJ, Hanif J, Washband S *et al:* The effect of previous antibiotic therapy on the bacteriology of the tonsils in children. *International Journal of Clinical Practice* 1999;53: 96-98.

TEMPOROMANDIBULAR JOINT

Anatomy

- Each joint is a pressure-bearing double synovial joint and constitutes a compound joint involving three or more bones.

Components

- Temporal articular surface: squamous part of temporal bone.
- Mandibular condyle.
- Synovial membrane: lines all internal joint surfaces (except for articular surfaces and disc), contributes to nourish and lubricate avascular surfaces, has bactericidal properties.
- Articular capsule: encloses articular surfaces.
- Articular disc: very low coefficient of friction and compensates for lack of congruence between articular surfaces.
- Joint ligaments: strengthen capsule laterally and medially.

Vasculature

- Arterial supply: predominantly from superficial temporal artery, also deep auricular branch and masseteric branch of maxillary artery.
- Venous drainage: via temporomandibular veins into retromandibular vein of pterygoid plexus.

Innervation of temporomandibular joint (TMJ)

- Motor: mandibular division of trigeminal nerve via auriculotemporal nerve.
- Sensory: auriculotemporal nerve, masseteric nerve, posterior deep temporal nerve.

Joint compartments

- Condyle articulates with the articular disc to form the disc-condyle complex that functions mainly for hinge and rotational movement.
- Disc-condyle complex in turn articulates with the temporal bone that functions principally in gliding or translatory motion.

Principle Movements of the Mandible Allowed by the Joint

- Forward-backward movement.
- Opening-closing movement.
- Lateral movement.

Clinical Evaluation

History (cardinal symptoms)
- Preauricular pain.
- Aggravating factors.
- Joint noise (popping and clicking).
  - Onset of the clicking
  - When the click occurs.
  - What symptoms are present when not clicking.
- Limitation of movement.
- History of emotional and environmental stresses.
- History of medications patient may be taking.
- History of rheumatologic disease (e.g., fibromyalgia).
- History of trauma (e.g., mandibular fracture).
- History of orthodontic or orthognathic procedures.

Physical examination
- Assessment of facial appearance and symmetry.
- Mandibular movements and excursions.
- Bite evaluation.
- Evaluation of associated muscle groups (e.g., pain in sternomastoid, temporalis, pterygoids).
- Assessment of joint noises with movement.

Special diagnostic studies
- Conventional radiograms and TMJ tomography.
- Arthrography.
- CT.
- MRI (procedure of choice).
- Arthroscopy.

Temporomandibular Joint Disorders

- 10 million people suffer from TMJ disorders (TMD).
- TMD encompasses two groups of patients: those with true TMJ disorders and those with primary involvement of the masticatory muscles (myofascial pain-dysfunction [MPD] syndrome).
- Establishing the proper diagnosis is often difficult because a variety of conditions unrelated to the TMJ often produce signs and symptoms similar to TMD.

Applied Anatomy

- The TMJ consists of a movable condyloid process and its articulating counterpart, the articular eminence, which forms the anterior aspect of the glenoid fossa.
- The articulating surfaces are lined with fibrous connective tissues (FCT).
- The condyle has a layer of hyaline cartilage beneath its layer of FCT. This layer of cartilage is an

important growth site for the mandible; damage to this layer effects mandibular growth and morphology, as well as growth of the maxilla and midface.

- The TMJ has a disc interposed between its articulating surfaces. This disc acts as a shock absorber and allows the condyle to undergo rotational and translational motion.
- Of note, a patient's bite ultimately determines the final position of the condyle (an important point to remember when treating TMJ disorders).
- The left and right TMJ are joined by the mandible, thus unilateral disorders often lead to bilateral joint disease.

Diseases and Disorders

- The TMJ is susceptible to the same conditions that affect other joints in the body; in addition, there may be internal derangements of the intraarticular disc.
- In general, the treatment of TMJ disorders parallels the treatment of other joints in the body. However, functional and anatomic differences unique to the TMJ sometimes mandate variations to the therapy.

Congenital and Developmental Anomalies

- Because the condyle plays an important role in mandibular growth, congenital agenesis, condylar hypoplasia, or condylar hypoplasia can produce severe facial deformity.

Condylar agenesis
- Congenital.
- Coronoid process, ramus, parts of mandibular body also possibly absent.
- Often associated with abnormalities of internal and external ear, temporal bone, facial nerve.
- Usually unilateral.

Physical examination and investigations
- Mandible deviates to the affected side.
- Severe malocclusion is present.
- Radiographs show condylar deficiency.

Treatment
- Early treatment helps limit the degree of deformity.
- Objectives are to reestablish normal ramal height and restore the missing growth site.
- When less severe, distraction osteogenesis is used.
- When large portion on condyle and ramus is absent, a costochondral graft is used to reconstruct the TMJ.

- Orthodontic therapy, orthognathic surgery, otoplasty, and soft tissue and bone grafts are often necessary for facial augmentation.

Condylar hypoplasia
- May be congenital, but usually results from trauma, infection, irradiation during postnatal growth period.
- Diagnosis based on a history of progressive facial deformity during growth period (frequently with an associated history of trauma).

Physical examination and investigations
- The decreased condylar growth produces a characteristic facial deformity.
- The affected side demonstrates a short mandibular body, fullness of the face, and deviation of the chin to the affected side.
- The contralateral face appears flat with an elongated mandible.
- Malocclusion is present.
- Radiographs show condylar deformity and antegonial notching.

Treatment
- When recognized during the growth period, replacement of the condyle with a costochondral graft is used; otherwise, distraction osteogenesis is used.
- Orthodontic therapy is often necessary to establish normal occlusion.

Condylar hyperplasia
- Unknown etiology.
- Characterized by a slowly progressing, unilateral overgrowth of the mandible.
- Produces facial asymmetry during the second decade of life when one condyle continues to grow after the contralateral side has stopped growing.

Physical examination and investigations
- Radiographs show a normal condyle with an elongated neck or a symmetrically enlarged condyle.
- Facial asymmetry with deviation of the chin to the unaffected side is present.
- Cross-bite malocclusion is present.
- Prognathic appearance is present.

Treatment
- Treatment depends on whether the condyle is still growing, which can be determined by scintigraphy.
- If growth is still occurring, condylectomy is performed.
- If growth has ceased, orthognathic surgery preceded by orthodontic alignment of the teeth is the treatment of choice.

Traumatic Injuries

- The condyle is one of the most frequent sites of fracture after trauma to the mandible.
- Associated with a fracture are preauricular pain and tenderness and difficulty in opening the mouth.
- In a unilateral fracture the jaw will deviate to the affected side when opening the mouth. In bilateral fractures, no deviation is noted, but frequent anterior open-bite deformities often occur. Diagnosis is based on physical and radiographic findings.

Treatment

- Intracapsular condylar fractures are treated by short periods of maxillomandibular fixation (approximately 3 weeks).
- In adults, maxillomandibular fixation is the treatment of choice unless the malposed segment interferes with jaw function, there are no occluding teeth on the involved side, or the condyles processes are fractured bilaterally and grossly displaced.
- In children, closed reduction and fixation is the treatment of choice unless surgical repositioning is necessary to prevent subsequent growth deformity
- Other conditions may require open reduction and fixation or a joint prosthesis.

Dislocation

- In a dislocated jaw, the mandible is fixed in an open position, with only the most posterior teeth contacting.
- Three forms of dislocation can be distinguished based on the frequency of dislocations: single acute, chronic recurrent, and chronic persistent.
- Only the last two categories may require surgical treatment.

Treatment

- Single acute dislocations are treated by manual reduction supplemented by the use of local anesthesia, intravenous sedation, or general anesthesia.
- Chronic recurrent dislocations are treated by injecting a sclerosing agent into the TMJ capsule and ligament to produce scarring and contraction of the stretched tissues. Capsulorrhaphy produces a similar effect and is also a treatment option.
- Chronic persistent dislocations are treated using a variety of techniques from temporal myotomy to the placement of traction wires through the angle of the mandible. Occasionally, direct manipulation of the condyles or condylectomies is necessary.

Ankylosis

- Most common causes of ankylosis are trauma and rheumatoid arthritis. Congenital abnormalities, infection, and neoplasm are other causes of TMJ ankylosis.
- It is important to differentiate between true ankylosis, which involves the joint, and false ankylosis, which involves extraarticular structures. Examples of false ankylosis include depressed fractures of the zygomatic arch or scarring from surgery.
- Radiographs show condylar deformity and either a narrowing or irregularity of the joint space or obliteration of the normal bony morphology.

Treatment

- Three basic principles:
  - A new joint should be established at the highest possible point on the ramus to maintain maximal ramal height and to minimize postoperative shift of the mandible.
  - Interposition materials should be used to avoid fusion of parts.
  - Long-term physical therapy should be followed postsurgery.

Arthritis

- Most frequent abnormal condition affecting TMJ.

Infectious arthritis

- Rare.
- Associated with systemic diseases: gonorrhea, syphilis, tuberculosis; develops as an extension of local infections or results from blood-borne organisms.
- Clinically: signs of local inflammation and limited jaw movement.
- Radiographs: initially negative; later may show bone destruction.

Treatment

- Treat with antibiotics, hydration, pain control, and jaw movement restriction.

Traumatic arthritis

- Characterized by TMJ pain, tenderness, limitation of jaw movement.
- Radiographs: negative or show a widening of joint space caused by intraarticular edema or hemorrhage.
- May retard growth of mandible in children.

Treatment

- NSAIDS, heat, soft diet, jaw movement restriction.

Rheumatoid arthritis

- Clinically: bilateral pain, tenderness, swelling; limitation of jaw motion.
- Radiographs: initially negative; with progression, articular surface of condyle destroyed and joint space obliterated (an anterior open bite may occur).
- In children, mandibular growth retardation and facial deformity possible result of such destruction.
- Patients at risk for ankylosis.

Treatment

- Antiinflammatory drugs used during acute exacerbations.
- Jaw exercises used to prevent loss of motion.
- Treatment of systemic disease as per rheumatology; may include corticosteroids, methotrexate, ant-TNFα monoclonal antibody, hydroxychloroquine, gold, penicillamine.
- Surgery possibly necessary if ankylosis develops.

Degenerative arthritis

Primary

- Seen in older patients and associated with normal aging.
- Onset insidious.
- Symptoms mild and complaints from patients rare.

Secondary

- Caused by trauma or chronic clenching.
- Occurs in younger patients.
- Symptoms of pain, joint tenderness, clicking, crepitation, and limitation of jaw movements more severe than symptoms of primary degenerative arthritis.
- Condition usually unilateral.
- Radiographs: flattening, lipping, osteophyte formation, erosion of articular surface of condyle.

Treatment

- Medical therapy includes NSAIDS, soft diet, limitation of jaw movement, and a bite appliance. If medical therapy fails to relieve symptoms after 6 months and radiographic studies show bony changes, then surgical intervention may be indicated.
- When performing surgery, remove the least amount of bone necessary to produce a smooth articular surface; this helps minimize continued resorptive changes.

Neoplasms

- Rare.
- Benign tumors (common): chondroma, osteochondroma, osteoma.
- Benign tumor (rare): myxoma, fibrous dysplasia, synovialoma, chondroblastoma, osteoblastoma, synovial hemangioma.
- Malignant tumors (even rarer): fibrosarcoma, chondrosarcoma, multiple myeloma.
- Clinically: pain, limited jaw movement, difficulty in occluding teeth.
- Biopsy necessary to establish a definitive diagnosis.

Treatment

- Surgery is the treatment of choice.
- Most malignant neoplasms are not radiosensitive.

Internal Derangements

Classification

- Anterior disc displacement with reduction on opening mouth, characterized by clicking or popping sounds.
- Anterior disc displacement without reduction on mouth opening, characterized by locking.
- Disc adhesion to articular eminence, characterized by limited mouth opening resulting from inability of condyle to translate.
- Caused by trauma, lateral pterygoid spasm, alterations in frictional properties of joint.
- Most common symptom: pain.
- Diagnosis: history and physical; confirmed by MRI visualization of the disc position.

Treatment

- Anterior disc displacement with reduction on opening the mouth
  - Painless click and no jaw dysfunction: no treatment.
  - Clicking and pain: NSAIDs, bite-opening appliance, muscle relaxant when associated with lateral pterygoid spasm.
  - Persistent pain and clicking unresponsive to medical therapy: disc repositioning via surgery.
- Anterior disc displacement without reduction on opening the mouth
  - Surgery is urgent because degenerative changes in the disc and condyle can occur.
  - If the disc cannot be repositioned or repaired, it should be replaced with auricular cartilage or dermal grafts.
  - Arthroscopic lysis of adhesions and joint lavage can be used to restore disc mobility, thereby reducing pain and increasing joint function. Note that the disc is not returned to its normal position with this procedure.
- Disc adhesion to the articular eminence
  - Treated with arthroscopic lysis or arthrocentesis to restore normal disc mobility.

Myofascial Pain Dysfunction Syndrome

- Psychophysiologic disease involving the muscles of mastication.
- Characterized by poorly localized, dull, aching, radiating pain that becomes acute during jaw use and mandibular dysfunction that usually involves a limitation of jaw opening.
- Usually unilateral.
- Tenderness in muscles of mastication a hallmark.
- Begins as functional disorder, but leads to organic changes in TMJ, masticatory muscles, dentition.
- Stress-related disorder: hypothesized that a centrally induced increase in muscle tension results in muscle fatigue and spasm, which produce pain and dysfunction.
- May also be associated with myofascial pain symptoms in other areas of the body, especially head and neck region.

Treatment

- Muscle relaxation exercises, bite block, local anesthetic blocks, NSAIDS, muscle relaxants.

Selected References from the Recent Literature

1. Anonymous: National Institutes of Health Technology Assessment Conference on Management of Temporomandibular Disorders. Bethesda, Maryland, April 29-May 1, 1996. Proceedings. [Review] [0 refs]. *Oral Surgery, Oral Medicine, Oral Pathology, Oral Radiology, & Endodontics* 1997;83:49-183.
2. Baker GI: Surgical considerations in the management of temporomandibular joint and masticatory muscle disorders. [Review] [31 refs]. *Journal of Orofacial Pain* 1999;13: 307-312.
3. Blank LW: Clinical guidelines for managing mandibular dysfunction. [Review] [57 refs]. *General Dentistry* 1998;46: 592-597.
4. Bush FM, Harkins SW, Harrington WG: Otalgia and aversive symptoms in temporomandibular disorders. [Review] [91 refs]. *Annals of Otology, Rhinology & Laryngology* 1999;108: 884-892.
5. Carlsson GE: Epidemiology and treatment need for temporomandibular disorders. [Review] [25 refs]. *Journal of Orofacial Pain* 1999;13:232-237.
6. Dao TT, Lavigne GJ: Oral splints: the crutches for temporomandibular disorders and bruxism. [Review] [199 refs]. *Critical Reviews in Oral Biology & Medicine* 1998;9:345-361.
7. Davidoff RA: Trigger points and myofascial pain: toward understanding how they affect headaches. [Review] [159 refs]. *Cephalalgia* 1998;18:436-448.
8. Dimitroulis G: Temporomandibular disorders: a clinical update. [Review] [37 refs]. *BMJ* 1998;317:190-194.
9. Dionne RA: Pharmacologic treatments for temporomandibular disorders. [Review] [55 refs]. *Oral Surgery, Oral Medicine, Oral Pathology, Oral Radiology, & Endodontics* 1997;83:134-142.
10. Dworkin SF: Behavioral and educational modalities. [Review] [24 refs]. *Oral Surgery, Oral Medicine, Oral Pathology, Oral Radiology, & Endodontics* 1997;83:128-133.
11. Forssell H, Kalso E, Koskela P et al: Occlusal treatments in temporomandibular disorders: a qualitative systematic review of randomized controlled trials. [Review] [55 refs]. *Pain* 1999;83:549-560.
12. Frediani F: Typical and atypical facial pain. [Review] [25 refs]. *Italian Journal of Neurological Sciences* 1999;20:S46-S48
13. Frost DE, Kendell BD: Part II: the use of arthrocentesis for treatment of temporomandibular joint disorders. [Review] [24 refs]. *Journal of Oral & Maxillofacial Surgery* 1999;57: 583-587.
14. Goldberg MB: Posttraumatic temporomandibular disorders. [Review] [27 refs]. *Journal of Orofacial Pain* 1999;13: 291-294.
15. Goldstein BH: Temporomandibular disorders: a review of current understanding. [Review] [97 refs]. *Oral Surgery, Oral Medicine, Oral Pathology, Oral Radiology, & Endodontics* 1999;88: 379-385.
16. Graff-Radford SB: Facial pain. [Review] [43 refs]. *Current Opinion in Neurology* 2000;13:291-296.
17. Kropmans TJ, Dijkstra PU, Stegenga B et al: Therapeutic outcome assessment in permanent temporomandibular joint disc displacement. [Review] [50 refs]. *Journal of Oral Rehabilitation* 1999;26:357-363.
18. LeResche L: Epidemiology of temporomandibular disorders: implications for the investigation of etiologic factors. [Review] [78 refs]. *Critical Reviews in Oral Biology & Medicine* 1997;8:291-305.
19. Marbach JJ, Raphael KG: Future directions in the treatment of chronic musculoskeletal facial pain: the role of evidence-based care. [Review] [44 refs]. *Oral Surgery, Oral Medicine, Oral Pathology, Oral Radiology, & Endodontics* 1997;83:170-176.
20. Milam SB: Failed implants and multiple operations. [Review] [103 refs]. *Oral Surgery, Oral Medicine, Oral Pathology, Oral Radiology, & Endodontics* 1997;83:156-162.
21. Sessle BJ: The neural basis of temporomandibular joint and masticatory muscle pain. [Review] [22 refs]. *Journal of Orofacial Pain* 1999;13:238-245.
22. Sessle BJ: Neural mechanisms and pathways in craniofacial pain. [Review] [25 refs]. *Canadian Journal of Neurological Sciences* 1999;26 Suppl 3:S7-S11.
23. Stohler CS: Muscle-related temporomandibular disorders. [Review] [66 refs]. *Journal of Orofacial Pain* 1999;13:273-284.
24. Stohler CS: Craniofacial pain and motor function: pathogenesis, clinical correlates, and implications. [Review] [131 refs]. *Critical Reviews in Oral Biology & Medicine* 1999;10: 504-518.
25. Tenenbaum HC, Freeman BV, Psutka DJ et al: Temporomandibular disorders: disc displacements. [Review] [29 refs]. *Journal of Orofacial Pain* 1999;13:285-290.
26. Wallace DJ: The fibromyalgia syndrome. [Review] [83 refs]. *Annals of Medicine* 1997;29:9-21.
27. Zarb GA, Carlsson GE: Temporomandibular disorders: osteoarthritis. [Review] [47 refs]. *Journal of Orofacial Pain* 1999;13:295-306.

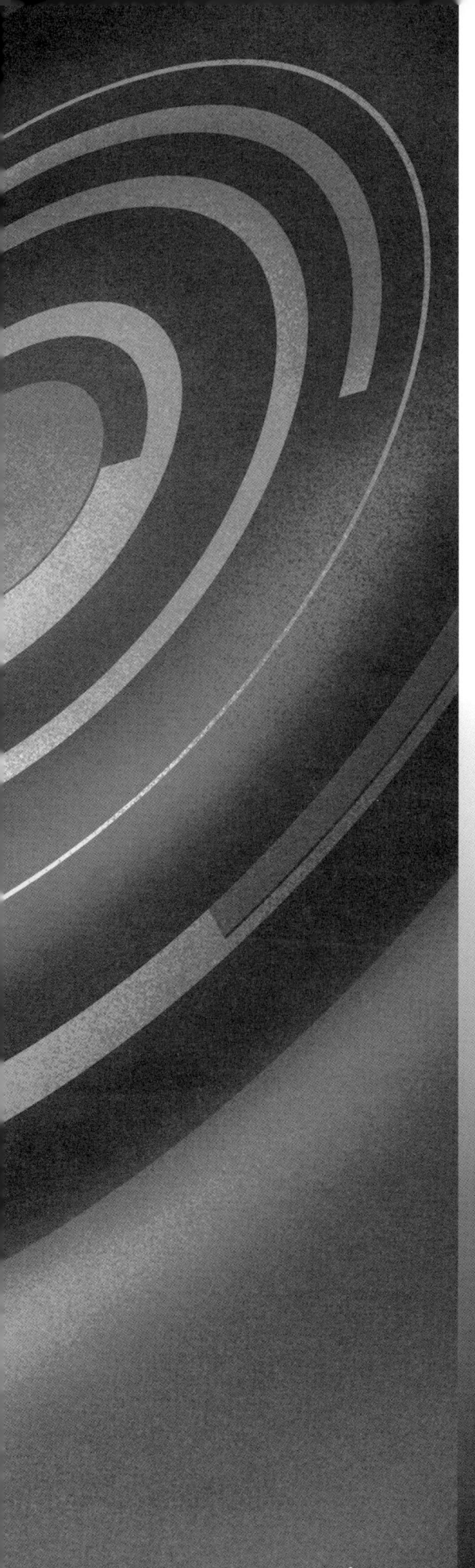

Laryngology

STRIDOR

Definition
- In Latin, means a "harsh, creaking sound."
- Audible noisy respiration caused by obstruction of airflow.

Etiology
- Inspiratory: supraglottic.
- Biphasic: glottis or subglottis.
- Expiratory: trachea/bronchi.

Inspiratory
- Pediatric causes of stridor (60% of stridor in children is localized to the larynx, 15% to the trachea, and 5% to the bronchi).
- Laryngomalacia accounts for 60% of congenital causes of stridor in children and is the most common cause of stridor in the neonate. It is caused by redundancy or weakness of the supraglottis (epiglottis, aryepiglottic folds, arytenoids). It is characterized by inspiratory stridor. Endoscopy may reveal an omega-shaped epiglottis and collapse of the supraglottis during inspiration. The disorder is benign and resolves within 6-24 months.
- Epiglottitis: an infectious supraglottitis caused by *Haemophilus influenza*. Treatment includes:
  - Evaluation of patient in the OR instead of the ER .
  - Intubation with bronchoscopy and tracheotomy sets at bedside.
  - A second-generation cephalosporin (e.g., cefuroxime).
  - Steroids used adjunctively.
  - Incidence decreased significantly with the advent of the *H. influenzae* vaccine.
- Pierre-Robin sequence (micrognathia, cleft palate, glossoptosis). Stridor when supine secondary to collapse of tongue posteriorly.
- Unilateral vocal cord paralysis.

Biphasic
- Croup (laryngotracheobronchitis) is the most common cause of stridor in the pediatric population. Croup is associated with viral upper respiratory infections (URIs) and is associated with a barking cough with inspiratory or biphasic stridor.
- Foreign bodies must always be considered, particularly if stridor is acute in onset and if the appropriate history is given. Because most foreign bodies are radiolucent, rigid bronchoscopy plays both a diagnostic and therapeutic role.
- Neoplasms:
  - Hemangioma is the most common head and neck neoplasm in children. Stridor is typically inspiratory or biphasic. Subglottic hemangiomas are more common in females (2:1) and occur more frequently on the left side. It should be suspected if a patient has a cutaneous hemangioma and stridor.
  - Lymphangiomas can cause airway compromise and stridor secondary to intraoral or laryngeal extension.
  - Recurrent respiratory papillomatosis is the most common benign neoplasm of the larynx in children and commonly presents with hoarseness, change in voice, or airway obstruction.
- Subglottic stenosis occurs when the airway is narrowed to <4 mm in diameter and can be congenital or acquired (usually from prior prolonged intubation).
- Laryngocele.
- Laryngeal web.
- Trauma.
- Allergic reactions.

Expiratory stridor
- Vascular compression
  - Innominate artery: If the innominate artery arises to the left of its normal position, it may then cross from left to right, anterior to the trachea, resulting in tracheal compression.
  - Vascular ring: A double aortic arch encircles the trachea and esophagus. Both limbs of the arch may be vascular, or one may be vascular and the other a fibrous remnant.
  - Vascular sling: The left pulmonary artery passes between the trachea and esophagus, compressing both.
- Laryngotracheal foreign body.
- Esophageal pathology leading to compression of the trachea.
- Tracheobronchial neoplasm.
- Tracheomalacia.

Causes in adults
Similar algorithm as in children, but bilateral vocal cord paralysis and neoplasms are more common in the adult.

Investigations (diagnosis)
- Diagnosis is made definitively by endoscopy. Flexible nasopharyngoscopy can assess the airway from the nasal passages to the level of the vocal cords, and possibly subglottis. Bronchoscopy evaluates the trachea and bronchi.
- Plain radiographs can be useful in identifying radiopaque foreign bodies, tracheal deviation, compression, or vascular abnormalities. Lateral neck films can be particularly useful. "Thumbprint" sign present in epiglottitis, "steeple sign" is present in croup.
- CT scans can aid in the evaluation of compressive airway lesions but cannot image the trachea along its long axis.

INFECTIOUS DISORDERS OF THE LARYNX AND TRACHEA

In general, for acute airway obstruction, follow the ABCs of resuscitation.

Croup: Laryngotracheobronchitis

- Most common cause of upper airway obstruction in children age 6 months to 6 years.
- Typically presents in children 1-3 years of age.
- Viral illness: parainfluenza and influenza viruses

Symptoms
- Fever.
- Prodromal URI.
- Barking cough.
- Hoarseness.
- Biphasic stridor.

Investigations
- Anteroposterior view of neck = "steeple sign" (narrowing of subglottic airway).
- Laryngoscopy/bronchoscopy: only in rare cases in which intubation is required or when anatomic abnormality is suspected.

Treatment
- Humidified air (cool).
- Corticosteroids.
- Racemic epinephrine.
- Intubation only in last resort, because subglottic stenosis is a risk in these children because of the inflamed subglottic airway. A leak should be maintained around the cuff.

If croup is recurrent and/or associated with failure to thrive, child should be investigated for anatomic airway abnormality.

Epiglottitis

- Bacterial supraglottitis.
- Most common in children age 2-7; however, epidemiology changing since the introduction of the *Haemophilus influenzae* Type B (HiB) vaccine.
- Prior to introduction of vaccine HiB was the major pathogen. Currently seeing more cases caused by nontypeable *H. influenzae* or *Streptococcus* species.

Clinical presentation
In child, tends to be acute onset.
- High fever.
- Tachycardia.
- Inspiratory stridor.
- Child sitting in "sniff" position to maintain airway.

- In adult, symptoms possibly less acute.
- May only complain of severe odynophagia with pain being in the region of the epiglottis.

Physical exam
- In child, physical exam of the upper airway deferred for fear of provoking airway obstruction.
- In adult, minimal findings typically seen in oral cavity/oropharynx.
- Indirect laryngoscopy or flexible laryngoscopy able to be performed if patient is stable.

Investigations
- If patient is stable, can obtain lateral soft tissue of neck, which will show widening of the epiglottic shadow (thumbprinting).
- Blood culture.

Treatment
In child
- Brought to OR.
- Anesthesiologist applies gas anesthetic with mask.
- When patient asleep, direct laryngoscopy and intubation performed.
- Culture supraglottis performed.
- Head and neck surgeon in the OR with bronchoscopy and tracheostomy setup.
- Admitted to ICU.
- IV second-generation cephalosporin (e.g., cefuroxime, cefotaxime) administered.
- IV steroids may be of benefit.
- Extubation based on presence of leak around balloon and/or fiberoptic laryngoscopy.

In adult
If severe as in child and if airway stable:
- Admitted to monitored bed.
- IV antibiotics administered.
- IV corticosteroids administered.

Bacterial Tracheitis

- Serious infection in children.
- Develops as a complication of URI (e.g., croup).
- Can be difficult to distinguish from croup.
- Diagnosis suggested by increasing severity of croup-type symptoms with fever and leukocytosis.
- Bacteria: *Staphylococcus aureus, H. influenzae, Streptococcus pyogenes, Moraxella catarrhalis*.
- Diagnosis made on bronchoscopy.
- Treatment by intubation or tracheostomy to allow for suctioning.
- Antibiotics based on culture results.
- May be complicated by pneumonia (60%) or acute airway obstruction.

Recurrent Respiratory Papillomatosis

- Viral infection of airway (larynx and/or trachea)
- Typically presents in children age 2-5, rarely in adults.
- Presentation at earlier age = poorer prognosis.
- Caused by infection by human papilloma virus (a DNA virus), mainly types 6 and 11.
- In pediatric patients, virus transmitted via genital tract of mothers with active genital condylomata: intrapartum, ascending, transplacental.
- Child: presents with hoarseness, stridor.
- Diagnosis: made with endoscopy and biopsy.
- Larynx: 100%; trachea: 17%-26%; pulmonary: 1%.

Treatment

- Endoscopy and debulking with CO_2 laser is mainstay of treatment.
- Argon laser is used for bronchial lesion.
- Care must be taken to avoid opposing raw mucosal surfaces during surgery.
- Pulsed dye laser targets the vasculature of the papilloma and may be as effective as CO_2 laser.
- Complications of lasers include glottic/subglottic stenosis, tracheoesophageal fistula, pneumothorax, airway fires, and facial burns.
- Systemic therapies have been tried, including systemic interferon, methotrexate, and indoles.
- Alpha-interferon has been used as an adjunct or on its own for therapy. It may give temporary or, more rarely, permanent regression (37%). It is associated with toxicities, including fever, fatigue, headache, nausea, and elevated liver function tests.
- Indole-3-carbinol alters estrogen metabolism and leads to a complete regression of papillomas in approximately 33% of patients. The only side effect is dyspepsia, and it is cheaper than interferon.
- Intralesional cidofovir has been used as an adjunct to laser debulking.
- Tracheotomy should be avoided if possible to prevent stomal seeding.
- The natural course is that as the child ages, the papilloma tend to regress; this is less aggressive in adults.

Tuberculosis

- May be secondary to pulmonary or gastric tuberculosis (TB); in children, may be primary to the larynx.
- Symptoms: hoarseness, dysphagia, odynophagia, cough, and weight loss.
- Posterior glottis most common site of involvement.
- Diagnosis on endoscopy = exophytic or ulcerative lesion.
- Biopsy sent for acid-fast stain, culture, pathology.
- Treatment: anti-TB therapy with triple antibiotics

BENIGN VOCAL CORD LESIONS

Presentation

- Hoarseness.
- Airway compromise.
- Pain.

Diagnosis

- Visualization: flexible fiberoptic laryngoscopy or direct laryngoscopy.

Pathology

Nodules

- Bilateral, occur at junction of anterior and middle third of cords.
- More common in prepubescent children.
- Patients are "voice abusers": "teachers, preachers, speakers."
- Occur secondary to mucosal injury at site of maximum amplitude of true vocal cord vibration.
- Acute stage: trauma leads to submucosal edema and swelling.
- Chronic stage: hyalinization of Reinke's space (the loose, subepithelial connective tissue layer ending at the junction of the squamous and respiratory epithelium on free margin of cord) and thickening of epithelium.

Management

- Good hydration, control of gastroesophageal reflux disease (GERD).
- Primary treatment: voice therapy.
- Surgical treatment (microdissection and excision) considered with persistence of symptoms and nodules after trial of voice therapy (3 months).

Capillary ectasia

- Dilated vessels on vocal cords secondary to voice abuse.
- More common in female singers who present with minor hoarseness after voice use.
- Treated primarily with voice therapy.
- Can be surgically coagulated with laser.

Polyps

- Pedunculated or sessile lesions arise only on true vocal cord.
- 90% Unilateral.
- Occur at junction of middle and anterior third of the vocal cord.
- Risk factors: female, tobacco use, hypothyroidism.

Types
Mucoid
- Translucent, avascular, broad base.
- Arises in Reinke's space.

Angiomatous
- Red, protuberant, may be multinodular.
- Occurs secondary to acute, explosive voice abuse, resulting in subepithelial hemorrhage.

Transitional
- Tortuous vessels in gelatinous substrate.

Management
- Elimination of provoking factors.
- Voice therapy.
- Evacuation of acute hemorrhage: possibly successful in preventing progression to chronic polyp
- Well-suited to CO_2 laser ablation.
- Postoperative care: voice rest and antireflux medication.

Reinke's edema (bilateral diffuse polyposis)
- Seen in middle-age patients, typically voice abusers and smokers. Rarely caused by severe hypothyroidism.
- Accumulation of (edema) in lamina propria (Reinke's space) between epithelium of cord and vocal ligament.
- Treatment: voice therapy, smoking cessation. (If this fails and voice is not acceptable, physician may incise mucosa, aspirate the edema, and excise excess mucosa.)

Glottic sulcus (may be congenital or acquired)
- Epithelial-lined pocket whose lip parallels the vocal cord. Surface epithelium adhered to vocal ligament.
- Seen in vocal abusers.
- Voice is hoarse, with limited high-pitch range and diplophonia.
- May be related to intracordal cyst.
- Treatment: voice therapy. Excision difficult. Careful hydrodissection with excision of the sulcus lips and any invaginated mucosa without any damage to vocal ligament; may need fat injection.

Intracordal cysts
Mucoid retention cysts
- Arise from obstruction of mucous gland duct, secondary to trauma.
- Originate just below free margin of cord with medial extension.

Epidermoid cysts
- Inclusion cysts that collect keratinous debris.

- Thought to originate either from congenital rest of epithelium within cord or from surface epithelium that is covered over by healing after trauma.

Treatment
- Large mucoid inclusion cyst may be unroofed.
- Smaller cysts (both types) excised using microflap technique, in which superficial epithelium is carefully dissected from the surface of the cyst; the cyst is identified and resected, with the epithelial flap returned to position.

Contact granuloma or ulcer
- Arises posteriorly over the vocal process of the arytenoid.
- History of laryngopharyngeal reflux (LPR).
- Chronic cough or throat-clearing.
- Prior intubation.
- Voice abusers.
- Smoking: exacerbating factor.

Management
- Anti-GERD regimen.
- Voice therapy.
- Surgical excision: last resort for persistent lesion.
- Botox injection into lateral crico-arytenoid muscle after surgical excision; decreases chances of granuloma recurrence.

Hemangioma
Infants
- Subglottic: originates posteriorly (more common on left), then increases circumferentially to occlude airway.
- Cutaneous hemangioma in 50% of infants.
- Subglottic hemangioma in 1%-2% of children with cutaneous hemangioma.
- Presents within first 6 months of life with biphasic stridor that is increased with agitation, URI.
- May present as recurrent croup.
- May progress to episodic cyanosis, failure to thrive.
- Female:male ratio = 2:1.
- Diagnosed on endoscopy = unilateral sessile, compressible lesion.
- Biopsy to be avoided because of hemorrhage.
- Typically of the capillary type.

Clinical course
- Proliferates rapidly at 8-18 months.
- Involutes over 5-8 years.
- Complete regression in 50% at 5 years, 70% at 7 years.

Treatment
Watchful waiting
- If lesion is small, without airway compromise.

Tracheotomy
- Indicated in cases of critical airway narrowing.

Oral corticosteroids
- Work only in proliferative phase.
- Prednisone 4 mg/kg/day × 4 weeks
- Taper over 2 weeks.
- 75% response rate; recurrence in 40%; may initiate second round of treatment.
- May maintain long-term use at 1 mg/kg/day, although complications of long-term steroid use must be considered; patient will require surveillance by a pediatrician.

CO₂ laser
- Staged excision widely used.
- Risk of subglottic stenosis.
- Tracheotomy not required postoperatively if not required preoperatively.

Open resection
- Via laryngofissure.
- Considered by some to be treatment of choice for selected large lesions.
- Long-term sequelae of laryngofissure in this population unknown.

Alpha-interferon
- Used when other treatments failed.
- Dose: 3×10^6 IU/m^2 s.c. Q.D. until 50% regression achieved.

In adult
- Typically at or above the glottis.
- Usually of the cavernous type.
- Patients present with hoarseness.
- Generally advise no treatment unless it progresses to involve other laryngeal structures leading to obstruction.
- If treatment required, corticosteroids or radiation therapy.
- CO₂ laser avoided because of cavernous pathology type.

Granular cell tumor (granular cell myoblastoma)
- Represents only 2.5% of laryngeal tumors.
- Originates from Schwann cells.
- Small, sessile, solitary, and gray.
- Associated with overlying *pseudoepitheliomatous hyperplasia*. If biopsy not deep enough, lesion can be mistaken for *squamous cell carcinoma*.
- Differential diagnosis: TB, syphilis, blastomycosis.
- Histology: pink, granular cytoplasm (periodic acid–Schiff [PAS]-positive granules).
- Treatment: endoscopic excision.

Chondroma
- Cartilaginous tumor typically arising from the posterior plate of the cricoid.
- Presents with hoarseness, dyspnea, neck mass, dysphagia.
- Manifests a slow growth pattern.
- Difficult to differentiate chondroma from low-grade chondrosarcoma.
- Diagnosed with plain views, which show subglottic lesion with or without calcification, CT scan
- Endoscopic biopsy.
- Treated with excision via laryngofissure in benign or low-grade lesions, total laryngectomy in high-grade sarcomas.

Amyloidosis
- May be primary or secondary to a neoplasm (e.g., multiple myeloma).
- Histology: apple-green birefringence with Congo red stain.
- Deposition sites: larynx > trachea > bronchus.
- Submucosal lesion of the true vocal cords or vestibular folds.
- Treated with conservative excision but recurrence common.

Sarcoidosis
- Systemic granulomatous disease, affects submucosal larynx (1%-5%).
- Sites: Mainly supraglottis. Epiglottis > aryepiglottic fold > false cords > subglottis; true vocal cords rarely involved.
- Histology = noncaseating granulomas.
- Serum ACE I levels no longer considered sufficiently accurate for diagnostic purposes.
- Process tends to regress spontaneously.
- Recurrent laryngeal neuropathy can cause hoarseness.

Wegener's granulomatosis
- Systemic disease: necrotizing granulomas and vasculitis.
- Friable granulomas or ulcerations common in the subglottis.
- Histology: giant cells, epithelioid granulomas, and necrotizing vasculitis.
- Systemic treatment: corticosteroids and cyclophosphamide.

Neurofibroma
- Rare, Schwann cell tumors of aryepiglottic fold.
- Female:male ratio = 2:1; full neurofibroma workup indicated.

Other lesions
- Include rhabdomyoma (can be confused with granular cell tumor or rhabdomyosarcoma), lipoma, and pleomorphic adenoma.

SACCULAR CYSTS AND LARYNGOCELES

- Both types of lesions arise from the saccule.
- Saccule: Arises vertically off the anterior end of the ventricle. Lined by pseudostratified columnar epithelium.

Saccular Cyst

- No communication between cyst and laryngeal lumen.
- Lateral saccular cyst: extends posterosuperiorly into false cord and aryepiglottic fold.
- Anterior saccular cyst: extends medially and posteriorly into laryngeal lumen from between true and false cords. More common than lateral cyst.

Symptoms

- In children: may cause stridor, cyanosis, altered cry.
- In adult: hoarseness. If large, may present as laryngocele (see below).

Physical examination

- Anterior cyst: submucosal mass extending from anterior ventricle and overhanging anterior part of vocal cord.
- Lateral cyst: submucosal swelling in aryepiglottic fold and false cord.

Investigations

- CT scan.

Treatment

- Neonate or pediatric patient: endoscopy, with aspiration, with or without marsupialization. May need tracheotomy.
- Adult: endoscopic removal. External approach for large cysts.

Laryngocele

- Communicates freely with laryngeal lumen.
- Internal: Extends posterosuperiorly into false cord and aryepiglottic fold.
- External: Extends superiorly into neck through thyrohyoid membrane via the orifice of the superior laryngeal nerve.
- Combined: Has clinical features of both external and internal laryngoceles.
- *Laryngopyocele:* infected laryngocele.
- Association exists between laryngocele and laryngeal cancer.

Etiology

- Increased transglottic pressure.
- Carcinoma or other obstructing lesion.

- More common in fifth and sixth decades of life.
- Male > female.

Clinical manifestations

Symptoms

- Hoarseness.
- Neck swelling.
- Stridor.
- Dysphagia.
- Sore throat.
- Snoring.
- Cough.

Physical examination

- Submucosal mass in aryepiglottic fold/false cord (internal).
- Neck mass (air-filled; will gurgle with compression) (external).

Diagnosis

- CT scan: air-filled mass.

Treatment

- Surgical excision: follow external sac through thyrohyoid membrane (may need to excise portion of thyroid cartilage). Excise sac as close to orifice as possible.

FUNCTIONAL VOICE DISORDERS

- Result from abuse or misuse of the vocal apparatus in the presence of normal structure and physiology.
- May also occur secondary to a maladaptive response to a physical condition.
- Very common forms of voice disorders.
- Typically treated with speech therapy.

Morrison *et al* (1986) have described four types of laryngeal abnormalities observable on physical exam with endoscopy associated with the various forms of functional voice disorders. These are referred to as muscle tension dysphonias (MTDs):

- MTD 1: Open posterior commissure.
- MTD 2: Plica ventricularis: approximation of false cords.
- MTD 3: Partial anterior/posterior contraction of the supraglottis.
- MTD 4: Complete supraglottic closure.

Six types of functional voice disorders have been characterized and classified.

1. Vocal Abuse Syndromes (five subtypes)

A. Tension-fatigue syndrome

- Long-standing fluctuant/intermittent symptoms.
- Symptoms include vocal fatigue, decreased range, and pain with speaking.

- Associated with vocal abuse or other myofascial pain disorders (e.g., TMJ).
- Voice quality may be harsh, strained, and associated with harsh glottal attacks
- Associated with all the MTDs.

B. Bogart-Bacall syndrome
- Long-standing fluctuant/intermittent.
- Symptoms include vocal fatigue, breaks, pitch, and resonance abnormalities
- Presents as low-pitched speech fundamental frequency and poor breath support for speech.
- Seen in professional singers; a good technique for singing but a bad technique for speaking.
- Associated with MTD 1 and 3.

C. Vocal nodules
- Chronic, fluctuant.
- More common in females.
- Most common functional voice disorder in children.
- Seen in vocal abuse, singing "out of range."
- Symptoms include vocal breaks, fatigue, decreased range, and pitch and resonance abnormalities.
- Voice breathy and possibly associated with hard glottic attacks.
- Associated with MTD 1 and 3.

D. Polypoid degeneration (Reinke's edema)
- Chronic, stable.
- Female predominant.
- Associated with smoking, severe hypothyroidism.
- Symptoms include fatigue, decreased range, and pitch and resonance abnormalities.
- Polypoid degeneration seen on fiberoptic exam along with MTD 2, 3, and 4.

E. Vocal process ulcer/granuloma
- Acute, intermittent.
- Symptoms include fatigue and pain with speaking.
- Voice quality strained, with hard glottal attacks and a low speech fundamental frequency.
- Seen in patients with poor breath support, chronic throat clearing and coughing, GERD, postintubation, and vocal abuse.
- Associated with MTD 3.

---

2. Conversion Aphonia/Dysphonia
- Sudden onset, may have precipitating event.
- Associated with MTD 1 and 3.

---

3. Habituated Hoarseness
- Chronic, stable.
- Usually after vocal surgery or laryngitis.
- Associated with GERD.

- Voice quality breathy, raspy; may manifest diplophonia.
- Associated most commonly with MTD 2, occasionally with 3 and 4.

---

4. Inappropriate Falsetto
- Developmental in males (failure of voice change with puberty).
- Sudden onset in females.
- Abnormally high pitch.
- Not associated with MTD.

---

5. Postoperative Dysphonia
- Severe dysphonia after vocal surgery.
- Symptoms include fatigue and pain with speech.
- Voice strained, harsh; associated with hard glottal attack.
- Associated with MTD 2 and 4.

---

6. Relapsing Aphonia
- Associated with severe psychopathology.
- Stable, voice "comes and goes."
- Associated with MTD 1.

Issues Unique to the Management of the Professional Voice

1. The image of professional voice users, such as actors and singers, is often intimately related to an identifiable vocal sound. Therefore, considerable anxiety and psychological issues can surround even minor changes or problems with their voices. As their physicians, we must remain cognizant of these additional factors and the "stigma" of even a perceived voice problem.
2. Even minor problems can be particularly apparent in a professional voice user given the extreme demands they place upon their voices.
3. The evaluation of a professional voice user should include the following issues:
    - Professional status and voice goals.
    - Amount and nature of voice training.
    - Performance commitments.
    - Performance environment (e.g., exposure to tobacco smoke).
    - Rehearsal practices.
    - Abusive habits during speech and singing. (These patients may be very aware of their voice abuse, but their mechanics of breathing and voice production must be carefully evaluated for technical errors that can be corrected.)
    - General health status (e.g., obesity, allergy, GERD, dental disease).
4. Factors that lead to vocal strain/fatigue in professional voice users:

- Long hours of practice/voice use.
- Shouting/screaming on stage.
- Speaking/singing over background music/noise.

5. Professional voice use requires adaptation to many different environments. The changes in loudness, pitch, and overall voice quality can lead to significant voice abuse.

6. Occupational hazards can include costumes, masks, and makeup that can affect or inhibit voice production. In addition, stage smoke, dust, and other irritants can be significant factors contributing to voice problems.

7. The lifestyle of a professional voice user must be taken into account during their evaluation. Voice production/use can be required for long periods and can be extremely strenuous. In addition, the professional voice user typically must travel extensively and live in many temporary environments (climate changes, changes in allergens other irritants).

8. The competitive nature of their profession leads these patients to place demands on themselves that cause vocal strain and abuse.

9. The required emotional range required for professional voice users to perform on stage may translate into a more volatile personality in life.

SPASMODIC DYSPHONIA

Classification
- Adductor spasmodic dysphonia.
- Abductor spasmodic dysphonia.

Etiology
- An action-induced laryngeal motion disorder. Most cases represent manifestations of primary dystonia (symptoms are enhanced with use of the affected body part, and the region may appear normal at rest), but many are secondary to other neurologic entities.
- In one study of primary laryngeal involvement, 16% had spread to another part of the body.
- Dystonias may be primary (sporadic or genetic) or secondary.
- Secondary dystonias are associated with a variety of genetic neurodegenerative conditions (e.g., Wilson's disease, Huntington's disease, progressive supranuclear palsy). Other causes of secondary dystonias include complications of medications (antipsychotics, antiemetics, anti-Parkinsonian). Rare causes include post-traumatic, postinfectious, vascular, and neoplastic syndromes.

Signs and symptoms
Adductor spasmodic dysphonia (87%)
- Irregular hyperadduction of the vocal folds.

- Exhibition of a choked, strained-strangled voice quality with abrupt initiation and termination, resulting in short breaks in phonation.
- Reduction in volume and monotone.
- Vocal tremor frequently observed with a slow speech rate and decreased smoothness of speech.
- Speech intelligibility generally decreased.
- May exhibit compensatory pseudo-abductor spasmodic dysphonia, resulting in whispering

Abductor spasmodic dysphonia (12%)
- Breathy, effortful voice quality with abrupt termination (breathy breaks).
- Results in aphonic whispered segments of speech.
- Voice reduced in loudness and vocal tremor often observed.
- Speech intelligibility generally decreased.
- Some patients exhibit a combination of adductor and abductor signs and are classified as mixed.
- Laboratory investigations are typically normal.
- All patients should have a complete neurological evaluation.

Treatment
Botulinum toxin
Adductor spasmodic dysphonia
- Dose based on titration and can range from 0.1-10 U per thyroarytenoid muscle injection, may be unilateral or bilateral.
- Performed percutaneously through the cricothyroid membrane and into the thyroarytenoid-vocalis muscle complex using EMG for optimal needle placement.
- Can also be injected via an indirect laryngoscopic approach. Onset of response to the toxin appears delayed (mean = 9.1 days), but degree of benefit and duration of efficacy appears comparable with EMG technique.
- Improved speaking by 60%-100% of normal function, with a mean of 90% with a duration of effect from 3-4 months.

Adverse effects
- Mildly breathy dysphonia for less than 2 weeks (45%).
- Mild choking on fluids for the first several days (22%).
- Hyperventilation and dizziness while trying to speak while hypophonic.

Abductor spasmodic dysphonia
- EMG-guided percutaneous injection into PCA muscle.
- Patient instructed to sniff, which uses the PCA maximally, resulting in a burst of activity on the EMG and helping to identify the correct site of injection.
- 0.5-5 U used; may need to repeat one to four times to weaken one or both PCAs.
- Return to mean maximal functional performance of 70% of normal.

Adverse effects

- Brief choking on fluids without aspiration, and mild stridor.
- No significant breathing difficulties, even in cases in which both PCAs were injected.
- No role exists for systemic pharmacotherapy.

Other

- Despite initial favorable reports, recurrent laryngeal nerve sectioning has fallen out of favor. By 3 years, only 36% of patients had some persistent improvement, and only 3% achieved a persistent normal voice. Of the 64% with failed voices at 3 years, 48% were worse than before surgery. Recent literature suggests benefits from selective sectioning of branches of the recurrent laryngeal nerve as it enters the thyroarytenoid (TA) muscle.

LARYNGEAL INTUBATION TRAUMA

Incidence

- 4%-13% in adults.
- 0.5%-13% in neonates.

Classification

Direct injury

- Lacerations, abrasions
  - ▫ Most will heal without intervention.
- Arytenoid dislocation/subluxation
  - ▫ Hoarseness: most common symptom.
  - ▫ Impaired vocal fold mobility.
  - ▫ Odynophagia: most common sign.
  - ▫ Other signs: absence of a jostle sign (movement of the arytenoid on the abnormal side caused by contact with the normal side during adduction in cases of vocal fold paralysis).
  - ▫ Asymmetric vertical position of the vocal processes.
  - ▫ Absence of increasing length with increasing pitch.
  - ▫ Decreased mobility on palpation during DL.
  - ▫ Studies: laryngeal EMG (differentiates between arytenoid vs. nerve pathology)

Pressure injury

- Edema
- Erythema
- Ulceration
- Necrosis
- Granulation tissue formation
- Scar formation
- Vocal fold paralysis.

Treatment

- Voice therapy: rarely effective.
- Early closed reduction: preferably in 48 hours of traumatic dislocation.

- Steroid injection.

Pressure injury

Pathogenesis

- The ET tube exerts the most pressure on the posterior glottis, the arytenoids, and the posterior cricoid cartilage.
- When pressure of tube exceeds capillary pressure of laryngeal mucosa, ischemia results in irritation, inflammation, congestion, and edema in a few hours.
- Continued ischemia leads to erosion and ulceration.
- Continued erosion and ulceration lead to deep stromal necrosis, perichondritis, chondritis, and cartilage necrosis.
- Histologic evaluation reveals active inflammatory injury with lymphocyte infiltration. Minor damage will heal by epithelial regeneration.
- Moderate damage results in squamous metaplasia and healing by secondary infection with granulation tissue formation.
- Severe damage leads to fibrous tissue and eventually scar tissue formation (glottic/subglottic stenosis).

Contributing factors

- Duration of intubation.
- Size of tube.
- Cuff pressure.
- Composition of tube.
- Prior state of larynx.
- Movement of the tube.
- Gastroesophageal reflux.
- Presence of nasogastric tube.
- Poor general health.

Clinical signs and symptoms

- Immediate obstruction secondary to granulation tissue.
- Onset of obstruction in hours secondary to subglottic reactive edema.
- Voice changes secondary to edema and granulation tissue.
- Slowly increasing obstruction (dyspnea, stridor) secondary to posterior glottic or subglottic stenosis.
- Edema, erythema, granulation tissue, ulceration on immediate postextubation examination.
- Chronic granuloma, healed fibrous nodules, interarytenoid adhesion, healed furrows, posterior glottic stenosis, subglottic stenosis, vocal fold paralysis on later examination.

Treatment

- Limit duration of intubation.
- Early tracheotomy for prevention (within 2 weeks of intubation).

- Tracheostomy if airway narrowed from granulation or stenosis.
- Others suggest endoscopic excision of obstructing granulation tissue.
- Control of GERD.

 UNILATERAL VOCAL CORD PARALYSIS

Etiology
In children
- Neurologic disorders: Arnold-Chiari a common cause of bilateral VC paralysis from herniation of the cerebellum and kinking of the medulla oblongata through the foramen magnum; however, may also present with unilateral VC paralysis.
- Surgical trauma (post–TE fistula repair, postcongenital heart repair).
- Birth trauma: accounts for 20% of all cases of VC paralysis.
- Idiopathic.

In adults
- 75% of vocal cord paralysis is unilateral.
- The left side is more frequently paralyzed than the right side because of the longer course of the recurrent laryngeal nerve.
- 90% caused by a peripheral lesion.
- Causes of laryngeal paralysis include neoplastic, traumatic, neurologic, and idiopathic conditions.
- Malignant neoplasms (36%) causing paralysis originate from the lung, thyroid, larynx, and esophagus.
- Trauma: surgical (25%) (neck, cardiothoracic), external.
- Idiopathic: 13%.
- Neurologic etiologies include poliomyelitis, pseudobulbar palsy, ALS, MS, and bulbar palsy. Vascular etiologies include Wallenberg's syndrome from infarction of PICA distribution.

Clinical symptoms
In children
- Stridor: vocal cord paralysis the second most common cause of stridor in children after laryngomalacia.
- Cyanosis.
- Weak cry.
- Hoarseness.
- Cough.
- Aspiration.
- In children with unilateral VC paralysis, airway usually adequate; these patients may present with minimal aspiration or weak voices but will eventually compensate for the deficit and will not require any airway intervention.

In adults
- Weak, breathy voice.
- Change in pitch.
- Chronic aspiration.
- Choking.

Diagnosis
History
- Trauma.
- Recent URI.
- Smoking/ethyl alcohol (EtOH).
- Other neurologic symptoms.

Physical exam
- Indirect laryngoscopy.
- Flexible nasopharyngolaryngoscopy.
- Laryngeal EMG allows analysis of the electrical activity generated by motor units. It helps to differentiate between joint abnormalities (e.g., cricoarytenoid joint fixation, arytenoid subluxation) and neurologic/myopathic abnormalities. The thyroarytenoid and cricothyroid muscles have the easiest access, and information about the superior and recurrent laryngeal nerve can be obtained by testing these two muscles. In a patient with myopathy, no change in frequency of firing will occur; however, there is a decrease of the amplitude of the muscle action potential. In a situation of neuropathy, there is a decrease in frequency of firing; however, the amplitude is normal. Fibrillation potentials show loss of neural innervation that can develop 1-3 weeks after an injury. Polyphasic reinnervation potentials indicate reinnervation but do not indicate the timing of recovery and may also indicate synkinesis.
- CT scan with contrast from skull base to superior mediastinum, to evaluate for neoplasms.

Treatment
Considerations
- Duration of symptoms.
- Degree of impairment.
- Presence of anatomic defect or prior surgery.
- Potential for recovery.
- Comorbidities and life expectancy.
- Vagal injuries with lateralization, marked bowing, atrophy, and loss of abductor and adductor function.
- Vocal demands.
- Function warrants early intervention.
- Need for a permanent vs. reversible procedure.

Options
- No therapy, allowing for spontaneous recovery.
- Speech therapy.
- Vocal fold injection.
- Medialization thyroplasty.

- Arytenoid adduction.
- Reinnervation.

Evaluation
- Aspiration: warrants early intervention.
- Videostroboscopy particularly helpful with severe dysphonia
  - Assessment of glottic closure and gap.
  - Assessment of mucosal wave patterns.
- Electromyography
  - Assessment of potential for recovery.
  - Helpful in determining choice of procedures.
- Direct laryngoscopy
  - Palpation of the vocal process and joints to rule out immobility.
  - Evaluation for webs or stenoses.

Vocal cord injection
Routes
- Percutaneous with fiberoptic flexible laryngoscopy.
- Transoral with direct laryngoscopy.

Temporary medialization
- Autologous fat.
- Collagen.
- Gelatin sponge (Gelfoam).

Permanent medialization
- Teflon (rarely used).

Procedure
- Ideally performed under local anesthesia.
- Can be performed with general anesthesia and jet ventilation.

Standard transoral procedure
- After local anesthetic applied, direct laryngoscope is introduced.
- Two injections are performed *lateral to the vocalis muscle.*
- Injection made with Bruening pistol syringe.
- First injection at level of vocal process; second injection at junction of anterior and middle thirds of the vocal cord.

Percutaneous injection
- Can inject through an anterior approach through the cricothyroid membrane, angling the needle laterally and posteriorly while passing it superiorly, or through the thyroid cartilage.
- Visualize cord with flexible fiberoptic laryngoscopy.

Complications
- Overinjection, managed with immediate removal through a mucosal incision or wait and watch.
- Underinjection.

- Inappropriate placement in vocalis.
- Loss of mucosal wave.
- Subglottic injection leading to stenosis.
- Teflon granuloma (excise).

External approaches: medialization thyroplasty (Isshiki Type I)
- Potentially reversible.
- May not adequately address a large posterior glottic chink or vocal cords at different levels.

Indications
- Vocal cord paralysis.
- Significant bowing and wasting of the cord.
- Loss of glottic tissue secondary to resection (e.g., partial cordectomy for cancer).

Advantages
- Allows more precise, anatomic correction of defect.
- Potentially reversible.
- Subperichondrial, therefore no disruption of mucosal wave.

Disadvantages
- Technically more difficult.
- Possibility of dislodged prosthesis.
- Patient subjected to open procedure.

Technique
- Local anesthetic preferred.
- Expose thyroid cartilage lamina.
- Create perichondrial window (5-8 mm posterior to vertical line, superior edge at level of vocal cord).
- Elevate perichondrium off inner aspect of lamina.
- Place prosthesis.
- May use preformed templates to determine ideal size.
- May use preformed silastic or hydroxyapatite prostheses or cut silastic block to size.
- A slight degree of overcorrection advised.

Complications
- Violation of mucosa.
- Wound infection.
- Implant migration or extrusion.
- Airway obstruction.

Arytenoid adduction
Indications
- Reduction of large posterior glottic chink where silastic implant is minimally effective.
- Different level of TVC causes bowing and drooping of paralyzed side.
- High CN X injury.
  - External branch of SLN innervating cricothyroid and RLN paralyzed.

- ❑ Downward displacement of vocal process in adduction.
- ❑ Upward displacement during abduction.
- Other common indications include intrathoracic malignancies.
- Can be performed separately or with Type I thyroplasty.
- Contraindicated in any patient with possible recovery of nerve function.

Procedure
1. After injecting local anesthetic, expose the thyroid cartilage at posterior margin.
2. Make a division along the attachment of the inferior pharyngeal constrictor muscle.
3. Perform a lateral reflection of the inner perichondrium and pyriform recess mucosa.
4. Incise the PCA posterior to the muscular process and the disarticulate cricoarytenoid joint.
   - Early prolapse of the arytenoid into the laryngeal introitus can occur due to disarticulation of the cricoarytenoid joint. Thus, not all practitioners perform this maneuver.
5. Identify the muscular process of the arytenoid cartilage.
6. Place a suture around the muscular process and pass it inferiorly to the thyroid ala.
7. Secure the suture at a point on the anterior surface of the ipsilateral ala:
   a. Two thirds distance of vertical height of cartilage.
   b. 6-10 mm from the anterior commissure.
8. Secure with microplate or nonabsorbable sutures.
9. Others perform a thyrotomy window and direct sutures through it.

Complications
- Laryngospasm.
- Violation of piriform mucosa = termination of procedure.
- Opening of cricoarytenoid joint = long-term ankylosis; thus procedure is permanent.
- Seroma.
- Hematoma.
- Significant airway edema (5%-10%).
- Local infection.

Outcome
- Improvement occurs in hoarseness, dyspnea, and decreased aspiration.
- Cadaveric studies indicate a reduction in distance between vocal processes and 3.5 mm vertical displacement (caudal) of the vocal process without change in vocal fold length.
- Combined medialization laryngoplasty and arytenoid adduction.

- Superior glottic efficiency.
- Superior sound production.

Bilateral vocal cord paralysis
Classification
- Abductor paralysis: glottic chink at posterior commissure 2-3 mm
- Adductor paralysis: cords at maximal abducted position.

Etiology
- Congenital: Hydrocephalus, meningomyelocele, Arnold-Chiari malformation, meningocele, encephalocele, cerebral agenesis, nucleus ambiguus dysgenesis, myasthenia gravis, neuromuscular disorders.
- Acquired
- Traumatic: external—blunt or penetrating.
- Surgery: thyroidectomy, cardiothoracic, skull base (rarely bilateral).
- Intubation
   - ❑ Disarticulation of arytenoids.
   - ❑ Bilateral nerve palsy from balloon pressure.
   - ❑ Posterior glottic stenosis.
- Neoplastic: thyroid carcinoma, esophageal carcinoma, laryngeal carcinoma, bronchogenic carcinoma.
- Neurologic
   - ❑ Cortical: vascular, traumatic
   - ❑ Subcortical: poliomyelitis, pseudobulbar palsy, amyotrophic lateral sclerosis, multiple sclerosis, encephalitis, bulbar palsy.
- Infectious: syphilis.
- Toxic: Vinca alkaloids, insecticide poisoning.
- Idiopathic.

Clinical presentation
- Abductor paralysis: stridor, airway obstruction.
- Adductor paralysis: aphonia, aspiration.
- Patients with bilateral vocal cord paralysis typically with good voice; main problem: airway compromise from an inability to abduct the vocal folds.
- Commonly present with airway obstruction during upper respiratory tract infections.

Evaluation
- Laryngoscopy and/or videostroboscopy
   - ❑ Above nodose ganglion: cords in abducted position (both recurrent and superior laryngeal nerves out).
   - ❑ Below nodose ganglion: cords in paramedian position.
- Laryngeal EMG
   - ❑ Innervation: quiescent tracing at rest, increased firing with voluntary motor activity.
   - ❑ Denervation: fibrillation potentials and positive sharp waves, decreased frequency of muscle firing.
   - ❑ Reinnervation: polyphasic motor potentials.

- CXR.
- CT with contrast and/or MRI scan: head, neck, and upper chest-tracing course of vagus and recurrent laryngeal nerves.
- Spirometry.
- Direct laryngoscopy
  - Palpation of arytenoids: rule out arytenoid fixation.
  - Rule out subglottic stenosis.
- Bronchoscopy: rule out tumor.

Treatment
Tracheotomy
- Almost always necessary as an initial procedure to improve the airway.
- Offers immediate relief of the airway obstruction without making the residual voice worse.
- In most cases, can be occluded the majority of the time, and uncapped at night, when exercising, and during URIs.
- Disadvantages: creation of a stoma with cosmetic and long-term care implications.

Surgical lateralization. Multiple techniques have been described to remove the arytenoid cartilage and/or lateralize the paralyzed vocal fold to improve the glottic airway. In general, all of these techniques improve the airway at the expense of worsening the quality of the voice and possibly increasing the potential for aspiration. In potentially reversible cases, lateralization is generally postponed for 6 months. A tracheotomy may be required during this period. The maximum success rate for any procedure is generally 70%.
- **Arytenoidectomy**
  - Involves the removal of part or all of the arytenoid cartilage to create a posterior glottic chink large enough to allow adequate ventilation. In general, an opening of 4 mm is considered adequate for normal adults, whereas a chink of 6 mm or more will likely result in problems with breathiness and aspiration.
  - May be accomplished endoscopically, using microsurgical techniques or CO_2 laser, or via an anterior thyrotomy or lateral approach.
  - The endoscopic approaches depend partially on scar contracture to keep the vocal cord lateralized, whereas the external approaches generally use a suture to fix the vocal process in the lateralized position (Woodman).
  - Endoscopic laser arytenoidectomy is currently the most common approach used.
  - Procedure for endoscopic arytenoidectomy:
1. Perform the procedure under general anesthesia, introducing a flame-resistant tube through a tracheostomy.

2. Suspend an adult Dedo laryngoscopy and bring an operating microscopy with a 400-mm lens into position.
3. Use a CO_2 laser in the continuous-pulse mode to vaporize the arytenoid, beginning at the vocal proceeding in a superior direction.
4. Vaporize the mucoperichondrium over the corniculate cartilage and the apex of the arytenoid to expose the underlying cartilage. Then vaporize the cartilage sequentially.
5. Next, vaporize the mucosa and perichondrium overlying the superior aspect of the body of the arytenoid.
6. Remove the interior aspect of the body of the arytenoid by working from lateral to medial down to the underlying cricoid cartilage. Medially, the muscular and vocal processes remain.
7. Lastly, vaporize the vocal process with a small portion adjacent vocalis muscle. Begin the mucosal cut 2-3 mm in front of the vocal process and bevel it posterolaterally to create a triangular notch in the glottic airway.
8. Take care to avoid injury to the mucosa in the interarytenoid area because scar contracture in this area may lead to further airway stenosis.
9. Routine use of perioperative tracheotomy, antibiotics, and antireflux medications is advocated.
   - Postoperative care:
     - Routine tracheotomy care is initiated.
     - A diet is introduced when the patient can swallow comfortably.
     - Some aspiration is expected. The use of a supraglottic swallow may assist with eating.
     - When the mucosal defect is healed, decannulation may be entertained.
   - Vocal cord lateralization (arytenoidopexy)
     - Involves displacing the vocal fold and arytenoid without surgical removal of tissue. Can be done endoscopically with a suture passed around the vocal process of the arytenoid and secured laterally. Has a relatively high failure rate.
- **Cordotomy**
  - A transverse incision is made with the CO_2 laser through the vocal cord and thyroarytenoid muscle immediately anterior to the vocal process. Postoperative contracture of the cut thyroarytenoid muscle results in a wedge-shaped widening of the posterior glottis, maintaining airway patency. The release of the vocal cord from the arytenoid minimizes dysphonia and decreases risk of aspiration.
- **Nerve muscle transposition**
  - Introduced by Tucker in 1976, this procedure involves grafting a neuromuscular pedicle (based on the omohyoid and ansa hypoglossi) to the

posterior cricoarytenoid muscle in an attempt to recover adductor function. Tucker's success rate of 80% has not been duplicated by other surgeons. Critics of the procedure claim that postoperative scarring results in movement of the arytenoid by the extralaryngeal musculature.

Management of bilateral vocal fold paralysis with weak voice and aspiration

This an unusual condition, and methods effective with unilateral adductor paralysis (Teflon injection, thyroplasty, arytenoid adduction) are not effective in this setting. Usually, a more definitive procedure to confront the problem of aspiration is necessary. A narrow-field laryngectomy is the most effective method of preventing aspiration, but it eliminates the larynx as an organ of communication. Reversible procedures to prevent aspiration include the epiglottic sew-down, surgical approximation of the vocal cords, and tracheal diversion procedures.

 GLOTTIC STENOSIS

Etiology
- Trauma
  - External (blunt, penetrating).
  - Internal (intubation, radiation, burn).
- Infection
  - Diphtheria.
  - Syphilis.
  - Mycobacteria.
- Inflammation
  - Wegener's granulomatosis.
  - Sarcoid.
  - Relapsing polychondritis.
- Neoplasm
  - Benign.
    - Intrinsic (e.g., papilloma).
  - Malignant (usually iatrogenic postradiation or laser therapy).

Diagnosis
- The following factors regarding the stenosis must be identified:
  - Location.
  - Dimensions.
  - Degree of fibrosis
  - Vocal cord mobility
  - Functional impairment.
- These factors are determined using the following evaluations:
  - Laryngoscopy.
  - Bronchoscopy.
  - Flow/volume loop.
  - CT (fine cuts of the larynx).

Treatment
Acute
- Initiate treatment as soon as possible (some consider 3-10 days postinjury as ideal).
- Endoscopy: for granulomas or granulations.
- Open repair for blunt or penetrating trauma.

Chronic
Supraglottic
- Usually from blunt trauma directed posterosuperiorly.

Pathology
- Epiglottis adherent to posterior or lateral walls.
- Fracture of the hyoid with or without displacement.
- Horizontal web running from posterior wall to epiglottis.
- Postcricoid/hypopharyngeal stenosis.

Treatment
- Transhyoid (anterior pharyngotomy with or without lateral pharyngotomy).
- Hyoid fracture (reduce or excise).
- Lyse adhesions/webs.
- Repair with
  - Undermine mucosa and direct repair.
  - Superiorly based mucosal flaps.
  - Free skin or mucosal grafts.
  - Free radial forearm flap if full thickness loss.

Laryngeal Inlet Stenosis

Pathology
- Posterior displacement of epiglottis and hyoid.
- With or without fracture of the thyroid notch.

Treatment
- Perform a laryngofissure.
- Incise the thyrohyoid membrane.
- Excise the base of the epiglottis.
- Incise the anterior fascia, perichondrium, and cartilage in an inverted "V."
- Elevate the laryngeal surface of the perichondrium off the incised cartilage.
- Resect the inverted "V" cartilage.
- Incise the remaining perichondrium in the midline, creating two flaps.
- Turn the mucosal flaps outward and sew them to the anterior surface of the perichondrium.

Glottic Stenosis

Anterior glottic stenosis
- Etiology of *anterior glottic stenosis* is typically external trauma to the thyroid cartilage, surgical removal of

mucosa overlying anterior surface of both vocal cords, or endotracheal trauma

Treatment
Endoscopic procedure
- If scar does not extend below inferior end of true vocal cord.
- Normal posterior commissure.
- Excision of scar endoscopically with microinstruments or CO_2 laser.
- Keel placed and stabilized with wires or sutures.

External laryngofissure
- Height greater than 5 mm subglottic extension.
- Laryngeal inlet extension.
- Fracture of thyroid cartilage leading to decreased AP length of glottis.
- Failed endoscopic treatment.
- Resection of scar with retention of mucosa.
- Skin and/or mucosal grafts with stents.

Posterior glottic stenosis
- Usually arises from intubation trauma, occasionally from arthritis.

Classification
- Class I: Interarytenoid adhesion with posterior sinus.
- Class II: Posterior commissure stenosis.
- Class III: Posterior commissure stenosis with unilateral cricoarytenoid ankylosis.
- Class IV: Posterior commissure stenosis with bilateral cricoarytenoid ankylosis.

Evaluation
- Must be differentiated from bilateral vocal cord paralysis with:
  - EMG.
  - Direct laryngoscopy with palpation of arytenoids.

Treatment
Class I
- Division of web.
- Fingercot splint × 2 weeks.

Class II (posterior commissure stenosis)
Endoscopic
- Incise: knife or laser
- Posterior micro-trap door flap if less than 3-4 mm (e.g., from interarytenoid or postcricoid region).
- If greater than 3-4 mm, soft keel × 4-6 weeks, which widens the mucosa with subsequent micro-trap door flap.

External Approach
- Used with height greater than 3-4 mm.

- Laryngofissure.
- Incise scar.
- Superiorly based mucosal flap.

Class III
- Laryngofissure with resection of scar.
- If one arytenoid mobile, no further resection.
- Mucosal flap or graft.

Class IV
- Arytenoidectomy (see section on bilateral vocal cord paralysis).

Complete glottic stenosis
- Severe injury.
- Laryngofissure.
- Scar excision with mucosa retention.
- Split skin or mucosal graft.
- Stent 4-8 weeks, then keel × 2 weeks.

Epiglottic flap
- Used in:
  - Severe glottic stenosis with greater than 50% reduction in glottic A-P dimension.
  - Glottic and subglottic stenosis.
  - Glottic and supraglottic stenosis.
    - Laryngofissure.
    - Excision of scar with mucosa retention.
    - Division of median thyroepiglottic ligament.
    - Epiglottis pulled inferiorly to the anterior cricoid and sutured in place, leading to an increased anterior commissure.

Subglottic Stenosis

Children
- Etiology most commonly from endotracheal intubation.
- Between 1% and 8% of children who have undergone intubation develop subglottic stenosis.

Symptoms
- Most common: biphasic stridor, worse with feeding or URI.
- Hoarseness: may or may not be present.
- Delayed growth.

Investigations
- AP and lateral neck.
- PA and lateral chest.
- CT or MRI.
- Bronchoscopy: if stenosis severe, may require a tracheotomy; postbronchoscopy steroids.
- Grade of stenosis determined with bronchoscopy (according to cotton):
  - Grade I: 0%-50% stenosis.

- ❑ Grade II: 51%-70% stenosis.
- ❑ Grade III: 71%-99% stenosis.
- ❑ Grade IV: no detectable lumen.
- ▪ Swallowing evaluation for aspiration.
  - ❑ Modified barium swallow or flexible endoscopic evaluation of swallowing (FEES).

Adult

- ▪ Endoscopic repair indicated in:
  - ❑ Adult without glottic pathology.
  - ❑ < 10 mm height (> 4 mm repair requires a tracheostomy).
  - ❑ CO_2 laser excision of superior surface of the scar and submucosal scar.
  - ❑ Inferiorly based mucosal flaps to resurface.
- ▪ External repair
  - ❑ Subglottic stenosis with mature submucosal scar *without* need for cartilaginous support:
    - • Resection of scar, buccal mucosa or split skin grafts, stent.
  - ❑ Subglottic stenosis with mature submucosal scar *with* need for cartilaginous support:
    - • Add autogenous cartilage graft (costal cartilage, septal cartilage with mucosa will provide up to 3 cm of augmentation without the need for a stent but cannot be used in children).
- ▪ Alternative repairs
  - ❑ Subglottic stenosis, with or without anterior glottic stenosis, with or without tracheal stenosis
    - • Pedicled flap, body of hyoid with periosteum pedicled to stylohyoid muscle.
      - ○ Interposed vertically into the defect and sutured.
      - ○ Stent only if epidermal graft required.
      - ○ Versatile single-stage procedure.
      - ○ Limited augmentation.
      - ○ Prone to granulation formation.
    - • Ipsilateral thyroid lamina with ipsilateral and contralateral perichondrium pedicled on sternothyroid
      - ○ Stent 1-6 weeks.
      - ○ Single stage procedure with a larger piece of cartilage and perichondrium (to minimize granulations).
    - • Clavicular perichondrium pedicled to sternocleidomastoid, up to 8 × 4–cm stent, gives rise to rigid bone formation.
  - ❑ Severe subglottic stenosis with or without glottic stenosis
    - • Division of posterior cricoid lamina with or without interarytenoid muscle.
    - • Can place anterior and posterior interposition grafts.
    - • Stent × 3 months.

If above techniques fail:

- ▪ Partial cricoid resection with thyrotracheal anastomosis.
  - ❑ 1 cm of normal lumen below glottis is required.
  - ❑ Complications include recurrent laryngeal nerve injury or dehiscence.
- ▪ Laryngeal release
  - ❑ May be needed for cricoid resection with thyrotracheal anastomosis or for tracheal stenosis repair.

Techniques

1. Incision of annular ligaments = 2.5 cm.
2. Superior mobilization of trachea from thorax with transection of left mainstem bronchus with end to side anastomosis with right mainstem bronchus = 6 cm
3. Infrahyoid release of larynx with transection of sternohyoid, omohyoid, and thyrohyoid muscles at the level of superior border of thyroid cartilage and division of greater cornu of thyroid cartilage. Risks damage of superior laryngeal nerve. Results in 5 cm of length.
4. Suprahyoid release (preferred). Transect mylohyoid, geniohyoid, genioglossus; expose pre-epiglottic space. Transect insertion of stylohyoid = 5 cm + 1-2 cm with postoperative neck flexion.

 FOREIGN BODIES

Esophageal Foreign Bodies

Epidemiology

- ▪ Approximately 1500 deaths annually from complications.
- ▪ Most often in children; coins most frequent, followed by food.

Diagnosis

- ▪ Adults: have more straightforward history (fishbones, dentures, meat and meat bones).
- ▪ Can lead to stricture of the esophagus or may be associated with an existing stricture (often the initial presentation of cancer is esophageal obstruction).
- ▪ Symptoms:
  - ❑ Adults frequently have dysphagia, drooling, vomiting, or chest pain, and occasionally airway symptoms.
  - ❑ Children often have vomiting and odynophagia and airway symptoms.
- ▪ Type and description of foreign body important to know (to prepare for removal).

Site of obstruction

- ▪ Upper and lower esophageal sphincter.
- ▪ Coins most commonly in postcricoid are or esophageal inlet. Disk-shaped objects often in cervical

esophagus distal to the cricopharyngeus or at inferior constrictor.

Investigations
- Chest x-ray: anteroposterior and lateral.
- Esophagogram possibly helpful (but to be avoided in those who might aspirate).

Treatment
- Can try conservative treatment, particularly in adult, if stable. Intravenous valium, glucagon may allow for passage of foreign body (particularly a food bolus).
- Most often removal under anesthesia through a rigid endoscope.
- Small disk-shaped batteries: emergencies; they contain alkaline materials that can cause caustic burns.
- With a rigid esophagoscope, physician must find the object, grasp with forceps, advance scope over object, and remove entire apparatus (to protect proximal mucosa).
- Patient reexamined endoscopically for second fiberoptic bronchoscopy (FB), mucosal injury, tears.

Complications
- Perforation.
- Mucosal tears.
- Stricture.
- Tracheosophageal fistula (TEF).

Tracheobronchial Foreign Bodies

Epidemiology
- Three thousand deaths annually.
- Early diagnosis and treatment essential.
- Can be associated with chronic respiratory symptoms (recurrent pneumonia, pulmonary abscess).
- Incidence highest in very young children (most commonly peanuts).

Diagnosis
Symptoms
- Many clinically normal.
- Some patients with intermittent wheezing.
- Cough.
- Decreased breath sounds on auscultation.
- Stridor.

Investigations
- Chest radiographs during inspiratory and expiratory phase to look for differential expansion, atelectasis, hyperinflation, or opaque foreign bodies.

Treatment
- Perform bronchoscopy with rigid endoscope in children.
- In adults, use flexible endoscope.

- Rapid induction with mask, insert laryngoscope; then if no object, pass bronchoscope with forceps, then remove as one unit.
- Reexamine for other FB (5% incidence) and injury to the mucosa.
- Observe for 12-24 hours.

Complications of foreign body
- Airway obstruction.
- Cough.
- Stridor.
- Granuloma formation.

Complications of bronchoscopy
- Airway obstruction.
- Laryngeal edema.
- Bleeding.
- Postoperative laryngospasm.
- Undetected second FB.

Controversies
- Rigid vs. flexible endoscopes (flexible technically more difficult to remove foreign body but may avoid the risk of anesthesia).
- Role of corticosteroids (reduce traumatic edema but may mask symptoms of undiagnosed FB).

 ## GASTROESOPHAGEAL REFLUX DISEASE (GERD)

- Otorhinolaryngology patients seem to have patterns and mechanisms of GERD that are different from those typically seen by the gastroenterologist. Most otolaryngology patients deny heartburn and regurgitation. The failure rate of medical management is high (35%).
- GERD may be a factor in the development of laryngeal carcinoma and laryngeal stenosis.

Etiology and pathogenesis
- The antireflux barrier consists of four lines of defense: (1) the lower esophageal sphincter (LES), (2) esophageal acid clearance, (3) epithelial resistance, and (4) the upper esophageal sphincter (UES). In addition, salivary and gastroduodenal function substantially influence antireflux mechanisms. Thus the integrity of the antireflux barrier is inexorably tied to the process of deglutination and digestion. Failure of this barrier leaves one susceptible to GERD.

Clinical manifestations
- The most common symptom: hoarseness: 70%.
- Chronic cough: 50%.
- Globus pharyngeus: 47%.
- Heartburn or regurgitation: 43%.
- Chronic throat clearing: 42%.

- Dysphagia: 35%.
- Note: 57% of patients deny having heartburn or regurgitation.

Investigations

- Standard diagnostic test for GERD (i.e., barium swallow, acid perfusion test, and radionuclide scan) are of limited use when dealing with the otolaryngologic manifestations of GERD.
- The majority of diagnoses are made clinically. This is due to the poor sensitivity of these tests.
- Ambulatory 24-hour double-probe pH monitoring is the most sensitive and specific test for GERD; its role in diagnosing GERD is increasing as experience with the technique grows.

Management

- After 6 months of antireflux management, 85% of patients have resolution of their symptoms. The remaining 15% have recalcitrant symptoms despite aggressive therapy consisting of lifestyle and dietary modification and ranitidine.
- Of the patients who respond to management, approximately one half respond within 3 weeks to 3 months; the other half respond by 6 months.
- Many patients who fail medical management with H_2 blockers benefit from proton pump inhibitor therapy at acid-suppressive doses (e.g., omeprazole 20 mg 2-4× daily). Those who fail on medical therapy may be candidates for an endoscopic or open fundoplication.

Selected References from the Recent Literature

1. Altman KW, Wetmore RF, Marsh RR. Congenital airway abnormalities in patients requiring hospitalization. *Archives of Otolaryngology—Head & Neck Surgery* 1999;125:525-528.
2. Bath AP, Panarese A, Thevasagayam M *et al*: Paediatric subglottic stenosis. *Clinical Otolaryngology & Allied Sciences* 1999;24:117-121.
3. Benninger MS, Gillen JB, Altman JS. Changing etiology of vocal fold immobility. [Review] [15 refs]. *Laryngoscope* 1998;108:1346-1350.
4. Carding PN, Horsley IA, Docherty GJ: A study of the effectiveness of voice therapy in the treatment of 45 patients with nonorganic dysphonia. [Review] [77 refs]. *Journal of Voice* 1999;13:72-104.
5. Carr MM, Nguyen A, Poje C *et al*. Correlation of findings on direct laryngoscopy and bronchoscopy with presence of extraesophageal reflux disease. *Laryngoscope* 2000;110: 1560-1562.
6. Casper JK, Murry T. Voice therapy methods in dysphonia. [Review] [58 refs]. *Otolaryngologic Clinics of North America* 2000;33:983-1002.
7. Choi SS, Zalzal GH. Changing trends in neonatal subglottic stenosis. *Otolaryngology—Head & Neck Surgery* 2000;122: 61-63.
8. de Jong AL, Kuppersmith RB, Sulek M *et al*. Vocal cord paralysis in infants and children. [Review] [86 refs]. *Otolaryngologic Clinics of North America* 2000;33:131-149.
9. Esclamado RM, Carroll WR. Repair of a complete glottic-subglottic stenosis with a fibular osseocutaneous free flap. *Archives of Otolaryngology—Head & Neck Surgery* 1997;123: 877-879.
10. Ford CN. Advances and refinements in phonosurgery. [Review] [77 refs]. *Laryngoscope* 1999;109:1891-1900.
11. Francois M, Dumont A, Narcy P. Longitudinal survey of voice quality after pediatric laryngotracheoplasty. *International Journal of Pediatric Otorhinolaryngology* 1997;40: 163-172.
12. Gardner GM. Posterior glottic stenosis and bilateral vocal fold immobility: diagnosis and treatment. [Review] [85 refs]. *Otolaryngologic Clinics of North America* 2000;33:855-878.
13. Gavilan J, Cerdeira MA, Toledano A. Surgical treatment of laryngotracheal stenosis: a review of 60 cases. *Annals of Otology, Rhinology & Laryngology* 1998;107:588-592.
14. Giannoni C, Sulek M, Friedman EM *et al*. Gastroesophageal reflux association with laryngomalacia: a prospective study. *International Journal of Pediatric.Otorhinolaryngology* 1998;43: 11-20.
15. Goldberg AN. Endoscopic postcricoid advancement flap for posterior glottic stenosis. *Laryngoscope* 2000;110:482-485.
16. Graham J: The effect of stents on mucosal wound healing [letter]. *International Journal of Pediatric Otorhinolaryngology* 2000;53:169-171.
17. Halstead LA. Gastroesophageal reflux: A critical factor in pediatric subglottic stenosis. *Otolaryngology—Head & Neck Surgery* 1999;120:683-688.
18. Hanson DG, Jiang JJ: Diagnosis and management of chronic laryngitis associated with reflux. [Review] [24 refs]. *American Journal of Medicine* 2000;108(Suppl 4a):112S-119S.
19. Harries ML. Laryngeal framework surgery (thyroplasty) [editorial]. [Review] [14 refs]. *Journal of Laryngology & Otology* 1997;111:103-105.
20. Harrill WC, Stasney CR, Donovan DT: Laryngopharyngeal reflux: a possible risk factor in laryngeal and hypopharyngeal carcinoma. *Otolaryngology—Head & Neck Surgery* 1999;120:598-601.
21. Havas TE, Priestley J, Lowinger DS. A management strategy for vocal process granulomas. *Laryngoscope* 1999;109: 301-306.
22. Hillel AD, Benninger M, Blitzer A *et al*. Evaluation and management of bilateral vocal cord immobility. [Review] [34 refs]. *Otolaryngology—Head & Neck Surgery* 1999;121:760-765.
23. Hoasjoe DK, Franklin SW, Aarstad RF *et al*. Posterior glottic stenosis mechanism and surgical management. *Laryngoscope* 1997;107:675-679.
24. Hoeve LJ, Kuppers GL, Verwoerd CD. Management of infantile subglottic hemangioma: laser vaporization, submucous resection, intubation, or intralesional steroids? *International Journal of Pediatric Otorhinolaryngology* 199742:179-186.
25. Holinger LD. Histopathology of congenital subglottic stenosis. *Annals of Otology, Rhinology & Laryngology* 1999108: 101-111.
26. Irving RM, Epstein R, Harries ML. Care of the professional voice. [Review] [23 refs]. *Clinical Otolaryngology & Allied Sciences* 1997;22:202-205.

27. Isshiki N. Mechanical and dynamic aspects of voice production as related to voice therapy and phonosurgery [editorial]. [Review] [51 refs]. *Otolaryngology—Head & Neck Surgery* 2000;122:782-793.

28. Isshiki N. Mechapnical and dynamic aspects of voice production as related to voice therapy and phonosurgery. [Review] [51 refs]. *Journal of Voice* 1998;12:125-137.

29. Kuhn J, Toohill RJ, Ulualp SO *et al.* Pharyngeal acid reflux events in patients with vocal cord nodules. *Laryngoscope* 1998;108:1146-1149.

30. Lano CFJ, Duncavage JA, Reinisch L *et al.* Laryngotracheal reconstruction in the adult: a ten year experience. *Annals of Otology, Rhinology & Laryngology* 1998;107:92-97.

31. Lesperance MM, Zalzal GH. Laryngotracheal stenosis in children. [Review] [25 refs]. *European Archives of Oto-Rhino-Laryngology* 1998;255:12-17.

32. Ludemann JP, Hughes CA, Noah Z *et al.* Complications of pediatric laryngotracheal reconstruction: prevention strategies. *Annals of Otology, Rhinology & Laryngology* 1999;108: 1019-1026.

33. Lundy DS, Casiano RR, Shatz D *et al.* Laryngeal injuries after short-versus long-term intubation. *Journal of Voice* 1998;12: 360-365.

34. Massie RJ, Robertson CF, Berkowitz RG. Long-term outcome of surgically treated acquired subglottic stenosis in infancy. *Pediatric Pulmonology* 2000;30:125-130.

35. McGuirt WFJ, Little JP, Healy GB. Anterior cricoid split. Use of hyoid as autologous grafting material. *Archives of Otolaryngology—Head & Neck Surgery* 1997;123:1277-1280.

36. McMurray JS: Medical and surgical treatment of pediatric dysphonia. [Review] [35 refs]. *Otolaryngologic Clinics of North America* 2000;33:1111-1126.

37. Milczuk HA, Smith JD, Everts EC. Congenital laryngeal webs: surgical management and clinical embryology. *International Journal of Pediatric Otorhinolaryngology* 2000; 52:1-9.

38. Mishra S, Rosen CA, Murry T: Acute management of the performing voice. [Review] [14 refs]. *Otolaryngologic Clinics of North America* 2000;33:957-966.

39. Monnier P, Lang F, Savary M: Cricotracheal resection for pediatric subglottic stenosis. International Journal of Pediatric.Otorhinolaryngology.1999.Oct.5 49 Suppl 1:S283-S286.

40. Morrison MD, Nichol H, Rammage LA. Diagnostic criteria in functional dysphonia. *Laryngoscope* 1986;94:1-8.

41. Moungthong G, Holinger LD. Laryngotracheoesophageal clefts. *Annals of Otology, Rhinology & Laryngology* 1997;106: 1002-1011.

42. Cotton RT. Management of subglottic stenosis. [Review] [34 refs]. *Otolaryngologic Clinics of North America* 2000;33: 111-130.

43. Murry T, Rosen CA: Vocal education for the professional voice user and singer. [Review] [10 refs]. *Otolaryngologic Clinics of North America* 2000;33:967-982.

44. Perkins JA, Inglis AFJ, Richardson MA. Iatrogenic airway stenosis with recurrent respiratory papillomatosis. *Archives of Otolaryngology—Head & Neck Surgery* 1998;124: 281-287.

45. Picerno NA, Bent JP, Hammond J *et al.* Is tracheotomy decannulation possible in oxygen-dependent children? *Otolaryngology—Head & Neck Surgery* 2000;123:263-268.

46. Rahbar R, Valdez TA, Shapshay SM. Preliminary results of intraoperative mitomycin-C in the treatment and prevention of glottic and subglottic stenosis. *Journal of Voice* 2000;14:282-286.

47. Ramig LO, Verdolini K. Treatment efficacy: voice disorders. [Review] [181 refs]. *Journal of Speech, Language, & Hearing Research* 1998;41:S101-S116.

48. Richter JE, Hicks DM: Unresolved issues in gastroesophageal reflux-related ear, nose, and throat problems [editorial; comment]. *American Journal of Gastroenterology* 1997;92:2143-2144.

49. Rimell FL, Dohar JE. Endoscopic management of pediatric posterior glottic stenosis. *Annals of Otology, Rhinology & Laryngology* 1998;107:285-290.

50. Roger G, Denoyelle F, Garabedian EN. Disorders of laryngeal mobility in children. [Review] [8 refs]. *Pediatric Pulmonology Supplement* 1997;16:105-107.

51. Rosen CA. Phonosurgical vocal fold injection: procedures and materials. [Review] [19 refs]. *Otolaryngologic Clinics of North America* 200033:1087-1096.

52. Rosen CA, Murry T: Nomenclature of voice disorders and vocal pathology. [Review] [20 refs]. *Otolaryngologic Clinics of North America* 2000;33:1035-1046.

53. Rovo L, Jori J, Brzozka M *et al.* Minimally invasive surgery for posterior glottic stenosis. *Otolaryngology—Head & Neck Surgery* 1999;121:153-156.

54. Roy N, McGrory JJ, Tasko SM *et al.* Psychological correlates of functional dysphonia: an investigation using the Minnesota Multiphasic Personality Inventory [published erratum appears in J Voice 1998 Jun;12(2):following 261]. [Review] [48 refs]. *Journal of Voice* 1997;11:443-451.

55. Rubin JS, Lieberman J, Harris TM. Laryngeal manipulation. [Review] [29 refs]. *Otolaryngologic Clinics of North America* 2000;33:1017-1034.

56. Saunders MW, Thirlwall A, Jacob A *et al.* Single-or-two-stage laryngotracheal reconstruction; comparison of outcomes. *International Journal of Pediatric Otorhinolaryngology* 1999;50: 51-54.

57. Shaker R. Protective mechanisms against supraesophageal GERD. *Journal of Clinical Gastroenterology* 2000;30:S3-S8.

58. Sichel JY, Dangoor E, Eliashar R *et al.* Management of congenital laryngeal malformations. [Review] [65 refs]. *American Journal of Otolaryngology* 2000;21:22-30.

59. Silva AB, Lusk RP, Muntz HR. Update on the use of auricular cartilage in laryngotracheal reconstruction. *Annals of Otology, Rhinology & Laryngology* 2000.109:343-347.

60. Sataloff RT: Evaluation of professional singers. [Review] [54 refs]. *Otolaryngologic Clinics of North America* 2000;33: 923-956.

61. Stolovitzky JP, Todd NW, Cotton RT et al. Autoimmune hypothesis of acquired subglottic stenosis: lack of support at time of surgical repair in children. *International Journal of Pediatric Otorhinolaryngology* 1997;38:255-261.

62. Veivers D, Laccourreye O. Supracricoid partial laryngectomy for severe laryngeal stenosis. *Archives of Otolaryngology—Head & Neck Surgery* 2000;126:663-664.

63. Verneuil A, Berke G. Improved method of insertion of a Montgomery T-tube. *Laryngoscope* 1999;109:1351-1353.

64. Walner DL, Stern Y, Gerber ME et al. Gastroesophageal reflux in patients with subglottic stenosis. *Archives of Otolaryngology—Head & Neck Surgery* 1998;124:551-555.

65. Wolf M, Yellin A, Talmi YP *et al.* Acquired tracheoesophageal fistula in critically ill patients. *Annals of Otology, Rhinology & Laryngology* 2000;109:731-735.

66. Woo P. Laryngeal electromyography is a cost-effective clinically useful tool in the evaluation of vocal fold function [see comments]. [Review] [11 refs]. *Archives of Otolaryngology—Head & Neck Surgery* 1998;124:472-475.

67. Yellon RF: The spectrum of reflux-associated otolaryngologic problems in infants and children. [Review] [34 refs]. *American Journal of Medicine* 1997;103:125S-129S.

68. Zalzal GH. Posterior glottic stenosis. *International Journal of Pediatric Otorhinolaryngology* 199949(Suppl 1):S279-S282.

69. Zalzal GH, Choi SS, Patel KM. Ideal timing of pediatric laryngotracheal reconstruction. *Archives of Otolaryngology—Head & Neck Surgery* 1997;123:206-208.

70. Zeitels SM. Phonomicrosurgery I: principles and equipment. [Review] [68 refs]. *Otolaryngologic Clinics of North America* 2000;33:1047-1062.

71. Zeitels SM, Hochman I, Hillman RE. Adduction arytenopexy: a new procedure for paralytic dysphonia with implications for implant medialization. [Review] [110 refs]. *Annals of Otology, Rhinology, & Laryngology Supplement* 1998;173:2-24.

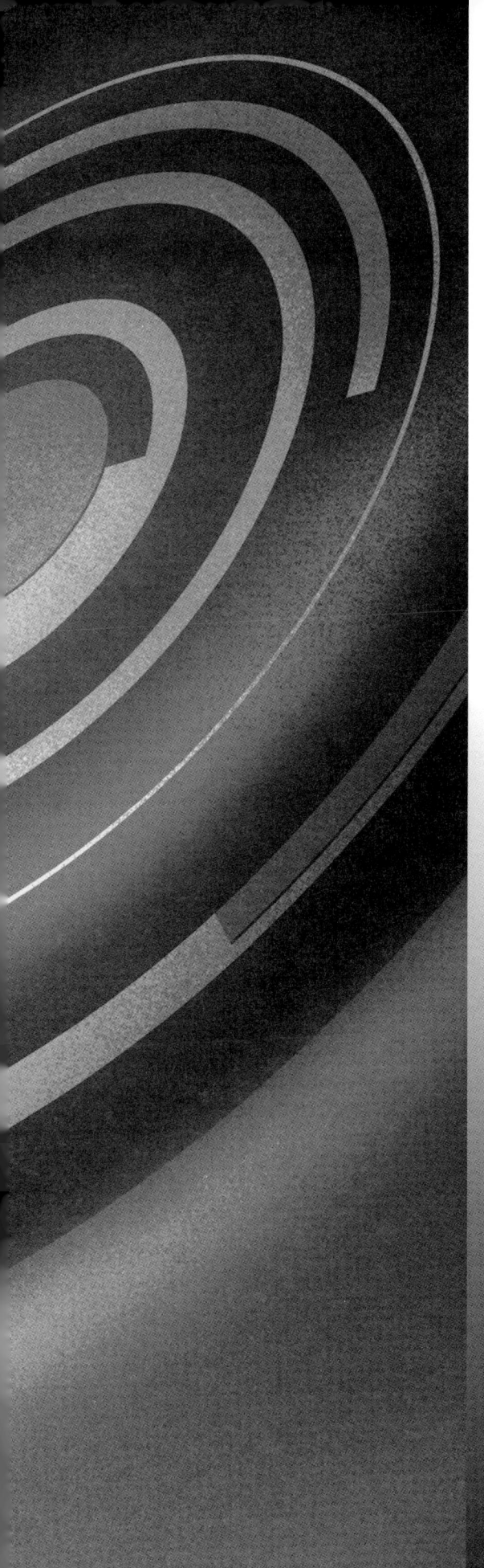

Disorders of the Head and Neck

SURGICAL MANAGEMENT OF THE AIRWAY

Crycothyroidotomy

Definition

- Creation of an opening in the cricothyroid membrane to create a patent airway.

Indications

- Acute airway obstruction secondary to an obstructive lesion that precludes intubation.

Contraindications

- Anatomic barrier (mass) preventing access to the cricothyroid membrane.

Technique

1. Identify cricoid cartilage and inferior border of thyroid cartilage.
2. Infiltrate with local anesthetic (if time permits).
3. Incise straight down and through cricothyroid membrane using a horizontal incision over the middle portion of the membrane.
4. Dilate incision using scissors, hemostat, or tracheal dilator.
5. Pass an endotracheal tube into airway.
6. Convert to formal tracheostomy when patient is stable.

Complications

- Bleeding.
- Tube displacement.
- Infection.
- True vocal cord damage.
- Subcutaneous emphysema.
- Subglottic or tracheal stenosis.
- Note: Cricothyroidotomy should not be used for long-term intubation because of laryngeal trauma

Open Tracheotomy/Tracheostomy

Definition

- A procedure designed to gain access to the tracheobronchial tree for purposes of providing ventilation. Technically a tracheo*stomy* involves creating a permanent stoma, whereas a tracheo*tomy* refers to incising the trachea; however, today the terms are used interchangeably.

Indications

- Airway obstruction.
- Prolonged ventilation (>1 week).
- Pulmonary toilet.

Contraindications

- No absolute contraindications. If the procedure is being performed on a patient with a stable airway (e.g. an intubated patient), coagulopathy should be reversed prior to performing a tracheostomy.

Technique

1. The patient's head is extended.
2. The lower midline of the neck is infiltrated with 1% lidocaine with epinephrine.
3. A *horizontal* incision is made halfway between the sternal notch and cricoid cartilage; a *vertical* midline incision may also be used.
4. Dissection is carried down to the strap muscles, which are then bisected in the midline.
5. If encountered, the thyroid isthmus may be:
   - Mobilized superiorly.
   - Mobilized inferiorly.
   - Transected with Bovie cautery.
   - Transected and ligated.
6. The balloon of the endotracheal tube in temporarily deflated and the trachea is incised below the second tracheal ring (typically between the second and third tracheal ring).
7. Vertical incisions are made.
8. An inferiorly based cartilaginous Bjork flap may be constructed and sutured to the skin.
9. The endotracheal tube is withdrawn under direct visualization.
10. A cuffed tracheostomy tube (no. 6 to no. 8 in an adult) is inserted and sewn to the skin.
11. The incision should not be closed or should be closed only loosely. A tight closure predisposes to subcutaneous emphysema and pneumothorax.
12. The tube may be changed every 5-7 days. Depending on the need for ventilation, a noncuffed, fenestrated tube may be placed.
13. A Passy-Muir one-way valve may be placed on the tube to allow for speech

Complications

Immediate complications

- Apnea secondary to loss of hypoxic drive; treatment with ventilation.
- Bleeding; controlled with cautery and/or suture ligation.
- False passage.
- Pneumothorax/pneumomediastinum (incidence = up to 4% in adults and 10%-15% in children) results from direct injury to the pleural apices or to high negative inspiratory pressures during the procedure. Small pneumothoraces may be observed with serial chest radiographs; larger pneumothoraces will require a chest tube.

- Injury to adjacent structures, including the recurrent laryngeal nerves, carotid artery, jugular vein, and esophagus.
- Postobstructive pulmonary edema; rare and typically transient.

Early complications (within first 24-48 hours)
- Early bleeding, minor bleeding controlled by packing. Major arterial bleeding typically results from one of the thyroid vessels and requires reexploration in the operating room with the airway secured by intubation.
- Obstruction.
  - May result from:
    - Mucous plugging: treated with suctioning with saline irrigation.
    - Tube displacement: the patient should be emergently intubated and the tube replaced in the operating room or at the bedside.
- Cellulitis: treated with parenteral antibiotics and opening of the wound.
- Subcutaneous emphysema: make sure wound is open.
- Pneumothorax/pneumomediastinum: as above.
- Atelectasis: occurs when tube is inserted beyond the carina.

Late complications
- Bleeding
  - Minimal bleeding may result from granulation tissue, which can be cauterized.
  - A significant bleed, particularly if pulsatile, must be regarded as a "sentinel" bleed, possibly indicating the formation of a *tracheo-innominate* fistula (incidence = 0.6%-0.7%, mortality may be as high as 80%). These patients must be evaluated with tracheoscopy/bronchoscopy to identify the source of bleeding, and possibly an arteriogram. If a fistula is identified, a thoracotomy and repair is emergently indicated.
  - If the patient presents with a catastrophic bleed, an endotracheal tube is placed with the tip distal to the bleeding site. Inflation of the balloon will prevent aspiration and may tamponade the bleed. If the balloon fails to tamponade the bleed, digital pressure within the wound should be applied while the patient is transported for a thoracotomy.
- Tracheomalacia
  - Stenosis: subglottic stenosis may result from a "high tracheostomy." Tracheal stenosis may result from excessive balloon pressure.
  - Tracheoesophageal fistula: may occur as a result of pressure from the tip of tracheostomy tube, particularly if a nasogastric tube is in place. Requires surgical repair with interposition of a muscle flap and temporary jejunostomy.

- Persistent tracheocutaneous fistula: may respond to simple resection of the edges and subsequent granulation or may be repaired with a multilayer closure.

Percutaneous Tracheostomy
- This technique is performed in an ICU setting.

Indications
- Prolonged intubation.

Contraindications
- Coagulopathy.
- Distortion of neck anatomy caused by trauma or mass.

Technique
- Several commercially available kits may be used. All use slightly different techniques, which can be summarized as follows.
- A 1.5- to 2-cm incision is made over the second or third tracheal ring after the area is prepped and infiltrated with local anesthetic with epinephrine.
- The trachea is identified with a needle or via blunt dissection.
- A guidewire is passed into the trachea.
- The trachea around the guidewire is dilated, the tracheostomy tube is inserted over the guidewire, and the guidewire is removed.
- The risk of creating a false passage may be minimized by performing the procedure over a bronchoscope.
- The complications of this procedure are similar to those seen with an open technique, with the exception of an increased risk of creating of a false passage leading to loss of the airway. The mortality rate resulting from this procedure is approximately 0.5%.

 TRACHEAL STENOSIS

Etiology
- Congenital.
- Acquired: trauma, tracheostomy, intubation.

Clinical presentation
- Narrow stenosis and/or a long-segment stenosis will present in the newborn or early infancy.
- Less-severe stenosis and/or shorter-segment stenosis may present in later infancy or early childhood.
- Symptoms include:
  - Stridor: biphasic or expiratory.
  - "Atypical asthma."
  - Recurrent bronchitis/pneumonia.
  - Poor weight gain/poor feeding.

Investigations

- Endoscopy:
  - Should be performed under general anesthesia with spontaneous breathing.
  - Smallest bronchoscope (4.0 mm OD) may not pass through narrow stenosis, and use of a fiberoptic telescope may be required to estimate length of stenosis.
- MRI or CT scan will provide detailed views of trachea and accurately estimate length of stenosis. MRI scan provides slightly more definition.
- Bronchography with thin layer of contrast can be performed. However, there is a risk of the contrast material inducing inflammation and airway obstruction.

Treatment

Dilation

- Indicated for:
  - Soft granulation tissue.
  - Temporary relief of obstruction in premature or medically unstable patient who will ultimately require an open repair.
- Currently, dilation performed by a balloon catheter passed via bronchoscope and attached to saline-filled syringe.
- Progressively larger balloons are used.
- Balloon technique causes less soft tissue trauma than older, rigid bougie dilators.
- Complications include tracheitis, atelectasis, and pneumomediastinum.
- In appropriately selected patients, balloon tracheoplasty provides 90% short-term improvement and 50% long-term improvement.

Laser

- CO_2 laser indicated for elimination of soft granulation or a short segment of mature fibrosis.
- May be used in combination with dilation.
- Prone to failure in following situations:
  - Circumferential scarring.
  - Fibrosis >1 cm in vertical length.
  - Active bacterial tracheitis in the presence of a tracheostomy.
  - Tracheomalacia.
- Technique should involve creation of radial incisions maintaining interposed islands of mucosa.
- Mucosal flap may be elevated with lasering of the underlying fibrosis.

Stents

- May be placed endoscopically or via open approach.
- *Montgomery Silastic T-tube stent* may used to support soft tissue grafts and cartilage.
- Complications include:
  - Obstruction.
  - Granulation tissue formation.
  - Infection.
  - Malposition.
- *Expandable stents* made of stainless steel wire or polymers have been used in cases of unresectable malignancies and experimentally in animal models and humans with tracheal stenosis.
- In addition to the complications listed above, additional complications with these stents include perforation and extrusion.

Open repair

- Indicated in patients who fail more conservative management.

Tracheoplasty with autologous tissue

1. The trachea is exposed anteriorly and the extent of the stenosis is outlined endoscopically.
2. A vertical incision is made in the trachea exposing the stenosis.
3. Granulation tissue is resected and fibrous scar tissue is incised.
4. A costal cartilage graft is harvested from the fifth or sixth rib with preservation of the perichondrium on the anterior surface.
5. The cartilage graft is then fashioned to the appropriate size and placed in the tracheal incision, with the perichondrium on the luminal surface.
6. The graft is sutured in place using dissolvable sutures (e.g., Vicryl, Dexon).
7. Endotracheal intubation is maintained for 5-7 days.
- An Aboulker or T-tube stent may be used for longer-term support
- Some authors advocate the use of cardiac bypass, extracorporeal circulation, or distal intubation.
- Pericardium may be used in place of rib cartilage.
- Complications include:
  - Granulation tissue formation.
  - Breakdown of anastomosis.
  - Airway obstruction.
  - Infection.

Wedge resection

- Useful in localized stenosis involving one or two tracheal rings.
- Anterior wedge of trachea resected and primary closure performed.

Segmental resection

Used when tracheal stenosis involves <50% of the trachea length.
1. The length of the stenosis is defined endoscopically.
2. The stenotic portion is resected.

3. The reanastomosis is performed with submucosal sutures ties extraluminally.
4. A tension-free anastomosis must be achieved by:
   - Infrahyoid release.
   - Suprahyoid release.
   - Maintenance of neck flexion with chin-to-chest suture.
   - Intercartilaginous incisions.
   - Perihilar release.
   - Dissection of the pulmonary vessels.
   - Transplantation of the left mainstem bronchus.

- Complications include:
  - Granulation at anastomotic site (treated with laser bronchoscopy).
  - Anastomotic leak (treated with maneuvers to decrease tension).
  - Recurrent laryngeal nerve injury.
  - Aspiration.

Techniques for longer stenosis
- Slide tracheoplasty.
- Tracheal homografts.

CAUSTIC INGESTION

Incidence and epidemiology
Children
- Typically occur as accidental ingestion of cleaning agents.
- Volumes are variable because children usually cease ingesting a foul-tasting substance.
- Lye ingestions = 5000/year.

Adults
- Typically suicide attempts.
- Large volumes ingested.

Pathogenesis
Base solution (pH >7)
- Causes *liquefaction necrosis:*
  - Begins within seconds.
  - Only requires milliliters of a strong base (pH >12.5).
  - Edema and inflammation of the submucosa; leads to thrombosis and sloughing.
  - Necrosis of the underlying muscular layer.
  - Fibrosis or perforation of the deeper layer.
  - Delayed reepithelialization with or without stricture formation.
- Base in liquid form causes more damage than base in a granular form.

Acid (pH <7)
- Causes a *coagulation necrosis.*
- Injury takes longer to occur.
- Coagulum forms on the surface, which protects the deeper layers.

- As acid passes into stomach, may cause gastric injury.

Bleach (pH = 7)
- An irritant, does not "burn."

Clinical presentation
- Primary attention must be focused on the "ABCs," with focus on signs and symptoms of airway obstruction.
- Symptoms of hoarseness, dyspnea, and/or stridor suggest airway involvement.
- A flexible endoscopy may be performed to assess the upper airway *if* the patient is stable.
- If airway is stable, parenteral corticosteroids are indicated with observation in a monitored unit.
- If airway is not stable, intervention should include:
  - Direct or fiberoptic laryngoscopy with intubation.
  - Cricothyroidotomy or tracheostomy.
  - Blind nasotracheal intubation should be avoided to prevent further trauma.
- A chest x-ray is performed to evaluate for the presence of pulmonary infiltrates indicative of aspiration.
- Abdominal assessment should evaluate for epigastric tenderness and peritonitis indicative of a possible perforation.
- Once the patient is stabilized, assessment should be made of the upper digestive tract.
- Signs or symptoms of upper digestive tract involvement include:
  - Odynophagia/dysphagia.
  - Oral/pharyngeal erythema and/or ulceration.
  - Drooling.
  - Tongue edema.

Investigations and treatment
- As above for acute stabilization.
- If acid or granular base ingested in the absence of any of the above symptoms, the patient may be observed with gradual progression of diet. A barium swallow may be performed if the patient develops dysphagia.
- Esophagoscopy and/or gastroscopy are indicated in cases of granular base or acid if the patient is symptomatic, or in cases of liquid base ingestion.
- Esophagoscopy should be performed within 24-48 hours of injury. Esophagoscopy earlier than 24 hours may underestimate injury, and endoscopy later than 48 hours increases risk of perforation.
- Treatment is based on the findings on endoscopy.
  - *First-degree injury (mucosal erythema):* no treatment required.
  - *Second-degree injury (mucosal erythema with noncircumferential exudates):* Treat with anti-reflux regimen and gradual advance in diet.

❑ *Third-degree injury: Focal mucosal erythema with circumferential exudates:* Sucralfate and anti-reflux medications. Tube feeds are recommended until dysphagia resolves.

❑ *Third-degree injury: Diffuse mucosal erythema with circumferential exudates WITHOUT transmural necrosis:* requires the performance of gastrostomy for feeding and, if needed, retrograde dilatation.

❑ *Third-degree injury: Diffuse mucosal erythema with circumferential exudates WITH transmural necrosis or frank perforation:* requires the performance of an esophagectomy and/or partial gastrectomy with delayed esophageal reconstruction. Delayed reconstruction can be performed with a free jejunal or colonic transfer or gastric pull-up.

- All patients with second- and third-degree injuries managed conservatively should undergo a barium swallow at 3 weeks postinjury for evaluation of stricture.

 ESOPHAGEAL DIVERTICULA

Zenker's Diverticulum (Pharyngoesophageal Diverticulum)

Definition

- A pulsion diverticulum that occurs at a naturally occurring dehiscence between the inferior constrictor of the pharynx and the cricopharyngeal muscle (Killian's dehiscence).

Incidence and epidemiology

- Most common in countries whose populations originate from Northern Europe (e.g., North America, Australia); rare in Asians and Africans.
- Male:female = 2-3:1.
- Most frequently seen in adults in their seventh to eighth decades of life.
- Incidence in population undergoing contrast radiography = 1:1000. Symptomatic Zenker's diverticula occur with incidence of 2/100,000.

Pathophysiology

- A pulsion diverticulum of pharyngeal mucosa thought to originate because of dysfunction of the cricopharyngeal muscle. Abnormalities in function may include:
  - ❑ Abnormal timing of cricopharyngeal contraction and relaxation.
  - ❑ Incomplete relaxation of the cricopharyngeus.
  - ❑ Elevated resting tone of the upper esophageal sphincter.
  - ❑ Loss of cricopharyngeal elasticity.
  - ❑ Cricopharyngeal myopathy or neuropathy.

Clinical presentation

- Dysphagia (sticking sensation of food).
- Regurgitation of undigested food.
- Halitosis.
- Audible gurgling with external compression.
- Cough: worse after eating and when supine.
- Aspiration leading to pneumonia or pulmonary abscess.
- Neck mass (in 90% of cases on left).
- Hemorrhage.
- Weight loss.

Investigations

- Contrast radiography (barium swallow).

Treatment

- Asymptomatic diverticula require no treatment.

Endoscopic surgery

- Increasingly popular because of more rapid resumption of oral intake and decreased hospitalization and morbidity.
- Used for small to moderate diverticula (<6 cm).
- A modified Weerda diverticuloscope is inserted, with the anterior blade in the esophagus and the posterior blade in the diverticulum. Spreading of the blades exposes the "party wall," or bridge of cricopharyngeus.
- The bridge is then divided using a GI stapler that simultaneously staples the two sides and incises. Electrocautery and laser were previously used with lesser success.

Open surgery

- The two main open procedures currently performed are *diverticulopexy with cricopharyngeal myotomy* or *diverticulectomy with cricopharyngeal myotomy.*
  1. A curvilinear incision halfway between the hyoid and clavicle is made and subplatysmal flaps are elevated.
  2. The sternocleidomastoid muscle is retracted laterally.
  3. The omohyoid is divided or retracted and the remainder of the strap muscles is retracted medially.
  4. The carotid is retracted laterally.
  5. The thyroid may be reflected anteriorly with division of the middle thyroid vein, if necessary.
  6. The larynx and pharynx are retracted medially and rotated slightly.
  7. The retropharyngeal space is entered and blunt dissection and dissection along the anterior border of the prevertebral fascia will reveal the diverticulum, which is then dissected free.
  8. Depending on the position and size of the diverticulum, the recurrent laryngeal nerve may need to be identified.
  9. A cricopharyngeal myotomy is performed with care

not to violate the mucosa

10. The diverticulum is either excised or sutured to the superior prevertebral fascia (pexy). If excision is performed, a GI stapler is typically used. An older technique involves sharp excision and a suture closure with a Connell technique.
11. An NG tube is placed, as is a drain.
12. Oral liquid feeds are begun 24-48 hours after surgery if there is no evidence of a fistula.

Complications

- Mortality: 0%-10% with open procedure and 0%-1% with endoscopic procedure.
- Fistula (open procedure: typically close with conservative management and nutritional support)
- Mediastinitis: manifests with fever and tachycardia, treated with surgical exploration and drainage
- Recurrent laryngeal nerve paresis/paralysis.
- Hemorrhage.
- Esophageal stenosis (open procedure).
- Dental injury (endoscopic procedure).

Midesophageal Diverticula

- These are the most common esophageal diverticula.
- They are *traction* diverticula and occur secondary to granulomatous disease (tuberculosis, histoplasmosis).
- They are *rarely* symptomatic. When symptoms do occur, they are typically mild dysphagia or hemorrhage.
- Rarely require treatment.

Lower Esophageal Diverticula

- Also known as *epiphrenic diverticula*.
- These are pulsion diverticula and occur in the lower 10 cm of the thoracic esophagus.
- Typically associated with other esophageal disease.
- Rarely require specific treatment.

 ## TERATOMAS AND DERMOID CYSTS

Definition and etiology

- Teratomas and dermoid cysts are developmental anomalies involving pluripotential embryonal cells; they are alien to the site in which they arise. Several theories have been proposed to explain the existence of these lesions. Of the two most plausible, one suggests isolation of pluripotential cells occurring during embryogenesis and subsequent disorganized growth of these cells. The second theory holds that germ layers may be buried in deeper tissues at points of failed fusion lines.

Incidence

- Teratomas occur in 1:4000 births, with less than 10 affecting structures in the head and neck. They most commonly are found in the sacrococcygeal, mediastinal, retroperitoneal, and gonadal regions. Teratomas are usually evident early in patients at an early age, but no age group is immune. In the head and neck, the sites most commonly involved are the orbital region, nose, nasopharynx, oral cavity, and neck.

Pathology

- Teratomas and dermoid cysts are classified into four groups. This system recognizes both germ layer of origin and the complexity of tissue organization. Regardless of site, neurogenic tissue is a prominent feature of the lesion, especially in the head and neck area.

1. *Dermoid cysts* are the most common form of teratoma and are composed of ectoderm and mesoderm. They are covered with skin and contain epidermal appendages such as hair follicles. They may be cystic but more commonly have an adipose matrix. Most occur along lines of embryonic fusion. The true dermoid cyst and dermoid sinus contain skin appendages (hair follicles, sweat glands, and sebaceous glands). A true *dermoid cyst* may occur alone subcutaneously on the nasal dorsum superficial to the nasal bones without a cutaneous opening. Simple dermoid cysts therefore appear as slowly enlarging masses under the skin, which over time may deform the underlying structures. Histologically and surgically this lesion is easily removed by excision. The *dermoid sinus* with or without a cyst is an extensive lesion extending into nasal cartilage and bone, usually passing deeply at the level of the osteocartilaginous junction on the dorsum of the nose. Dermoid sinuses with or without sinus are most commonly occur in the orbital region (50%); 24% occur in the submental and submandibular regions, and 13% occupy the nose.
2. *Teratoid cysts* are composed of ectoderm, mesoderm, and endoderm. The lining of the teratoid cyst may range from simple stratified squamous epithelium to ciliated respiratory epithelium. Tissues from the three layers are poorly differentiated in these lesions.
3. *Teratomas* are composed of all three germ layers. In contrast to teratoid cysts, however, cellular differentiation is such that recognizable organs may be found in these masses.
4. *Epignathi* are lesions involving the highest form of differentiation; development of fetal organs and limbs may occur. They are rarely compatible with life.

   With regard to the nose, dermoid cysts and sinuses form in a potential space: the prenasal space that occurs between the developing nasal bones and cartilaginous capsule behind. A normal herniation of dura passes through the gap in the vault: the *foramen cecum*. The herniation is continuous with connective tissue, which forms the inner periosteal lining of the nasal bones, and this skin maintains a connection to underlying fibrous tissue or the cartilaginous nasal capsule. Epithelial elements may be pulled inward to form a sinus, which usually has hair protruding from the opening. The sinus may extend through the gap between the frontal bones superiorly beyond the cribriform plate to the dura, deeply to the basisphenoid and the nasal bones inferiorly (through fonticulus nasofrontalis), appearing as a bulging mass at the glabella, and septum.

Clinical presentation
- *Dermoid sinuses and cysts* are slightly more prevalent in males, and familial cases occasionally are seen. They are usually midline masses and most commonly present as a painless mass. Pain may be present if infection develops or if the mass enlarges significantly. The dermoid cyst with sinus is usually visible at birth. The opening is usually the osteocartilaginous junction of the dorsum. The occasional discharge of purulent material and the presence of a group of hairs at the opening are diagnostic. Although a sinus without cyst can occur, the tract is often narrowed, suggesting cystic formation proximal to the narrowing. Deep extension may be predicted when the nasal bones are splayed or true hypertelorism is present.
- *Teratomas* are usually present at birth. Maternal polyhydramnios is reported in 18% of cases. Teratomas frequently are quite large and can cause severe breathing and feeding difficulties. The overlying skin is normal.

Investigations
- CT with contrast and/or MRI. The major CT findings of a dermoid cyst and sinus include fusiform enlargement of the septum, a bifid appearance of the septum, widening or erosion of the nasal vault, destructive changes in the glabella or nasal bones, or a defect in the cribriform area.

Treatment
- Complete nasal excision is required for cure. Cauterization, injection of sclerosing agents, and limited dissection cause a high recurrence rate. Occasionally, a secondary infection is the presenting problem. An incision and drainage with antimicrobial treatment resolves the problem acutely, but a fistulous tract with drainage usually persists and requires removal. Although a horizontal elliptic incision for removal of the sinus opening is cosmetically desirable, a wide exposure with medial nasal osteotomies may be required and a Y incision with the vertical limb midline down the nasal dorsum

may be needed. An H-type incision is an alternative for an external ethmoidectomy. At the point where a dural connection is expected, a combined subfrontal approach is advisable.
- Teratomas present at birth may present major difficulties in management of the neonatal. Ultrasound allows these lesions to be diagnosed prenatally. Under these circumstances steps may be taken to protect the infant airway at birth. This may be accomplished via endoscopy to secure the airway while the neonate remains on fetal circulation. Teratomas should be excised as expeditiously as possible; encroachment on the airway is an ever-present danger. Encapsulization is common, facilitating complete removal. Recurrence following apparent total excision is rare.

 ## THYROGLOSSAL DUCT CYSTS

Etiology and embryology
- At 4 weeks a ventral (thyroid) diverticulum of endodermal origin forms between the first and second branchial arches; the obliterated invagination point is known as the *foramen cecum*. This diverticulum becomes the thyroid, descends caudally within mesodermal tissues, and may track superficial to, through, or deep to hyoid.
- At 4.5 weeks, connection between diverticulum and floor of pharynx begins to obliterate
- Thyroid remnants may persist along any part of the tract and may form cysts or fistulas.

Classification
- Commonly classified by location:
  - Base of tongue: 1%-2%.
  - Infrahyoid: 85%.
  - Suprahyoid: 8%.
  - Low neck: 5%.

Clinical symptoms
- Cystic, midline neck mass.
- Typically 2-4 cm.
- Elevate on protrusion of the tongue (deglutition) or swallowing.
- May rapidly increase in size or become tender when infected, such as after an upper respiratory tract infection (URI).
- Rarely fistulize to skin.
- Typically pediatric patient (second decade), although may present at any age.

Treatment
- Definitive treatment is surgical: Sistrunk procedure.
- Must remove cyst and tract to base of tongue, including middle third of hyoid bone (recurrence 3%)

- Failure to remove tract and hyoid segment results in recurrence as high as 30%.

Note:

1. Must confirm presence of normal thyroid (CT, MRI, ultrasound) prior to excision.
2. Thyroglossal duct cysts have been reported to contain carcinoma; adjunctive thyroidectomy in these cases remains controversial.

 ## LINGUAL THYROID

Definition

- Ectopic thyroid tissue found the base of tongue (foramen cecum).

Incidence and epidemiology

- Much more common in females.
- Often presents during pregnancy.

Pathogenesis

- Failure of descent of the thyroglossal duct from its origin in the floor of the pharynx during embryologic development.

Clinical presentation

- Cough.
- Dysphagia.
- Dyspnea.
- Change in voice.
- Hemorrhage.
- Infection.
- Asymptomatic mass at base of tongue. The mass is soft, dark, epithelial-covered vascular mass.

Investigations

- Thyroid scan: confirms the presence of ectopic thyroid and the presence or absence of other thyroid tissue in the neck.

Treatment

- Suppressive therapy is the mainstay of medical management. The goal of therapy is to suppress TSH levels and thereby remove the stimulus for gland enlargement. This approach is mandatory for patients with mild symptoms and for asymptomatic patients who have elevated TSH levels. It may also be warranted in asymptomatic euthyroid patients as a preventative measure. The patient is then monitored every 3 months with serial clinical examinations and thyroid function tests. More frequent examinations are necessary during periods of metabolic stress such as puberty or pregnancy.

A.

- Radiotherapy: Ectopic thyroid tissue can be ablated by a therapeutic dose of I^{131}. This results in unpredictable thyroid shrinkage and should be reserved for patients who refuse or are unfit for surgery.
- Excision: Indicated for patients who are symptomatic despite suppressive therapy for:
  - Neoplastic enlargement.
  - Hyperthyroidism.
  - Airway obstruction.
  - Dysphagia.
  - Dysphonia.
- Prior to embarking on surgery, a thyroid scan is necessary to determine of there is any other functioning thyroid tissue in the neck. The presence of normal thyroid tissue will assist in postoperative management.
- CT or MRI scans are helpful in determining the best surgical approach for total gland excision.
- Partial excision has been attempted; however, regrowth is common.
- Nasotracheal intubation or tracheostomy is necessary to secure an airway.
- Surgical excision can be performed transorally or through the neck with a midline or lateral pharyngotomy. The transoral approach classically involves a midline split of the chin, mandible, and tongue.
- Autotransplantation of thyroid tissue may be desirable in euthyroid patients. The tissue is moved by free graft into the anterior rectus sheath or under the strap muscles; 30% of patients remain euthyroid without replacement thyroxine.

 ## BRANCHIAL CLEFT ANOMALIES

Definition

- Branchial cleft anomalies include congenital cysts, sinuses, and fistulas that develop from residual components of the branchial clefts and pouches.

Incidence and epidemiology

- Branchial cleft anomalies comprise one third of congenital neck lesions.

Pathogenesis and pathology

- No definitive theory has been established. Incomplete closure of the branchial clefts and pouches, or failure of obliteration of the cervical sinus of His, are the prevalent theories.
- Pathology reveals them to be lined with stratified squamous epithelium with hair follicles, sweat glands, and sebaceous glands. Approximately 10% of cysts will be lined by a ciliated, columnar epithelium. The walls may contain hyaline cartilage. An inflammatory infiltrate is usually present.
- The anatomic relations of the various branchial cleft anomalies are determined by the structures that

develop from the individual branchial clefts, which become apparent beginning in the fourth week of development.

- Derivatives of the branchial arches are:
  - First arch: mandible, teeth, lining of mouth, anterior two thirds of tongue, head of malleus, body of incus, part of pinna, muscles of mastication, tensor tympani muscle, trigeminal nerve, facial artery.
  - Second arch: lesser horn of hyoid bone, anterior base of tongue, long process of the malleus and incus, stapes superstructure, majority of pinna, muscles of facial expression, facial nerve, stapedial artery.
  - Third arch: base of tongue, greater horn and body of hyoid, stylopharyngeus muscle, glossopharyngeal nerve.
  - Fourth and sixth arches: laryngeal cartilages, pharyngeal musculature, Vagus nerve, aortic arch, subclavian vessels.
- Derivatives of branchial pouches are:
  - First pouch: eustachian tube, tympanic cavity, mastoid air system.
  - Second pouch: Tonsillar fossa, palatine tonsil.
  - Third pouch: Pyriform sinus, inferior parathyroid, thymus.
  - Fourth pouch: Superior parathyroid, cervical esophagus.
- Derivatives of branchial grooves (clefts) are:
  - First cleft: external auditory canal.
  - Second to fourth cleft: degenerate.

Clinical presentation
- Patients will present with a cystic swelling, abscess, or draining sinus in the region of the anomaly.
- They may increase in size during URIs.
- Large cysts may present with dyspnea, stridor, or dysphagia.
- Smaller cysts may present in second or third decades of life.

Classification
First branchial cleft anomalies
- Uncommon: approximately 8% of branchial cleft anomalies.
- Always superior to hyoid (a second and third arch derivative).
- Fistula, if present, ends in external auditory canal (EAC) (a first cleft derivative).
- The cyst and its tract may course within the parotid gland.
- Variable relationship of the cyst/tract to the facial nerve.
- Two types:
  - **Type I:** first cleft defect:
  - "Duplication" of EAC found medial to concha, often in the postauricular crease.

  - Fistulous tract extends anteriorly and medially, paralleling the external auditory canal, to end at level of mesotympanum.
- **Type II**: first cleft and arch defect:
  - The cyst may be found below angle of mandible along anterior border of the sternocleidomastoid muscle (SCM).
  - The tract passes superiorly over angle of mandible.
  - The tract may pass medial or lateral to facial nerve.

Second branchial cleft anomalies
- Most common.
- Cysts are more common than fistulas or sinuses. The cyst may occur anywhere along the tract but is most common in the anterior triangle of the neck.
- The external opening, when present, is found along anterior border of the SCM, at the junction of its lower and middle thirds.
- The fistula tract, if present, ascends along the carotid sheath and crosses lateral to the CN XII and then IX, passes between the internal carotid and external carotid arteries, and enters tonsillar fossa.

Third branchial cleft anomalies
- Rare.
- The external opening, when present, is along anterior border of the SCM at junction of its lower and middle thirds (same as second cleft anomaly)
- The fistula, if present, ascends along the carotid sheath, posterior to the internal carotid artery and crosses lateral to the XIIth nerve, then turns medial to the internal and external carotid arteries, inferior to the CN IX, and lateral to the vagus nerve and enters into the pyriform sinus.

Fourth branchial cleft anomalies
- Theoretically possible but never definitively demonstrated.
- Would have external opening anterior border of the SCM in the lower neck.
- The tract would descend along carotid sheath and enter chest to pass under the aorta (left) or subclavian (right).
- The tract would then ascend in neck to cross lateral to CN XII, turn medial to the internal and external carotid arteries, inferior to CN IX, and then descend to enter cervical esophagus (a fourth arch derivative).

Treatment
- Antibiotics and cyst aspiration are indicated when an abscess is present.
- Surgical resection is the definitive treatment.
- When an opening is present in the neck, an ellipse is skin is excised with the tract.

- The tract is then followed and excised in its entirety.
- Step-ladder (multiple horizontal) incisions are recommended if further exposure is required.
- Excision of a Type I, first branchial cleft cyst may require facial nerve dissection.
- Excision of a Type II, first branchial cleft cyst may require superficial parotidectomy.

LYMPHANGIOMAS

- Lymphangiomas are congenital lesions that result from failure of the lymphatics to join the rest of the lymphatic system.
- *Lymphangioma simplex*: multiple, small, thin-walled spaces.
- *Cavernous lymphangiomas*: Larger cystic spaces surrounded by a fibrous adventitia.
- *Cystic hygromas*: Large lesions with lymphatic spaces of different sizes.
- Present as a soft, nontender, compressible neck mass that transilluminates.
- It may fluctuate in size with presence of URIs.
- CT scan and/or MRI scan will delineate its characteristics and extent.
- Surgical resection is indicated with symptoms of dyspnea or dysphagia, or with cosmetic deformity.
- The lesion tends to interdigitate between various structures and thus is difficult to resect in its entirety.

Hemangiomas

Definition

- Currently classified as benign vascular neoplasms.

Incidence and epidemiology

- Incidence in Caucasians is 10-12 times that seen in blacks and Asians
- Seen in 10% of white infants, 30% present at birth, 70% present within first few weeks of life.
- Female:male ratio = 3:1.

Pathophysiology and pathology

- Hemangiomas have *proliferation* and *involution* stages.
- In proliferative stage, hemangiomas are composed of proliferating, plump endothelial cells, that, in time, form vascular spaces and channels containing blood cells. During involution, mast cells infiltrate and secrete a variety of factors that precipitate involution.

Clinical presentation

- Patients with hemangiomas within the neck present with a soft to firm mass (increasing firmness during proliferative phase).

- Skin color may be normal or have a blue or red hue, depending on the level of proliferation and the distance from the skin.
- The lesions are compressible and may increase in size with crying.
- A cutaneous hemangioma is typically present somewhere on the body.
- Airway compromise may occur resulting in:
  - Hoarseness.
  - Stridor, worse with feeding or crying.
  - Cough.
  - Cyanosis.
  - Sleep apnea.
  - Failure to thrive.
- Other symptoms include ulceration and infection.
- A consumptive coagulopathy (Kasabach-Merritt phenomenon) is a rare complication.

Investigations

- MRI scan with enhancement is the imaging study of choice.
- Direct laryngoscopy may be indicated in cases of airway compromise.

Treatment

- Most hemangiomas will involute spontaneously beginning at 18-24 months of age and, if airway compromise is not present, will require no specific treatment.
- If the infant presents with an acute airway obstruction, intubation is indicated. If the lesion fails to respond to conservative treatment, a tracheostomy is indicated.
- Corticosteroids are effective at decreasing the size of hemangiomas. They are given orally during the proliferative phase. Intralesional steroids have been used in orbital hemangiomas.
- Interferon alfa-2a has proved helpful in cases of steroid failure.
- Surgical excision or laser treatment with pulsed-dye laser are indicated in cases of residual lesions that cause a persistent functional or cosmetic deficit.

Thymic Cysts

- Present as left-sided cystic swelling in the neck.
- They are typically unifocal, unilateral, and may form abscesses.
- Treatment is by excision.
- Diagnosis is made by the identification of Hassall's corpuscles on histologic assessment.

Congenital Torticollis

- Infants (1-8 weeks) present with hard mass within the sternocleidomastoid muscle, which will increase in size for 2-3 months.

- The mass involutes within 2-3 months, leaving a fibrous scar.
- The etiology is unclear.
- It typically occurs in the firstborn child.
- Treatment is physical therapy to prevent the formation of a restrictive scar.

Lipomas

- They are benign, encapsulated, fatty tumors that can present at any age.
- They are excised if the cause a cosmetic deformity.

Ranulas

Definition

- Cystic swelling of sublingual gland.
- Plunging ranula: extension of the ranula into the neck.

Pathology and pathophysiology

- A congenital ranula may develop secondary to failure of development of the salivary duct.
- Acquired: Trauma to the sublingual gland or duct is the most common acquired etiology for a ranula.
- Plunging ranula may form by passing through a dehiscence in the mylohyoid, via an ectopic gland, or via an anatomic association with the submandibular gland allowing the ranula to pass around the posterior border of the mylohyoid.

Clinical presentation

- Most typically presents as a painless, bluish cyst arising on the floor of the mouth.
- A plunging ranula will present as a neck swelling in a submandibular region, with (80%) or without (20%) an associated floor-of-the-mouth swelling.
- In the case of a plunging ranula, squeezing the neck mass will enlarge the lesion in the floor of the mouth.

Investigations

- MRI scan is the investigation of choice to delineate the extent of lesion and its association with normal structures.
- CT scan is an alternate form of imaging if MRI cannot be performed.

Treatment

- Excision of the cyst and the gland via a transoral route is the treatment of choice.
  - Trauma to the lingual nerve (paresthesias) and to Wharton's duct are the main complications.
  - Allows for obtaining specimen for pathology to rule out malignancy.

- Other options include:
  - Marsupialization:
    - Cyst is opened and edged tacked to surrounding oral mucosa.
    - Oldest technique but has 60%-90% recurrence rate.
  - Placement of silk suture or Seton:
    - A silk suture or Seton may be placed in the cyst and retained in place until the tract epithelializes.
  - Sclerosis with Bleomycin or OK-432 has been reported to be effective.
  - CO_2 laser may be used to resect the cyst and scar the gland to prevent recurrence.
  - For plunging ranulas, transoral resection of gland with drainage of cyst is primary treatment.
  - Persistence or recurrence of the cervical cyst requires a transcervical approach.

 BENIGN CERVICAL LYMPHADENOPATHY

Viral

- A large variety of viruses will cause a reactive lymphadenopathy, typically associated with URIs. This lymphadenopathy is typically symmetric and involves the anterior chain of lymph nodes.
- Epstein-Barr virus, cytomegalovirus, and Rubella will cause a pronounced symmetric lymphadenopathy that may also involve the *posterior triangle*. Hepatosplenomegaly is typically associated with these infections.
- Cervical lymphadenopathy is a frequent manifestation of HIV infection.
- Fine-needle aspiration should be considered in these patients to rule out lymphoma, Kaposi's sarcoma, or granulomatous infection if:
  - A single node is rapidly enlarging.
  - A newly tender node is present.
  - A node has enlarged with the development of systemic symptoms.
  - A single node greater >3 cm is present.

Bacterial

- URIs, ear infections, dental infections, and salivary gland infections may lead to a bacterial (suppurative) lymphadenitis.
- *Staphylococcus aureus* and *group A beta hemolytic streptococcus* are the most frequent pathogens.
- *Moraxella* and *Haemophilus influenzae* are also implicated.
- Anaerobic bacteria are responsible for approximately 20% of infections.

- Gram-negative bacteria, including pseudomonas, may be present in neonatal infections.
- **Cat-scratch disease**
  - A disorder characterized by cervical lymphadenopathy, mild fever, and other constitutional symptoms.
  - It affects young patients, less than 20 years old.
  - Occurs more in males.
  - A history of feline (kittens > older cats) contact is present in >90% of patients. Fleas are most likely the vector.
  - Pathogenic bacteria = *Bartonella henselae*, formerly classified as *Rochalimaea henselae*, (pleomorphic gram-negative bacteria).
  - Diagnosed with serologic testing by indirect fluorescent antibody assay for this organism.
  - Disorder is typically self limited.
  - CNS findings occur in 5% of patients with CSD and include headaches, mental status changes, seizures, myelitis, transient peripheral neuropathy, and retinitis.
  - The value of antibiotics has not been established definitively as being effective, but in general a 10-14–day course of one of the following antibiotics is indicated: rifampin, ciprofloxacin (not indicated in children), trimethoprim-sulfamethoxazole (TMP-SMX), and gentamicin, clarithromycin, azithromycin, or tetracycline.
- **Toxoplasmosis**
  - Infection caused by *Toxoplasma gondii* (intracellular protozoan).
  - Pathogen is ingested from poorly cooked meat.
  - Cervical adenitis, typically unilateral, occurs in 90% of cases; associated symptoms include fever, odynophagia, constitutional symptoms.
  - May be complicated by pneumonitis, myocarditis, and/or retinitis.
  - Diagnosed by serologic testing.
  - Treated with pyrimethamine or sulfonamides.

Mycobacterial Infection

- Cervical lymph node involvement may occur in cases of both typical and atypical mycobacterial (TB) infections.
- Atypical mycobacterial cervical adenitis (*Mycobacterium avium-intracellulare, Mycobacterium kansasii, Mycobacterium fortuitum,* and *mycobacterium haemophilum*) is responsible for approximately 60% of the cases of mycobacterial cervical adenitis. The infection is typically unilateral, with the skin overlying the adenitis being discolored. Definitive diagnosis is made by biopsy and culture. Treatment is generally not required. In cases in which skin breakdown and draining sinuses occur, surgical debridement and antibiotic therapy are indicated.

- *Mycobacterium tuberculosis* will typically cause bilateral cervical adenitis associated with pulmonary disease. Skin testing will be positive. Treatment is with antibiotics.

Tularemia

- *Francisella tularensis*—an aerobic, gram-negative, pleomorphic, and primarily rod-shaped coccobacillus—causes tularemia.
- Infections are rare (approximately 200/year).
- The bacteria are transmitted by ticks, rabbits, and rodents.
- It causes a variety of clinical syndromes, one of which is generalized lymphadenitis associated with constitutional symptoms.
- Diagnosis is by ELISA.
- Treatment is with intramuscular streptomycin. Levofloxacin may be effective.

Brucellosis

- Rare in the United States (100 cases/year); more pervasive in underdeveloped countries
- Caused by gram negative *Brucella* species.
- Transmitted via infected meat or nonpasteurized milk.
- Causes a multisystemic disease with manifestations, including fever, myalgias, acute arthritis, genitourinary infection, and generalized adenitis.
- Diagnosis is made by serologic assays.
- Treatment is with tetracycline (over age 9) or trimethoprim-sulfamethoxazole.

Noninfectious Inflammatory Cervical Adenitis

Kawasaki disease

- A potentially fatal medium vessel vasculitis.
- Occurs in children; peak incidence in the United States is at 2 years old.
- Tends to occur in epidemics.
- Clinical manifestations include:
  - Fever lasting more than 5 days and refractory to appropriate antibiotic therapy.
    - Polymorphous erythematous rash.
    - Nonpurulent bilateral conjunctival injection.
    - Oropharyngeal changes, including diffuse hyperemia, strawberry tongue, and swelling, fissuring, and erythema of the lips.
    - Peripheral extremity changes, including erythema, edema, induration, and desquamation of the hands and feet.
    - Nonpurulent cervical lymphadenopathy.
    - The major morbidity and mortality of this vasculitis is the development of coronary artery aneurysms.

- Diagnosis is made by the presence of the above-described clinical syndrome.
- Blood studies reveal findings of acute inflammation including elevations in the sedimentation rate and C-reactive protein. Thrombocytosis is present in the acute phase.
- Treatment is with intravenous gamma-globulin.

 DEEP NECK INFECTIONS

Anatomy of the Cervical Fascia

- The cervical fascia is divided into the superficial and deep layers.
- *Superficial cervical fascia*: sheet of fibrous connective tissue that completely encloses the head and neck and is contiguous with the fascia of the shoulder, thorax, and axilla. It contains the platysma muscle.
- *Deep cervical fascia.*
- Superficial layer: connective tissue layer that splits to enclose the trapezius, sternocleidomastoid (SCM), and the submandibular and parotid glands.
  - Superior extent = zygoma, mastoid process, external occipital protuberance.
  - Inferior extent = clavicle, scapula, and manubrium of the sternum.
  - Anterior extent = mandible and the hyoid bone.
- Middle layer: splits to enclose all visceral organs (larynx, pharynx, trachea, esophagus, thyroid gland). It also encloses the strap muscles anteriorly.
- Deep layer: circumferentially encloses the vertebral bodies and the paraspinal muscles.

Spaces

Retropharyngeal space
- A potential space that exists between the posterior aspect of the middle layer and the alar division of the deep layer.
- Extends from the base of skull to the tracheal bifurcation.
- Contains two lateral chains of lymph nodes that drain the nose, nasopharynx, soft palate, and paranasal sinuses.
- These two chains separated by a midline raphe, which is formed by the attachment of the superior constrictor muscle to the alar fascia.

Danger space
- A potential space that lies between the alar and prevertebral divisions of the deep cervical fascia.
- Extends from the base of skull to the level of the diaphragm.
- Lateral extent is confined by the fusion of the alar and prevertebral layers at the vertebral transverse process.

Prevertebral space
- A potential space that exists between the anterior surface of the vertebral bodies and the prevertebral division of the deep cervical fascia.
- Extends from the base of skull to the level of the coccyx.

Lateral pharyngeal (parapharyngeal) space
- A potential space between the superficial and middle layers of the deep cervical fascia. Inverted cone with apex attached to the hyoid bone.
- Petrous portion of the temporal bone forms the base.
- Medial border: lateral pharyngeal wall.
- Lateral border: superficial layer of the deep cervical fascia as it invests the mandible, internal pterygoid muscles, and parotid gland.
- Anterior border: pterygomandibular raphe.
- Posterior border: prevertebral (deep) and visceral layers (middle) layers of fascia in continuity with the carotid sheath, which pierces the cone at the apex to pursue a course into the mediastinum.
- The lateral pharyngeal space is divided into prestyloid and poststyloid compartments:
  - Anterior compartment contains fat, lymph nodes, "dumbbell tumor of parotid," internal maxillary artery, lingual nerve, inferior alveolar nerve, auriculotemporal nerve.
  - Posterior compartment contains carotid artery, internal jugular vein, sympathetic chain, cranial nerves IX, X, XI, XII.
- It communicates with the submandibular space along the inferior border.

Submandibular space
- Sublingual component: mylohyoid inferiorly, body of mandible laterally, floor of mouth mucosa superiorly.
- Submaxillary component:
  - In continuity with the sublingual space at the posterior edge of the mylohyoid muscle.
  - Lateral border is the anterior belly of the digastric.
  - Inferior border is the superficial layer of the deep fascia, connecting the mandible and the hyoid.

Anterior visceral space
- Is enclosed by the middle layer of the deep cervical fascia.
- Completely surrounds trachea, esophagus, and thyroid gland.
- Superior border at the hyoid.
- Inferior border at the level of the fourth thoracic vertebra in the superior mediastinum.
- Important in esophageal perforation.

Etiology of infection
- Odontogenic infection: affecting primarily the submaxillary space.

- Tonsillar and pharyngeal infections (seeding the lateral and retropharyngeal spaces).
- Upper aerodigestive tract trauma: both penetrating and iatrogenic (intubation, instrumentation) are fairly common, involving primarily the retropharyngeal space.
- Salivary gland infection.
- Sinusitis: primarily seeds the retropharyngeal space.
- Infected branchial cleft cyst.
- Infected thyroglossal duct cyst.
- Laryngopyocele.
- Mastoiditis leading to a Bezold's abscess.
- Tuberculosis infection of the cervical spine can lead to a prevertebral space infection.
- Direct seeding: intravenous drug use.
- Idiopathic: no specific source of infection (20%-50% of deep neck infections).

Bacteriology
- Usually reveals mixed aerobic and anaerobic organisms, often with a predominance of oral flora. The following bacteria may be found in various combinations.
  - Group A beta-hemolytic streptococcal species (*Streptococcus pyogenes*).
  - Alpha-hemolytic streptococcal species (*Streptococcus viridans, Streptococcus pneumoniae*).
  - *Staphylococcus aureus.*
  - *Fusobacterium nucleatum.*
  - *Bacteroides melaninogenicus, Bacteroides oralis.*
  - *Spirochaeta, Peptostreptococcus,* and *Neisseria.*
  - *Pseudomonas* species, *Escherichia coli,* and *H. influenzae* are occasionally encountered.

Clinical presentation
- Fluctuance and pointing are rare since the dawn of the antibiotic era.
- Fever.
- Pain and swelling are common and can guide the clinician in localizing the site of the infection.
- Dysphagia is more common when the lateral pharyngeal and retropharyngeal spaces are involved.
- Trismus is seen with involvement of the submaxillary space or anterior aspect of the lateral pharyngeal space.
- Dyspnea, stridor is seen if airway compromise.
- "Hot potato voice" associated with retropharyngeal abscess.
- **Ludwig's angina:** an anaerobic infection secondary to dental pathology specific to sublingual space, but can also involve the submaxillary space and the lateral pharyngeal space. Causes retrusion of tongue and airway compromise. The neck will manifest a "woody" hard edema.

Investigations
- Complete blood count: leukocytosis.
- Blood culture.
- Lateral neck film: look over C2. Soft tissue should be no wider than the thickness of C2 in child and no thicker than one third the width of C2 in the adult. Retropharyngeal involvement is suggested if the soft tissue is wider than normal. This study can also demonstrate foreign bodies, subcutaneous air (indicative of an anaerobic infection), air/fluid levels, and erosion of the vertebral bodies.
- CT scan with contrast is the investigation of choice for the evaluation of deep neck abscesses.
- Panorex: evaluate for dental pathology.

Treatment
- Airway has first priority:
  - Tracheostomy should be performed if any question of compromise exists.
  - Intubation may be used in selected cases in which the anatomy is not significantly distorted.
- Antibiotics:
  - Cephazolin and metronidazole or clindamycin are the first choices for antibiotic coverage, pending results of culture.
  - In some patients, particularly children, small abscesses may be managed with antibiotics alone. Failure to improve within 24-48 hours indicates the need for surgical intervention.
- Surgical drainage remains the treatment of choice in most patients, especially adults.
- Immune-compromised patients warrant prompt drainage.
- Retropharyngeal and prevertebral infections with a noticeable mass can be approached intraorally.
- The remainder of infections requires a transcervical approach.
- Recent evidence indicates that CT scan–guided aspiration and insertion of a drain may provide results equivalent to those obtained with surgical intervention.

Complications
- **Mediastinitis**
  - Most common from retropharyngeal space.
  - Associated with 35% mortality.
  - Requires drainage via a thoracic approach.
- **Horner's syndrome** with lateral pharyngeal space.
- CN IX, X, XI, XII neuropathy with lateral pharyngeal space infection
  - **Vernet's syndrome**: CN IX, X, XI
  - **Villarette's syndrome**: CN IX, X, XI, XII
- **Thrombophlebitis:**
  - Occurs in cases of lateral pharyngeal space abscesses.

- ❑ Manifests with spiking fever and facial edema.
- ❑ Diagnosis is confirmed with MRV.
- ❑ Treat with immediate exploration and internal jugular vein ligation.
- ❑ Erosion of the carotid system in lateral pharyngeal space abscesses.
- ❑ Treatment with immediate exploration and intraoperative angiography.
- ❑ Aspiration pneumonia with retropharyngeal and lateral pharyngeal abscesses.

PRIMARY NEOPLASMS OF THE NECK

Paragangliomas

Carotid body tumor
Definition
- Tumor arising from the paraganglia around the carotid artery bifurcation.

Etiology
- Carotid body tumors are the most common paragangliomas of the neck.
- 90% are sporadic.
- Overall, 10% of tumors are multicentric.
- 10% are familial, of these; approximately 25%-35% are multicentric. Patients with a family history of paragangliomas have a higher incidence of having an adrenal pheochromocytoma.
- 2% secrete catecholamines.

Pathology
- Paragangliomas derive from extraadrenal paraganglioma, which derive from neural crest cells.
- The paraganglia are distributed along vascular and neural structures.
- In the head and neck, paraganglia resemble carotid bodies.
- The tumors are composed of granule storing "chief cells" that form nests *(Zellballen)* in a highly vascular, fibrous stroma.
- 5% of tumors are considered malignant, demonstrating nodal metastases and invasion of local structures.

Clinical presentation
- Carotid body tumors most commonly present as an asymptomatic neck mass.
- Dysphagia, cough, or hoarseness are other symptoms.

Investigations
- MRI scan with contrast is the diagnostic test of choice.
- Arteriography will provide a definitive diagnosis. It is usually performed 24 hours prior to surgical resection to allow for embolization. Four-vessel arteriography allows for the identification of multicentric tumors.
- 24-hour urine for vanillylmandelic acid (VMA) and metanephrines are indicated in patients with symptoms of secretory tumors (tachycardia, hypertension, flushing, diaphoresis).

Treatment
- Surgical resection remains the treatment of choice.
- Preoperative embolization is generally indicated.
- Patients with secretory tumors require α- and β-adrenergic blockade.
- A transcervical approach is used. The external carotid is ligated for exposure. A subadventitial dissection is performed. Infiltration of the internal carotid with 1% lidocaine may prevent constriction.
- In large or recurrent tumors, plans for carotid ligation or bypass should be made.
- Patients who fail a balloon occlusion test should have a bypass performed prior to resection.
- Radiation therapy may be of some benefit in patients who cannot tolerate surgery.
- Conservative observation may be indicated for small tumors in the elderly.

Vagal Paragangliomas (Glomus Vagale)

- These paragangliomas may present along the skull base, in the jugular foramen, or just inferiorly at the nodose ganglion.
- The tumors present and are treated like glomus jugulare tumors (see Neurotology section).
- Vagal paragangliomas may present in the neck along the superior or recurrent laryngeal nerve. When presenting in the neck they are surgically resected.
- Other benign tumors presenting in the neck include schwannomas, neurofibromas, and lipomas.

SKIN CANCER OF THE HEAD AND NECK

Introduction

- Skin cancer is the most common human malignancy.
- Basal cell carcinoma (BCC) is the most common skin cancer (85%), followed by squamous cell carcinoma (10%). Melanoma accounts for approximately 5% of skin cancers but is responsible for 75% of skin cancer deaths.

Basal Cell Carcinoma

Etiology and risk factors
- BCC arises from basal cells.
- Risk factors include ultraviolet (UV) exposure, fair complexion, light hair, blue or green eyes, propensity to sunburn, exposure to carcinogens, chronic radiation damage, viral infection, immunosuppression, and genetic syndromes such as xeroderma pigmentosa and nevoid basal cell carcinoma syndrome (e.g., multiple BCCs, jaw cysts, bifid ribs, scoliosis, mental retardation, and frontal bossing).

Clinical manifestations (five clinical forms)
Nodular or nodular-ulcerative (most common form)
- Discrete, raised, circular lesion with rolled border and often with central necrosis.
- Easiest type to recognize and treat.

Morphealike or sclerosing
- Typified by macular, whitish, yellowish plaque with indistinct margins.
- Complete excision difficult due to ill-defined margins.

Superficial multicentric
- Consists of one or several red, scaling patches with irregular borders that gradually increase in size by peripheral extension.
- Relatively uncommon in head and neck; more common on trunk and extremities.

Pigmented basal cell carcinoma
- Less common.
- Characterized by brown pigmentation and may resemble pigmented nevus or melanoma.
- Behavior similar to nodular BCC.

Basosquamous cell carcinoma (keratotic basal cell carcinoma)
- Histologic features of both BCC and squamous cell carcinoma.
- More biologically aggressive than other types of BCC.

Histopathology
- Proliferation of monomorphic, basaloid-appearing cells; invading dermis; and formation of nests and lobules.
- Smooth, regular boundaries between nest of tumor cells and surrounding tissue.
- Palisading pattern to outer layer of cells in each nest.

Routes of spread
- BCC slowly growing, locally invasive neoplasm.
- Morpheaform and keratotic are more prone to recurrence.
- BCC most infiltrative and aggressive.
- BCC metastasis are rare; incidence less than 0.5%.

Squamous Cell Carcinoma

Etiology
- Squamous cell carcinoma (SCC) arises from epidermal keratinocytes.
- It commonly arises from sun-damaged skin or from a preexisting lesion such as chronic radiodermatitis, keratosis, chronic scars and ulcers, burn scars (e.g., Marjolin's ulcer), and other chronic inflammatory states.

Clinical presentation
- Usually presents as erythematous, ulcerated, crusting lesion.
- Usually elevated area of induration at lesion edge and may be inflammatory response in adjacent tissues.
- Can also present as thickened hyperkeratotic patch or area of crusting.
- Occasionally presents as nodular exophytic lesion.

Histopathology
- Masses of pleomorphic epidermal cells proliferating downward and invading dermis as small nests and single cells.
- Occasionally irregular borders between nests of tumor cells and surrounding normal tissue.
- Keratin formation by well-differentiated tumor cells; frequent mitosis.
- Histologic variations: adenoid, bowenoid, verrucous, spindle cell.

Routes of spread
- SCA may be actinically induced or arise de novo.
- Actinically induced lesions follow a more benign course with a low incidence of metastasis.
- De novo lesions are more aggressive and exhibit a higher metastatic potential.
- Regional metastatic spread is correlated with depth of invasion; lesions that penetrate Clark's level IV or V are associated with a 20% regional metastatic rate.

Nonsurgical Treatment for Nonmelanotic Skin Carcinoma

- Excisional surgery is primary treatment modality for melanotic skin cancer.
- Moh's surgery and excisional surgery are main modalities in treatment of BCC and SCC.
- For appropriately selected BCC and SCC, alternative modalities exist, including electrodesiccation and curettage, cryosurgery, and radiotherapy
- Most authorities recommend discontinuation of topical 5-fluorouracil cream in the treatment of BCC and SCC.

Electrodesiccation and curettage (EDC)

- From 92%-98% success rate for small, properly selected tumors in skilled hands.
- Indicated for small, previously untreated, nonaggressive tumors with well-defined borders, particularly in low-risk sites.
- Independent risk factors for recurrence: lesion size, location (Table 1).
- Keys to success: skill, experience of operator; appropriate use of sharp large and small curettes; appropriate selection of tumor; detailed instructions to patient regarding wound care.

Technique

- Cleanse skin with alcohol or antibacterial scrub; outline clinical margins of tumor; give local anesthesia.
- Debulk majority of tumor with large curette until normal feeling surrounding tissue is reached.
- Destroy residual tumor with electrodesiccation of wound periphery and base with 1-2–mm margins.
- Repeat curettage of wound base and periphery with large, then small, curette, followed by repeat electrodesiccation until normal tissue is felt.

- Administer final electrodesiccation followed by light curettage to remove char.
- Dressing placement.
  - Postoperative wound care stresses frequent cleansing (i.e., H_2O_2), minimization of infection (antibacterial ointment), and prevention of eschar formation to force wound to heal from base and minimize cosmetic defect.

Advantages

- Outpatient setting.
- Rapid with high cure rate.

Disadvantages

- Scarring.
- Delayed wound healing.
- Occasional bleeding.

Cryosurgery

- Cure rates comparable to EDC and excision for properly selected tumors (small, low-risk primary BCCs).
- Used less commonly in SCC.
- Best cryogen liquid nitrogen.
- Critical parameters: depth of freeze, width of freeze beyond margin of tumor, thaw time (i.e., marginal and total).
- Marginal thaw time at least 120 seconds in BCC.
- Thoroughness of cryonecrosis increased with double and triple freeze-thaw cycles.

Technique

- Outline clinical tumor with 2-5–mm margin.
- Anesthetize with local anesthetic.
- Cryoprobes or thermocouples placed to appropriate depth at margin of tumor.
- Tumor, surrounding tissue frozen, allowed to thaw; note marginal thaw time.
- Repeated at least once.
- Prefreezing curettage can be of benefit.

Advantages

- Excellent on tissue with fixed undersurface, such as cartilage that is not affected by the freezing.
- Useful in overall plan in patient with multiple BCCs.

Disadvantages

- Prolonged healing time of 3-10 weeks.
- Marked edema, wound necrosis, serous drainage in initial 2 weeks of healing.
- Hypopigmentation.
- Permanent hair loss in hair-bearing skin.

TABLE 1. Independent Risk Factors for Recurrence: Lesion Size, Location

Risk (Site)	Size (cm)	5-Year Recurrence Rate (%)
Low risk (trunk, neck, extremities)	all	3.3
Medium risk (scalp, forehead, malar)	<1.0	5.3
	>1.0	22.7
High risk (central face, ears, chin)	<0.6	4.5
	>0.6	17.6

Radiation therapy

- Once quite popular, now less common due to relative contraindications and several disadvantages.
- Specific concern for radiation chondritis and osteoradionecrosis (preventable by proper fractionation).
- Efficacy good, but only 63% have good cosmetic results (Table 2).

Advantages

- Useful as *primary therapy for small tumors* in elderly or debilitated patients who are poor surgical candidates.
- Useful for *palliation for large tumors* in elderly or debilitated patients who are poor surgical candidates.
- Useful *adjuvant* to excisional surgery for high-risk tumors.

Disadvantages

- Long length of treatment (2-6 weeks).
- Worse cosmetic result than EDC, cryosurgery, excisional surgery.
- Radiodermatitis and potential for secondary carcinogenesis (young patients).
- Tumors that recur after radiotherapy generally more aggressive, invasive, destructive than tumors that recur after other primary modalities.

Topical 5-fluorouracil cream

- 5-Fluorouracil and other topical agents have been reported to be useful in the treatment of superficial BCC.
- Multiple reports outline problems with these agents and recommend discontinuing their use. Deep foci of tumor can be concealed until dermal spread

TABLE 2. Results of Radiation Therapy

Size (cm)	5-Year Recurrence Rate (%)
<1	4
>1	10

occurs and the lesion is found to be larger than anticipated

- Topical 5-fluorouracil is effective in the treatment of actinically damaged skin and actinic keratoses, but *should not be used* as treatment for BCC or SCC (Table 3).

Moh's surgery for cutaneous cancer

- Moh's surgery should be considered as a primary modality in *all* tumors occurring in areas associated with high rate of recurrence (e.g., central face, nose, chin, ear) or areas of cosmetic importance (e.g., nose, lip, eyelid, helix of ear)
- Moh's surgery is best choice for recurrent tumors, incompletely excised tumors, or tumors with ill-defined borders.

Technique

- Moh's is usually performed under local anesthesia.
- The surgeon makes clinical outline of tumor.
- All gross tumor is removed with a scalpel or curette.
- The surgeon angles the scalpel blade at 45 degrees and carefully dissects a thin layer of tissue from the wound in the shape of a saucer with 1-3–mm lateral and deep margins.

TABLE 3. Selection of Treatment

	Low Risk: Trunk, Neck, Extremities	Medium Risk: Scalp, Malar, Forehead	High Risk: Central Face, Nose, Chin, Ear
NONAGGRESSIVE			
Nodular, superficial	<2.0 cm 1. EDC 2. Cryosurgery 3. XRT >2.0 cm 1. Moh's 2. Excision	<1.0 cm 1. EDC 2. Cryosurgery 3. XRT >1.0 cm 1. Moh's 2. Excision	<0.6 cm 1. EDC 2. Cryosurgery 3. XRT >0.6 cm 1. Moh's 2. Excision
AGGRESSIVE			
morpheaform, sclerotic, fibrosing, desmoplastic, keratotic	1. Moh's 2. Excision	1. Moh's 2. Excision	1. Moh's 2. Excision

EDC, Electrodessication and curettage; *XRT,* x-ray therapy.

- This layer is carefully oriented, divided into sections, and histologically examined as a frozen section.
  - Because the tissue specimen is flexible, it can be bent to incorporate the beveled edges into the deep margin.
  - Colored dyes are used to color-code the frozen sections, which correspond to a carefully drawn map of the surgical defect.
  - These dyes allow for exact anatomic orientation of each section on the microscope slide.
- The Moh's surgeon examines the tissue to determine if the margins are free.
- If residual tumor is seen, its exact location is marked on the corresponding location on the map of the patient.
- Only this area is reexcised and reevaluated by frozen section as above.
- This continues until all margins are negative.

Indications
- May be used to treat many different types of skin cancer.
- Main uses to be confined to:
  - Tumors for which maximal conservation of adjacent tissue may be important.
    - Tumors of eyelid, nose, ear, lip.
    - Tumors in young patients.
    - Tumors that potentially involve vital structures.
  - Tumors with high recurrence rates following standard skin cancer treatment.
    - Recurrent tumors.
    - Size >2 cm in diameter.
    - Tumors in high risk locations (e.g., H zone of face).
    - Tumors with poorly defined clinical margins.
    - Tumors with perineural invasion.
    - Immunosuppressed patients with SCC.
    - Poorly differentiated SCC.

Contraindications
- None.

Advantages
- Conservation of more normal surrounding anatomy.
- A 99% 5-year tumor cure rate for BCC compared with 90%-93% for standard excision.
- A 94% 5-year tumor cure rate for recurrent BCC compared with 60%-84% for standard excision.
- Increased rate to local control of large head and neck cutaneous SCC when compared with standard excision.

Disadvantages
- Requires a specially trained Moh's surgeon.
- Very time-consuming and labor-intensive procedure.

Reconstruction of Postexcisional Defects

General considerations
- Complete options for repair of facial defects include:
  - Primary closure.
  - Secondary intention.
  - Skin graft (e.g., split thickness, full thickness).
  - Flap repair (e.g., local, regional, microsurgical, distant staged).
- Methods used to classify local flaps:
  - Blood supply (e.g., random versus axial).
  - Configuration (e.g., rhomboid, bilobe).
  - Method of transfer (e.g., rotation, transposition, interpolation, advancement).

Local flaps
- Diagnosis should be made before and extent of lesion should be determined before flap coverage:
  - Can mask recurrence.
  - Can obscure positive margins.
- Incisions should be made in relaxed skin tension lines and should avoid unnecessary pull.

Anatomy
- Blood supply.
  - Branches of external carotid.
    - Facial.
    - Superficial temporal.
  - Branches of internal carotid.
    - Supraorbital.
    - Supratrochlear.
    - Zygomaticofacial.
    - Zygomaticotemporal.
  - Entry of blood supply to flap is usually random; width of base determines surviving length.
  - If flap has known vessels, length can be extended.

Facial nerve
- Exposed superficially.
  - Between lateral canthus and EAC.
  - Mandibular branch: between angle of mandible and mental foramen.

Types of flaps
- Some variation between classifications of flap types.

Pivotal (rotation, advancement, transposition, interpolation)
- Rotation
  - Semicircular; rotated into defect about arc; base not too narrow.
  - Best used to close triangular defect.
  - Designed immediately adjacent to defect.
  - Lymphatic drainage promoted by inferior base.
  - Simple:
    - Fill triangular defects.
    - Flap-size to defect-size ratio approximately 4:1.

- Ideal for medial canthal and cheek defects.
- Burow's triangles potentially necessary.
  □ V-Y:
  - Similar to simple with smaller arc.
  - Pivot in shape of V, closed in shape of Y.
  - Useful in nasal region.
  - Sometimes categorized as an advancement flap.
  □ O-Z:
  - Two opposing, inverted, semicircular rotation flaps.
  - Closes circular defect, final scar shape of Z.
  - Useful for lateral forehead defects.
- Advancement
  □ Flaps with a linear configuration are moved into a defect by sliding tissue adjacent tissue.
  □ Unilateral and bilateral advancement flaps may require Z-plasties or Burow's triangle excision at the base of the flap and may facilitate closure.
  □ Direction is directly perpendicular to base of flap.
    - Fusiform: takes shape of defect; skin undermined ~2 cm in both directions.
    - Rectangular: two parallel incisions extended away from defect in relaxed skin tension lines; flap extended into defect.
- Transposition (very versatile)
  □ A combination rotation-advancement flap that moves tissue about, fixed point into defect over intact skin to close defect.
  □ Simple: flap outlined adjacent to defect, elevated, transposed.
    - Nasolabial and glabellar regions best sites.
    - May require two-stage procedure to remove bridging skin.
  □ Bilobed: two transposition flaps.
    - Often at 90-degree angles to each other, can be less.
    - First lobe: approximately size of defect.
    - Second lobe: half width, three-quarter length.
    - Second donor site closed primarily.
  □ Rhombic: fills rhombic defect.
    - Flap equal to size of defect raised along one edge at 60-degree angle.
    - Transfers line of tension on closure to donor site.
  □ Z-plasty: often used for scar revision.
    - Two lines drawn from central member, which is rotated into relaxed skin tension line.
    - Changes direction of scar.
    - Lengthens scar area; gives more acceptable broken-line closure.
    - If angle is <60 degrees, must watch for tip necrosis.

- Interpolation
  □ A transposition flap in which the donor site is separate from the recipient site and the flap bridges over or passes under intact intervening skin.
  □ More dependent on axial blood supply.
  □ Typically requires second stage to sever and inset pedicle.
  □ May deepithelialize pedicle and place under intact intervening skin in one stage, in which case the flap is a *subcutaneous island flap*.
  □ Example: midforehead.

Hinge flaps
- Also referred to as trap-door flap, turn-in flap, turn-down flap.
- Linear or curvilinear flaps; pedicled on one border of defect, dissected in subcutaneous plane, and turned over on defect like page in book.
- Epithelial surface of flap turned deep to provide internal lining for facial defect that requires external and internal surface reconstruction.
- *Always* require second flap to cover exposed subcutaneous surface of hinge flap.
- Example: melolabial turn-in.

Tissue expansion (see Facial Cosmetics section)
- Can provide additional soft tissue for flap, has enhanced vascularity.
- High rate of complications.

Guidelines for local flap construction and selection
Rotation
- Frequently used in areas with convex surfaces or curved tension lines (e.g., malar cheek, temples, nasal dorsum, upper lip, scalp)
- Flap generally three to four times as large as defect.
  □ Single rotation: triangular or circular defects (e.g., eyelid, cheek).
  □ O-Z: circular wound (e.g., scalp).
  □ Glabellar: high nasal dorsum, medial canthus.

Transposition
- Frequently used in areas where it is advantageous to transfer tension away from the closure of the primary defect and into the repair of the secondary defect, such as the nasal tip and ala, inferior eyelid, and lips.
- Ideal parameters for the design and orientation of bilobe and classic rhombic flaps have been developed.
  □ Single lobe: circular defect (medial cheek, nasal ala, and tip).
  □ Bilobe: nasal dorsum and sidewall, temporal forehead.
  □ Rhombic: temporal forehead, lateral inferior, or medial cheek.

Interpolation
- Allow surgeon to bring tissue from sites near, but not immediately adjacent to, defect.
- Frequently used when no good options exist for movement of adjacent tissue into wound.
  - Midforehead: midface reconstruction, especially nasal.

Advancement
- Ideal guidelines for the design of A-T flaps have been developed: The height-to-base ratio should be 2:1.
- V-Y flaps useful to lengthen structure or region or to release contracture.
  - Single advancement: square defects, central forehead.
  - Double advancement: square defects, central forehead.
  - V-Y: eyelid, vermillion, nasolabial crease, columella.
  - A-T/O-T: central/temporal forehead, chin, lower lip.
  - Island pedicled: medial cheek near alar base.

Hinge
- Most commonly used to provide inner lining in full-thickness nasal or buccal defects.
- Melolabial turn-in: reconstruction of nasal lining.

Regions
Central forehead
- Must preserve hair line and eyebrows.
- Rectangular advancement flap: good use of relaxed skin tension lines.
- O-Z flap: good for moderate-sized defect.
- Large defect: may need multiple serial advancements, possibly with tissue expanders.

Temporal region
- Must preserve lateral canthus and hairline, temporal branch of facial nerve.
- O-Z flap often effective for small defects.

Medial canthus and cheek
- Glabellar and cheeks flaps most effective.
- Can use transposition or V-Y rotation flap.
- Cheek flaps preferred for large defects due to skin similarity.

Lateral cheek
- Must preserve parotid duct and branches of facial nerve.
- Rhombic and bilobed flaps most popular, but can use almost any flap.

Melanoma
Etiology
- Arises from melanocytes.
- Patients at greatest risk: those with family history of malignant melanoma; relative risk increases two to eight times.
- Fair complexion.
- Marked freckling (three times risk).
- Three or more blistering sunburns before 20 years of age.
- Some melanomas from precursor pigmented lesions, whereas others *de novo*; congenital melanocytic nevi and dysplastic nevi considered precursor lesions; cutaneous melanoma from preexisting lesion 50% of time.
- Incidence: 11 per 10,000 in Caucasian, with males more commonly affected than females.

Clinical features
- May be remembered by the mnemonic ABCD:
  - A = asymmetry.
  - B = border irregularity.
  - C = color variegation.
  - D = diameter greater than 6 mm.
- Progression of legions.
  - Tends to be sequentially in two directions.
  - In early phase, spread in plane parallel to skin surface; known as radial growth phase.
  - After period of time, growth changes to direction perpendicular to surface of skin; known as vertical growth phase.

Types of melanoma
- Melanoma in situ (lentigo maligna; precedes vertical growth phase.)
- Superficial spreading melanoma (most common).
- Acral lentiginous melanoma.
- Nodular.

Histopathology
- Nests of vacuolated melanocytic cells.
- Classification systems include Clark's and Breslow's.
  - Clark's classification:
    - Level I = confined to epidermis.
    - Level II = extension into papillary dermis.
    - Level III = expands papillary dermis, not into reticular dermis.
    - Level IV = infiltrates reticular dermis.
    - Level V = extension to subcutaneous fat.
      - Levels I and II in radial-growth phase with little capacity for metastasis.
      - Levels III-V in vertical-growth phase with higher metastatic risk.
  - Breslow's classification:

- Thickness as measured from the granular layer of the overlying epidermis (Table 4).
  - Specific lesions.
  - Cutaneous melanocytic lesions (benign).
    - Non-neoplastic hyperpigmentation (freckle, solar lentigo).
    - Benign neoplasms: proliferative melanocytes.
    - Congenital melanocytic nevi (size determines lifetime risk for melanoma).
    - Acquired melanocytic nevi.
      - Junctional nevi: melanocytes at dermal-epidermal junction.
      - Dermal nevi: melanocytes deep to junction.
      - Compound nevi: with junctional and dermal melanocytes.
      - Dysplastic nevi: larger and irregular; (+) melanoma association.

Malignant Neoplasms

Lentigo maligna (melanoma in situ)

- Known as Hutchinson's freckle.
- Large, flat heterogeneous pigmentation.
- 5%-33% progression to invasive melanoma.
- Isolated to epidermis and adnexal epidermis.
- Pleomorphic, variable atypical melanocytes.
- Treatment: complete excision with 99% survival.

Superficial spreading melanoma

- Most common (<50% of all melanomas).
- Most often in patients with risk factors (e.g., nevi, sun exposure).
- Flat and deeply pigmented.
- Nuclear pleomorphism and mitoses.
- Prolonged radial growth phase, metastasis with vertical phase.

Nodular melanoma

- Rare.
- 1-2-cm diameter with color variegation.
- Can exhibit pure vertical growth phase.
- Most aggressive form.

Acral lentiginous melanoma

- Predilection for nail beds, plantar, and palmar surfaces.
- Nonwhites > whites.

Variants

- Desmoplastic melanoma: vertical growth phase, spindle cells with fibrotic stroma.
- Neurotropic melanoma: perineural invasion and predilection for lip.

Diagnosis

- Excisional biopsy preferred.

TABLE 4. Breslow's Classification of Thickness

Stage	Size (mm)	5-Year Survival Rate (%)
1	<0.76	90
2	0.76-1.49	85
3	1.5-3.99	70
4	>4.0	50

  - Need sufficient tissue to allow for accurate staging.
  - Bevel away from tumor to fascial plane below subcutaneous layer.

Spread

- Patterns of spread
  - Most frequent site of metastasis: regional lymph nodes.
  - Patients with regional lymph node metastasis: 70%-85% chance of developing distant metastasis.
  - Strong correlation between Clark's levels, Breslow's thickness, and recurrence/mortality.
- Cervical spread:
  - <0.75 mm = approximately 0%.
  - >0.76 mm = 25% cervical metastases.
  - >1.5 mm = 56% cervical metastases.
  - >4.0 mm = 62% cervical metastases.
- Face, ear, anterior scalp draining to parotid lymph nodes.
- Posterior scalp to retro-auricular, occipital, posterior cervical nodes.
- Distant metastases.
  - With thickness >4.0 mm, see >70% with distant disease
  - Sites: skin, subcutaneous, liver, brain, bone, other nodal chains.
  - Distant disease with median survival = 6 months.

Staging

- Stage I = localized primary melanoma.
- Stage II = regional nodal disease.
- Stage III = disseminated disease.

Treatment

- Local resection is primary treatment of choice.
- Classic 3-5-cm margins are not recommended or required in head and neck region.
- Margins of 1 cm appear adequate in most cases.
- General recommendations with regard to the depth of lesion is:
  - Lesion 1 mm thick = 1-cm margin.
  - Lesion 1-2 mm thick = 1-2 cm margin.
  - Lesion 2-4 mm thick = 2-cm margin.
  - Lesion >0.4 mm thick = at least 3-cm margin.

- Margin size can be diminished depending on the site of lesion, and these therefore are guidelines.

Neck dissection

- If nodes are clinically positive nodes:
  - Neck dissection always indicated.
  - Main benefit in local and regional control.
  - Overall survival very poor (25% 5-year) in these cases.
- With clinically negative nodes, role for elective neck dissection controversial; current recommendations (based on incidence of occult metastases; see above):
  - Neck dissections are not required in lesions <0.75 mm in thickness or lentigo maligna melanoma.
  - Elective neck dissection in lesions 0.75-1.5 mm in thickness may be of value, especially when the lesion is on the thicker end of the spectrum, when the histologic type is nodular, when the lesion is ulcerative, or when long-term follow-up may be indicated.
  - Neck dissections should be performed when primary lesions are 1.5-4.0 mm thick.
  - Neck dissections offer the opportunity for improved local and regional control in patients with lesions >4.0 mm in thickness, but likely do not affect patient survival.

Radiation therapy

- May be adequate primary therapy in cases of lentigo maligna melanoma.
- May have role as adjuvant therapy in patients with more advanced disease (i.e., Breslow 3 or 4).
- Chemotherapy.
- Very limited role in management of disseminated disease.

Immunotherapy for melanoma

- Biological response modifier (BRM) therapy or immunotherapy has not been shown to be effective in treating melanoma. Clinical trials are being done to find biological therapies that are effective.
- Cytokines such as interferons and interleukins alone or in combination with cytostatic agents are primary BRM interventions. Secondary BRM interventions were introduced with the discovery of hybridoma technology in 1975, when the isolation of monoclonal antibodies of defined specificity became possible.
- Monoclonal antibodies are typically developed in a mouse host and are used to provide directed therapy. They have been used in several ways to evoke a clinical response:
- Activation of components of the immune system.
  - In all cases, the antigens against which the monoclonal antibodies are directed are expressed on both melanoma cells and normal tissue,

although in considerably greater proportion in the melanoma cells.
  - The most promising monoclonal antibodies are directed against glycolipid antigens on the melanocyte cell surface. In particular, the gangliosides GD2 and GD3 have proven to be the most potent activators of the immune system. Two other cell surface antigens that are currently involved in clinical trials are p97/gp95 and mCSP.
  - Once antibodies have been directed to the melanocytes, lysis can be mediated by antibody-dependent cellular cytotoxicity (ADCC) via leukocytes or complement-dependent cytotoxicity (CDC) via the serum.
- Drug delivery.
  - Antitumor agents can be delivered to tumor sites; monoclonal antibodies may be combined with recombinant cytokines or conjugated to radionuclides (for diagnosis and staging) or toxins (e.g., ricin for treatment).

Active immunization

- Antiidiotype vaccine (polyvalent melanoma vaccine derived from cultured melanoma cell lines)
- Example: immunization with a modified peptide from the gp 100 followed by high-dose IL-melanocyte-stimulating hormone and a monoclonal antibody to the CD3 T cell.

Prognosis

- 10-year survival data may be needed to accurately assess treatment efficacy.
- Prognosis of localized melanomas related to:
  - Thickness.
  - Type (nodular worse prognosis than other types).
  - Presence of ulceration (poorer prognosis on scalp and posterior neck).
  - Age (slightly worse in patients over 55).
- With spread to regional lymphatics, 5-year survival rate drops to 10%-20%, whereas similar patients with no lymphatic spread have an overall survival rate of 70%-80%.

Selected References from the Recent Literature

1. Ohno T. Autologous cancer vaccine: a novel formulation. [Review] [45 refs]. *Microbiology & Immunology* 2003;47: 255-263.
2. Srivastava A, Ralhan R, Kaur J. Angiogenesis in cutaneous melanoma: pathogenesis and clinical implications. [Review] [139 refs]. *Microscopy Research & Technique* 2003;60: 208-224.
3. Ramirez-Montagut T, Turk MJ, Wolchok JD *et al.* Immunity to melanoma: unraveling the relation of tumor immunity and autoimmunity. [Review] [55 refs]. *Oncogene* 2003;22: 3180-3187.

4. Streit M, Detmar M. Angiogenesis, lymphangiogenesis, and melanoma metastasis. [Review] [111 refs]. *Oncogene* 2003;22:3172-3179.

5. Soengas MS, Lowe SW. Apoptosis and melanoma chemoresistance. [Review] [181 refs]. *Oncogene* 2003;22:3138-3151.

6. Polsky D, Cordon-Cardo C. Oncogenes in melanoma. [Review] [48 refs]. *Oncogene* 2003;22:3087-3091.

7. Molife R, Hancock BW. Adjuvant therapy of malignant melanoma. [Review] [143 refs]. *Critical Reviews in Oncology-Hematology* 2002;44:81-102.

8. Medina JE, Ferlito A, Pellitteri PK *et al.* Current management of mucosal melanoma of the head and neck. [Review] [44 refs]. *Journal of Surgical Oncology* 2003;83: 116-122.

9. Palmowski M, Salio M, Dunbar RP *et al.* The use of HLA class I tetramers to design a vaccination strategy for melanoma patients. [Review] [44 refs]. *Immunological Reviews* 2002;188:155-163.

10. Bedrosian I, Gershenwald JE. Surgical clinical trials in melanoma. [Review] [34 refs]. *Surgical Clinics of North America* 2003;83:385-403.

11. Eggermont AM, van Geel AN, de Wilt JH *et al.* The role of isolated limb perfusion for melanoma confined to the extremities. [Review] [81 refs]. *Surgical Clinics of North America* 2003;83:371-384.

12. Kadison AS, Morton DL. Immunotherapy of malignant melanoma. [Review] [153 refs]. *Surgical Clinics of North America* 2003;83:343-370.

13. Ballo MT, Ang KK. Radiation therapy for malignant melanoma. [Review] [88 refs]. *Surgical Clinics of North America* 2003;83:323-342.

14. Brown CK, Kirkwood JM. Medical management of melanoma. [Review] [190 refs]. *Surgical Clinics of North America* 2003;83:283-322.

15. Pitman KT, Ferlito A, Devaney KO *et al.* Sentinel lymph node biopsy in head and neck cancer. [Review] [65 refs]. *Oral Oncology* 2003;39:343-349.

16. Tueche SG. Behavior of malignant melanoma with tonsil metastasis. [Review] [15 refs]. *Annales de Medecine Interne* 2002;153:136-138.

17. Essner R. Surgical treatment of malignant melanoma. [Review] [267 refs]. *Surgical Clinics of North America* 2003;83:109-156.

18. Zettersten E, Shaikh L, Ramirez R *et al.* Prognostic factors in primary cutaneous melanoma. [Review] [95 refs]. *Surgical Clinics of North America* 2003; 83:61-75.

19. Liu V, Mihm MC. Pathology of malignant melanoma. [Review] [94 refs]. *Surgical Clinics of North America* 2003;83:31-60.

20. Desmond RA, Soong SJ. Epidemiology of malignant melanoma. [Review] [74 refs]. *Surgical Clinics of North America* 2003;83:1-29.

21. Medina JE, Ferlito A, Brandwein MS *et al.* Current management of cutaneous malignant melanoma of the head and neck. [Review] [29 refs]. *Acta Oto-Laryngologica* 2002;122: 900-906.

22. Nestle FO. Vaccines and melanoma. [Review] [27 refs]. *Clinical & Experimental Dermatology* 2002;27:597-601.

23. Elbaum M. Computer-aided melanoma diagnosis. [Review] [37 refs]. *Dermatologic Clinics* 2002;20:735-747.

24. Rivers JK. Unusual melanoma types. [Review] [43 refs]. *Dermatologic Clinics* 2002;20:727-733.

25. Bystryn JC. Vaccines for melanoma. [Review] [23 refs]. *Dermatologic Clinics* 2002;20:717-725.

26. Cooper JS. Radiation therapy of malignant melanoma. [Review] [31 refs]. *Dermatologic Clinics* 2002;20:713-716.

27. Pavlick AC. Chemotherapy approaches to melanoma. [Review] [23 refs]. *Dermatologic Clinics* 2002;20:709-712.

28. Carucci JA. Mohs' micrographic surgery for the treatment of melanoma. [Review] [59 refs]. *Dermatologic Clinics* 2002;20:701-708.

29. Shapiro RL. Surgical approaches to malignant melanoma: practical guidelines. [Review] [165 refs]. *Dermatologic Clinics* 2002;20:681-699.

30. Swanson NA, Lee KK, Gorman A *et al.* Biopsy techniques: diagnosis of melanoma. [Review] [9 refs]. *Dermatologic Clinics* 2002;20:677-680.

31. Friedman RJ, Heilman ER. The pathology of malignant melanoma. [Review] [29 refs]. *Dermatologic Clinics* 2002;20: 659-676.

32. Rogers GS, Braun SM. Prognostic factors. [Review] [159 refs]. *Dermatologic Clinics* 2002;20:647-658.

33. Geller AC. Screening for melanoma. [Review] [88 refs]. *Dermatologic Clinics* 2002;20:629-640.

34. Rigel DS. The effect of sunscreen on melanoma risk. [Review] [21 refs]. *Dermatologic Clinics* 2002;20: 601-606.

35. MacKie RM. Risk factors for the development of primary cutaneous malignant melanoma. [Review] [22 refs]. *Dermatologic Clinics* 2002;20:597-600.

36. Bevona C, Sober AJ. Melanoma incidence trends. [Review] [61 refs]. *Dermatologic Clinics* 2002;20:589-595.

BENIGN LESIONS OF THE NOSE AND PARANASAL SINUSES

Epithelial Lesions

Papilloma
- Fungiform: occur on septum.
- Cylindric (<1%).
- Keratotic: occur in the nasal vestibule.
- Inverted (see below).

Histopathology
- Hyperplastic respiratory epithelium with exophytic/inverting growth pattern.
- Epithelium with or without keratin formation.
- Micromucinous cysts frequently present.

Symptoms
- Unilateral nasal obstruction.
- Incidental finding on exam.

Treatment
- Complete excision.

Ameloblastoma
Neoplasm of dental origin occasionally as mass in sinus
- Locally aggressive.
- 20% in maxilla, usually in region of third molar.

Histopathology
- Both follicular and plexiform pattern.
- Hallmark: enamel.

Treatment
- Complete excision with adequate margins.

Nonepithelial Lesions

Osteoma
- Frontal (80%), ethmoid (16%), maxillary (4%).
- More common in males.

Radiographic findings
- Sharply defined bony margins.
- Eburnated: uniformly radiodense.
- Cancellous: central core of cancellous bone (bony rim with radiolucent center).

Histopathology
- Densely sclerotic well-formed bone projecting out from cortical surface.

Symptoms
- Most often asymptomatic; picked up as incidental finding.

- If large, may cause headache, diplopia, sinus obstruction (mimics symptoms of frontoethmoid mucocele).

Treatment
- Asymptomatic: radiographic evaluation on periodic basis.
- Symptomatic: excision (if nasofrontal ostium obstructed, sinus should be obliterated with fat).

Ossifying fibroma
- Originate from periosteum or periodontal membrane.
- Peak incidence second to fourth decade of life.
- Most commonly involves mandible, then maxilla.
- More common in females than males.

Radiographic findings
- Well-demarcated with eggshell appearance.

Histopathology
- Woven or lamellar bone with smooth borders and rimming osteoblasts.
- Parallel birefringence with polarized light.

Treatment
- Enucleation.

Fibrous dysplasia
- Developmental maturation defect/fibroosseous metaplasia
- Most common in first decade of life.
- More common in females than males.
- Maxilla > mandible.
- 3% with Albright's syndrome (polyostotic bone lesions, cafe-au-lait spots, and precocious puberty).

Radiographic findings
- Poorly demarcated density, range from completely lucent to opaque (ground glass).

Histopathology
- Woven bone with feathery irregular borders, "Chinese characters."
- Random birefringence with polarized light.

Treatment
- Symptomatic only, usually osteotomies to reduce deformities.

Juvenile nasopharyngeal angiofibroma
- Exclusively in males.
- Presents around puberty.
- Usually arises from lateral wall of nasopharynx; frequently extends superiorly into sphenoid.

- If extends laterally though pterygomaxillary fissure into pterygomaxillary space, produces characteristic anterior bowing of posterior maxillary wall (Holman-Miller sign).

Signs and symptoms
- Nasal obstruction and bleeding.
- Tumor pale to beefy red, avoid biopsy.

Radiographic findings
- CT with contrast: enhancing mass.
- Angiography usually not necessary for diagnosis, utilized in preoperative embolization.
- Magnetic resonance imaging (MRI): Particularly useful if central nervous system (CNS) extension suspected.

Giant cell tumors
- Rare tumor.
- Peak incidence second to fourth decade of life.
- Most common location: premolar teeth.

Signs and symptoms
- Mass or deformity of maxilla.
- Pain, cortical bone perforation, loose tooth, paresthesia.

Radiographic findings
- Opacification of sinus with thinning and expansion of bone.
- CT: calcification in soft tissue.

Histopathology
- Multinucleated osteoclastic giant cells without malignant characteristics.

Treatment
- Resection with wide margins.

 INVERTING PAPILLOMA

Incidence and etiology
- Production of benign lesions (Schneiderian papillomas) due to proliferation of reserve cells in nasal reparatory mucosa (Schneiderian mucosa).
- Unilateral.
- Presents more often in men than women (3:1).
- Presents most commonly between 40-70 years of age.
- Transformation of up to 15% of inverting papillomas into malignant lesions (general transformation rate: 5%-7%).

Pathology
- Arises from lateral nasal wall and/or paranasal sinuses and invades underlying stroma (hence term *inverting*)

- Associated with human papillomavirus (types 6, 11)

Clinical manifestations
- Unilateral nasal obstruction with or without sinusitis.
- Rhinorrhea.
- Epistaxis.
- Nasal mass.
- Facial/sinus pain.
- Anosmia.
- Facial paresthesia/anesthesia.
- Epiphora.
- Trismus perhaps ominous sign of malignancy (invasion into masseteripterygoids).

Investigations
- CT scan (include coronal axis views).
- MRI to delineate tumor extent (e.g., if CNS involvement possible) and to distinguish disease from mucosal thickening.
- Biopsy.
- Culture for concomitant nasal pathogens in patients with obstructed sinuses.
- Consider angiography depending on the size and location of the lesion.

Treatment
- Difficult to remove completely; requires wide mucosal margins.
- Location of lesion to dictate approach and technique.
- Endoscopic wide ethmoidectomy with or without maxillectomy.
- Ethmoidectomy and medial maxillectomy via open (e.g., lateral rhinotomy, midface degloving) approach.
- Approach to depend on surgeon preference and skill, extent of disease, concern for malignancy.

Complications of treatment
- CSF leak.
- Dacryocystitis.
- Epiphora.
- Diplopia.
- Nasocutaneous fistula.
- Nasal collapse.
- Scarring.
- Frontal sinus mucocele.
- Radiation treatment considered ineffective and possibly induces carcinoma.

Prognosis
- High recurrence rate (up to 44%); possibly require multiple procedures to control disease.

- Must be vigilant for transformation of these benign growths into malignant lesions.

MALIGNANCIES OF THE NASAL CAVITY

Incidence and etiology
- Increasing incidence to 1:700,000 in eighth decade of life.
- Associations between development of carcinoma with exposures to following substances:
  - Nickel.
  - Chromium.
  - Hydrocarbons.
  - Isopropyl oils.
- People in professions at increased risk:
  - Woodworkers.
  - Boot and shoe workers.
  - Furniture makers.

Sites of tumors
- Maxillary sinus: 55%
- Nasal cavity: 35%
- Ethmoid: 9%
- Sphenoid, frontal sinus, septum: 1%

Signs and symptoms
- Early: Nasal obstruction, epistaxis, blood tinged sputum, unilateral tearing, nasal polyp.
- Late: Facial asymmetry, sensory changes, loose teeth, malposition of eye, bulge in hard palate, obstructed breathing, change in voice, trismus, ocular palsy, pain.

Evaluation
- History and physical exam.
- Lymphadenopathy, cranial neuropathies (IV, V, VI), otitis media.
- Nasal endoscopy.
- Ophthalmologic evaluation.
- Radiographic studies.
- High resolution CT in addition to MRI, magnetic resonance angiography (MRA) complementary.
- Angiography an option, although rarely used unless embolization to be considered.

Pathology
- No separate staging system for tumors arising in the nasal cavity.

Tumor Types

Squamous cell carcinoma
- Most common.
- Sites: lateral nasal wall, turbinates (50%).
- May not be able to tell lateral nasal wall from sinus origin.

- Septum: 9% of nasal malignancies, 20%-30% associated with other malignancies.
- Meatus, vestibule.

Therapy
- Wide excision with 1-cm margins; postoperative radiation therapy.
- High rate of ocular injury.
- Neck lymphadenectomy if palpable adenopathy.

Procedures
- Local resection with wide margins.
- Septectomy.
- Rhinectomy.
- Maxillectomy with or without orbital exenteration (with periosteal involvement).

Prognosis
- SCC of septum: 70% cure rate; worse prognosis with extensive disease or neck nodes.

Adenoid cystic carcinoma (ACC)
- 10% of nasal malignancies.
- Arises from minor salivary glands.
- Classic "Swiss cheese" histologic pattern.
- Low grade vs. high grade: important distinction with higher incidence of vascular invasion, distant metastases with high grade.
- Perineural invasion and spread common.
- Surgical excision treatment of choice.
- Prognosis: 60% 10-year survival rate.
- Late >10 years recurrence common.
- Role of radiotherapy controversial.

Adenocarcinoma (mucoepidermoid carcinoma and acinic cell carcinoma)
- Tends to be aggressive.

Papillary adenocarcinoma
- Most well localized.
- Tall columnar cell histology.
- Resemble colonic papillary carcinoma.

Sessile adenocarcinoma
- Greater invasive properties; alveolar mucoid variant.
- Most aggressive.
- Poorer prognosis.
- Histology: abundant mucin with nests of individual cells.
- Similar management strategy to SCC.

Sarcomas
- 1% of head and sarcomas; 15% of paranasal sinus tumors.
- Radiation: risk increase of malignant fibrous histiocytoma.

- Usually advanced at presentation.
- Surgical resection in addition to radiation therapy if:
  - Not rhabdomyosarcoma.
  - Positive margins (45% cure rate); neck dissection if positive nodes.

Rhabdomyosarcoma
- Treat with surgery, radiation, chemotherapy.

Chondrosarcoma
- Typically arise from posterior nasal septum.
- Difficult to tell benign from malignant.
- Grows slowly with late metastases.
- May extend intracranially with increased mortality.
- En bloc resection curative.

Other Malignant Lesions

Hemangiopericytoma
- Originates from capillary pericyte of Zimmerman, therefore arises wherever capillaries found.
- Has predilection for musculoskeletal system and skin.
- Typically presents as slowly expanding asymptomatic mass.
- Incidence equal in both sexes.
- Regarded as malignant neoplasm.
- Treatment: wide surgical excision with preop embolization.
- Role of radiation not clearly delineated.
- Rate of metastases reported ranges from 33%-57%.
- High rate of recurrence even after surgical excision.

Lymphoma
- Polymorphic reticulosis, lethal midline granuloma, idiopathic midline destructive lesion).
  - B cell or T cell.
  - Association with EBV.
  - 50% mortality.
  - Treat with radiation therapy.

Melanoma
- Rare, arises from septum and lateral nasal wall.
- Pigmented lesion.
- Treatment with local excision.
- Frequent local recurrence.

Esthesioneuroblastoma
- Rare neuroepithelial malignancy.
- Arises from olfactory epithelium in region of roof or upper lateral wall of nose (e.g., neuroectodermal tumor).
- Histology: undifferentiated small round epithelial cells, arranged in compact cellular aggregates, scant cytoplasm, dense nuclei, absent mitotic figures, secretory granules on erythema multiforme (EM).

- Tumor sometimes multicentric, one tumor above and one below cribriform plate.
- Surgery treatment of choice.
- Lateral rhinotomy alone for small tumors arising from lateral wall.
- Combined-approach craniofacial resection for tumors based superiorly or for larger tumors.
- Postoperative radiation for tumors with no intracranial extension possibly reduces local recurrence rates, but studies show it is likely not indicated.

Plasmacytoma
- Isolated plasma cell tumor.
- Must rule out systemic multiple myeloma or plasma cell leukemia. Total serum protein/albumin, CBC with differential, chest x-ray, skeletal survey, serum protein electrophoresis, urine for Bence-Jones protein.
- Biopsy to confirm diagnosis (may elicit significant hemorrhage).
- Surgical debulking possibly required in larger tumors.

 ## MAXILLARY SINUS MALIGNANCIES INCIDENCE AND ETIOLOGY

- Malignant tumors of the sinonasal tract constitute less than 1% of all malignancies in the body and about 3% of those arising in the upper respiratory tract.
- Maxillary sinus is the most common site of origin for malignancies of the sinonasal tract.
- Ratio of males to females is 2:1
- Nickel-refining processes have been implicated in the development of SCC and anaplastic carcinomas.
- Woodworkers exposed to hardwood dust suffer an increased incidence of adenocarcinoma of the ethmoid sinus. Other workers exposed to softwood dust show an increased incidence of SCC, anaplastic carcinoma, and adenocarcinoma.
- Tobacco smoking alone is not thought to be a significant etiologic factor.
- Tanning leather, mineral oils, chromium, isopropyl oils, lacquer paint, soldering and welding, and radium dial painting are thought to be etiologic factors.

Pathology
- SCC most common.
- Adenocarcinoma = 4%-8%; most common in ethmoid sinuses and nasal cavity.
- Adenoid cystic: account for 20% of all adenoid cystic tumors that occur in the head and neck.
- Mucoepidermoid extremely rare.

- Melanoma primary or metastatic: 1% of 20% that arise in head and neck.
- Olfactory neuroblastoma: rare tumor arising in olfactory epithelium.
- Undifferentiated carcinomas, teratocarcinomas.
- Rhabdomyosarcomas: 35%-45% occur in head and neck; 8% of those originate in sinonasal tract.
- Neurogenic sarcomas, leiomyosarcomas, fibrosarcomas.
- Angiosarcomas, hemangiopericytomas, osteogenic sarcoma.
- Chondrosarcomas, non-Hodgkin's lymphoma, extramedullary plasmacytoma, giant cell tumor.
- Metastatic tumor: renal cell carcinoma most common.

Classification
- Ohngren's line: divides maxillary sinus into infrastructure and suprastructure; line runs from medial canthus to angle of jaw.
  - T1: tumor confined to antral mucosa of infrastructure with no erosion or destruction of bone.
  - T2: tumor confined to antral mucosa of suprastructure with no erosion or destruction of bone, or to infrastructure with destruction of the medial or inferior walls only.
  - T3: involvement of skin, orbit, anterior ethmoid sinus, pterygoid sinus.
  - T4: invasion of cribriform plate, posterior ethmoids, sphenoid sinus, nasopharynx, pterygoid plate, pterygoid muscle, skull base.

Clinical manifestations
- Most common clinical presentation of tumors of the sinonasal tract includes symptoms that are identical to those caused by inflammatory sinus disease, such as nasal airway obstruction, pain, epistaxis, and nasal discharge.
- Regional and distant metastases are infrequent.
- Cervical metastases upon initial presentation occur in 10% of patients, distant metastases in 7%.
- Cranial neuropathies occur in 34% of patients.
- Proptosis, chemosis, extraocular muscle impairment, mass effect in the cheek, gingiva or gingivobuccal sulcus, and loose dentition also suggest the presence of a sinonasal tumor.

Investigations
- CT helps to evaluate bony architecture.
- MRI helps to differentiate adjacent soft tissue with different composition (e.g., secretions from tumor); also helps with issues pertaining to intracranial extension
- Angiography with or without balloon occlusion test if carotid resection contemplated.

- CT of chest and abdomen in tumors that spread hematogenously.
- LP/MRI brain if concern for tumors that extend to brain and spine.

Treatment
- Surgery: mainstay of treatment.
- Radiation as adjunctive modality when there are positive margins, perineural invasion, perivascular invasion, lymph node involvement, recurrent tumor.
- Radiation as lone modality for unresectable tumors, poor surgical candidates, lymphomas.
- Chemotherapy as palliative role and investigational as primary modality.
- T1-T2: maxillectomy or primary radiation.
- T3-T4: surgery with preoperative or postoperative radiation.

Adenocarcinoma
- Locally aggressive, therefore require aggressive surgical intervention.

Adenoid cystic
- Good local control with good short-term survival rate (5-year: 75%). However, high risk of late distant recurrence (15-year survival: 15%). Treatment is, therefore, controversial.
- In general, surgical resection with radiation for positive margins is a logical approach. The role of systemic chemotherapy at the time of primary treatment to try to decrease the incidence of distant metastases is unclear.

Cervical metastases
- Occurs in 25%-35% of cases.
- Carries poor prognosis.
- Neck dissection indicated with clinically palpable nodes.
- Ipsilateral neck dissection with preauricular area or inclusion of these areas in radiation field with T3 and T4 maxillary sinus malignancies.

Prognosis
- Varies on histopathology of tumor.
- 5-year survival rate for SCC of maxillary sinus 40%-50%.

 MALIGNANCIES OF THE FRONTAL, ETHMOID, AND SPHENOID SINUSES

Incidence and epidemiology
- Malignant diseases of the sinus <3% of head and neck cancers.
- Tumors of frontal and sphenoid sinuses extremely rare (<1% of sinonasal tumors).

- Present in fifth to seventh decades of life.
- Risk factors: see discussion of maxillary sinus carcinoma.

Clinical presentation
- Unilateral symptoms: epistaxis, obstruction, pain, discharge, dysthesias, visual changes.
- <10% with cervical metastases at presentation.
- 33% associated with cranial neuropathy.

Pathology
Tumors of epithelial origin
Squamous cell carcinoma
- More common on lateral nasal wall.
- 80% of sinus malignancies.
- Poorly marginated, destructive lesion.
- Associated with nickel exposure and wood-dust exposure.

Glandular tumors
- 10% of malignant sinus tumors, but majority involve maxillary antrum.
- Adenocarcinomas: rare (4%-8%), usually ethmoid sinuses, woodworker association.
- Minor salivary gland tumors.
- Slow growth; associated with bone expansion rather than erosion.
- Adenoid cystic (high-grade and low-grade histology).
- Mucoepidermoid extremely rare in sinuses; 25% with metastasis.

Melanoma
- Rare (<1% of H&N melanomas).
- Middle turbinates or septum > maxillary > ethmoid > frontal.
- Often presents with bleeding.
- High incidence of recurrence with 25% 5-year survival rate.

Esthesioneuroblastoma
- See Tumors of the Nasal Cavity.

Tumors of nonepithelial origin
Non-Hodgkin's lymphoma
- 8% of sinus malignancies.
- Treat with radiation and chemotherapy.

Other rare sinus tumors
- Fibrosarcoma
- Rhabdomyosarcoma (8%) = wide surgical resection and XRT.
- Leiomyosarcoma = smooth muesli tumors.
- Hemangiopericytomas = Zimmerman pericytes; 16% found in H&N.
- Extramedullary plasmacytoma.

Undifferentiated nasopharyngeal carcinoma
- See related discussion.

Diagnosis
Endoscopic evaluation of the nasal cavity and sinuses
- Radiologic evaluation
  - MRI: 95% of sinonasal tumors have intermediate intensity on T2, allowing differentiation between mucosal inflammation, polyps, or inspissated secretions; information on extension.
  - CT allows review of bony erosion.
- Intraoperative biopsy
  - After determination that tumor is not vascular.

Treatment
Surgical resection
- Lateral rhinotomy (maxillary, ethmoid, sphenoids).
- Midfacial degloving (maxillary, ethmoid, sphenoids).
- Bicoronal (frontal, intracranial).
- Approaches combined for craniofacial resection.
- Craniofacial resections usually required because these tumors tend to present at more advanced stages.

Contraindications
- Prevertebral fascia invasion.
- Cavernous sinus invasion.
- Carotid artery involvement.
- Optic chiasm invasion.
- Ocular involvement (invasion of the periorbita) may necessitate orbital exenteration.

Chemotherapy with surgery and XRT
- Induction chemotherapy with cycles of cisplatin and 5-fluorouracil in advanced tumors.
- XRT necessary with positive margins.
- Ocular complications vary with dose:
  - <3500 cGy (<5%).
  - 6000-7000 cGy (50%).
  - 8000 cGy (>85%).

Prognosis
- For most epithelial malignancies of sphenoid, ethmoid, frontal sinuses, 5-year survival rate still under 50%.

Selected References from the Recent Literature

1. Knott PD, Gannon FH, Thompson LD. Mesenchymal chondrosarcoma of the sinonasal tract: a clinicopathological study of 13 cases with a review of the literature. [Review] [30 refs]. *Laryngoscope* 2003;113:783-790.
2. Lee CF, Liu TC, Hsu CJ *et al*. Sinonasal adenocarcinoma: clinical study of nine cases in Taiwan. [Review] [27 refs]. *Acta Oto-Laryngologica* 2002;122:887-891.
3. Syrjanen KJ. HPV infections in benign and malignant sinonasal lesions. [Review] [134 refs]. *Journal of Clinical Pathology* 2003;56:174-181.

4. Loevner LA, Sonners AI. Imaging of neoplasms of the paranasal sinuses. [Review] [102 refs]. *Magnetic Resonance Imaging Clinics of North America* 2002;10(3):467-493.

5. Rinaldo A, Ferlito A, Shaha AR *et al.* Is elective neck treatment indicated in patients with squamous cell carcinoma of the maxillary sinus? [Review] [27 refs]. *Acta Oto-Laryngologica* 2002;122:443-447.

6. Yih WY, Stewart JC, Kratochvil FJ *et al.* Angiocentric T-cell lymphoma presenting as midface destructive lesion: case report and literature review. [Review] [53 refs]. *Oral Surgery, Oral Medicine, Oral Pathology, Oral Radiology, & Endodontics* 2002;94:353-360.

7. Kumar M, Fallon RJ, Hill JS *et al.* Esthesioneuroblastoma in children. [Review] [21 refs]. *Journal of Pediatric Hematology/Oncology* 2002;24:482-487.

8. Mra Z, Roach JC, Brook AL. Infectious and neoplastic diseases of the sphenoid sinus—a report of 10 cases. [Review] [18 refs]. *Rhinology* 2002;40:34-40.

9. Eisen MD, Buchmann L, Litman RS *et al.* Inverted papilloma of the sphenoid sinus presenting with auditory symptoms: a report of two cases. [Review] [14 refs]. *Laryngoscope* 2002;112:1197-1200.

10. Osguthorpe JD, Patel S. Craniofacial approaches to tumors of the anterior skull base. [Review] [50 refs]. *Otolaryngologic Clinics of North America* 2001;3:1123-1142.

11. Browne JD. The midfacial degloving procedure for nasal, sinus, and nasopharyngeal tumors. [Review] [12 refs]. *Otolaryngologic Clinics of North America* 2001;34: 1095-1104.

12. Rice DH. Endonasal approaches for sinonasal and nasopharyngeal tumors. [Review] [17 refs]. *Otolaryngologic Clinics of North America* 2001;34:1087-1093.

13. Osguthorpe JD, Richardson M. Frontal sinus malignancies. [Review] [23 refs]. *Otolaryngologic Clinics of North America* 2001;34:269-281.

14. Senior BA, Lanza DC. Benign lesions of the frontal sinus. [Review] [30 refs]. Otolaryngologic *Clinics of North America* 2001;34:253-267.

15. Sunderman FW, Jr. Nasal toxicity, carcinogenicity, and olfactory uptake of metals. [Review] [169 refs]. *Annals of Clinical & Laboratory Science* 2001;31:3-24.

16. Batsakis JG, Suarez P. Schneiderian papillomas and carcinomas: a review. [Review] [42 refs]. *Advances in Anatomic Pathology* 2001;8:53-64.

17. Reino AJ. Factors in the pathogenesis of tumors of the sphenoid and maxillary sinuses: a comparative study. [Review] [1186 refs]. *Laryngoscope* 2000;110:1-38.

18. Bertrand B, Eloy P, Jorissen M *et al.* Surgery of inverted papillomas under endoscopic control. [Review] [48 refs]. *Acta Oto-Rhino-Laryngologica Belgica* 2000;54:139-150.

NASOPHARYNGEAL CARCINOMA

Incidence and epidemiology

- In North American and European white populations, nasopharyngeal carcinoma (NPC) is relatively rare, with an incidence of 1 per 100,000. The incidence increases moderately (2-4 per 100,000) in people of African, North African, North American Inuit, and Polynesian (Filipino) descent.
- By contrast, the incidence is 30 per 100,000 in the area of southern China, with the highest incidence in the coastal regions and large cities, notably Hong Kong and Taiwan. First-generation descendants of emigrants from southern China to areas of low incidence, such as the United States, display a considerable decrement in incidence of NPC; however, at 15 per 100,000, this incidence is still markedly increased compared with the U.S. baseline. Such data imply that a combination of genetic and environmental factors is responsible for the increased susceptibility to NPC.
- Genetic analysis of many affected Chinese has revealed association with human leukocyte antigens (HLA)-A2, B17, and Bw46, with a twofold increase in the risk for NPC, suggesting that a gene imparting susceptibility to tumorigenesis is closely linked physically to these HLA loci. HLA association is not seen in North American patients. Familial NPC is almost invariably of type III histology. In sibling pairs afflicted with NPC, the risk associated with sharing HLA locus increased 21 times; the HLA region is on chromosome 6.
- The most striking environmental factors to be implicated in the pathogenesis of NPC are dietary. The southern Chinese and Taiwanese diets include many salt-preserved foods, most notably dried salted fish. There is a twofold to threefold increased risk of NPC associated with the frequent consumption of dried salted fish; this risk increases again twofold to tenfold as the age at onset of such consumption decreases.
- Finally, an epidemiologic association has been found between NPC and the presence of serum antibodies to components of EBV. Among both Chinese and North Americans with nonkeratinizing NPC, 80%-90% show abnormally increased antibody titers to EBV viral capsid antigen (VCA) and early antigen (EA).

Histopathological subtypes

- In 1979, the World Health Organization (WHO) defined NPC as carcinoma of squamous cell origin that can be subdivided on the basis of light microscopy into three types. Despite the diversity of morphologic features described above, electron microscopy has demonstrated ultrastructural characteristics of squamous cell lineage in all three categories.

Type I

- *Keratinizing squamous cell carcinoma* is characterized by the presence of intracellular bridges and prominent keratin formation. Its presence is similar to that of SCC in other areas of the aerodigestive tract. Type I carcinoma accounts for about 25% of NPC in the North American white population but accounts for only 1%-2% of NPC in endemic areas. This by far has the worse prognosis. The 5-year survival rate is 35%.

Type II

- *Nonkeratinizing squamous cell carcinoma* exhibits a definitive maturation sequence characteristic of squamous epithelium but displays no light-microscopic evidence of keratin formation. Type II is the least frequently encountered histological type of NPC and tends to be lumped together with type III NPC. The 5-year survival rate is 61%.

Type III

- *Undifferentiated carcinoma of the NPC (UCNT)* consists of cells of varying morphology that share common light microscopic features, including vesicular nuclei, prominent nucleoli, and syncytia (fused multinucleated giant cells). Type III NPC also has been referred to frequently as *lymphoepithelioma* because of the constant finding of intermixed strands or clumps of benign T cells within the tumor mass. Type III NPC accounts for more than 95% of all cases in endemic areas, whereas in lower-risk populations, such as the North American white population, this number decreases to about 60%. The 5-year survival rate is 61%.

Clinical manifestations

- Among head and neck cancers, NPC entails one of the poorest prognoses because of the primary tumor's proximity to the skull base and multiple vital structures, the invasive nature that typifies NPC tumor growth, the subtlety of early symptoms, and the difficulty of nasopharyngeal examination, which hamper early diagnosis.
- The complaints of patients with NPC are related to the location of the primary tumor and the degree and direction of spread. The patient with NPC most often presents with an asymptomatic *neck mass* located in the mandibular angle or just inferior to the mastoid tip; such a mass is evident in 70% of patients at presentation, a consequence of the relatively weak barriers to tumor spread into the parapharyngeal space. Further, the lymphatic channels of the nasopharyngeal epithelium communicate freely across the midline, and *bilateral cervical* metastasis by

way of the retropharyngeal nodes is frequent. In 33% of the patients the onset of unilateral hearing loss, aural fullness *(otitis media with effusion),* prompts them to seek medical attention. A tumor within the fossa of Rosenmüller may result in dysfunction of the adjacent eustachian tube with subsequent onset of serous otitis media. Other frequent complaints localizing to the nasopharynx include blood-stained nasal discharge from tumor laceration and recent onset of nasal obstruction secondary to tumor bulk.

- *Cranial neuropathy* results from superior or posterior extension of the tumor. Upward spread of the tumor through the foramen lacerum to the cavernous sinus leads to involvement of cranial nerves 5 and 6, which produces the most common deficits seen on initial presentation. Such extension frequently occurs in combination with spread to the foramen ovale or rotundum, leading to complaints of diplopia and pain or paresthesias involving the lower two-thirds of the face. Cavernous sinus involvement frequently causes paralysis of cranial nerves 3-6, as well as Horner's syndrome secondary to destruction of sympathetic nerve fibers in the carotid sheath. Tumor spread to the jugular foramen by the retroparotid route leads to deficits in cranial nerves IX, X, and XI; the adjacent cranial nerve 12 is also frequently involved.
- In North American patients with NPC the incidence of distant metastasis is <3% compared to 6% in other regions of the world. The bones are the most frequently involved sites in metastatic disease, followed by the lungs and liver.

Staging

- The most frequently used staging system in the United States is the American Joint Committee on Cancer (AJCC) system for all head and neck carcinomas:
  - Tis: carcinoma in situ.
  - T1: confined to one nasopharyngeal (NP) site, no visible tumor (biopsy [+] only).
  - T2: two NP sites involved, post/sup and lateral walls.
  - T3: tumor extends to nasal cavity or oropharynx.
  - T4: skull or cranial nerve invasion.
  - NX: nodes not assessed.
  - N0: no clinically (+) nodes.
  - N1: single node <3 cm.
  - N2: single node 3-6 cm.
  - N2b: multiple ipsilateral, all <6 cm.
  - N3a: multiple ipsilateral nodes, all <6 cm.
  - N3b: B clinically (+) nodes
  - N3c: contralateral clinically (+) nodes only
- The shortcoming of the AJCC classification is that it places 80% of all patients into stage IV on presentation. In addition, the precise extent of the NP primary is often difficult to determine clinically because

submucosal spread beneath normal-appearing mucosa is common. Other investigators have identified the major prognostic factors. These include length and symptomatology of disease, extension of tumor outside the NP, presence of low neck adenopathy, keratinizing histologic architecture, cranial nerve and skull base extension, and presence of distant metastases.

Diagnosis

- History (as above).
- Clinical exam: indirect or flexible fiberoptic nasopharyngoscopy.
- Biopsy.
- MRI with enhancement: documents extension, intracranial spread.
  - Immunologic: anti-EBV antibodies.
  - Antiearly antigen (e.g., IgA) and antiviral capsid antigen (e.g., IgG): overall (+)ve ~70%.
  - Antiearly antigen (e.g., IgA) and antiviral capsid antigen (e.g., IgG): (+)ve WHO II and III ~85%.
  - High incidence (>90%) in early and occult neoplasms (Stage I).
  - Sera tested using an antibody-dependent cell-mediated cytotoxicity (ADCC) assay directed against EBV: induced-membrane antigen complex shows that high titers in this assay correspond to an improved clinical prognosis in WHO II and III.

Treatment

- Radiation primary treatment modality.
- Primary tumor and upper echelon nodes treated using lateral, opposed portals.
- Small tumors: 6500 cGy (175-200 cGy/day).
- Large tumors: 7000+ cGy with electron beam supplement.
- Prophylactic irradiation of lower echelon nodes (e.g., 5000 cGy).
- Neck dissection: rarely necessary; used with control of primary site and persistent cervical disease.
- Local resection of residual tumor: limited role in selected persistent or recurrent tumors.
- Intracavitary radioactive seeds: may have role in primary therapy or may be reserved for treatment of recurrence.

Prognosis

- WHO I: 37% (3 years), 10% (5 years).
- WHO II and III: 65% (3 years), 50% (5 years).

 CARCINOMA OF THE ORAL CAVITY

Incidence

- 1 per 20,000 cases per year.
- Much more common in developing nations than in industrialized countries.

Etiology
- Tobacco use of any form (seen in 90% of patients with oral SCC).
- Alcohol (seen in 70%-80% of oral SCC), synergistic with tobacco.
- Ultraviolet light: lip.
- Betel nut and leaf chewing.
- Minor factors:
  - Poor oral hygiene.
  - Riboflavin deficiency.
  - Iron deficiency (achlorhydric iron deficiency = Plummer Vinson syndrome).
  - Recurrent *Herpetic stomatitis*.
  - Immune deficiency.

Pathology
- >90% SCC.

Premalignant lesions (for SCC)
- Leukoplakia.
- Erythroplakia (higher risk than leukoplakia).
- *Lichen planus*.

Squamous cell carcinoma
Gross pathology
Exophytic
- Seen least commonly, except on lip.
- Grow superficially.
- Metastasize later.

Ulcerative
- Most common type in oral cavity.
- More aggressive than exophytic.

Infiltrative
- Most commonly seen on tongue.
- Tends to infiltrate deeply with elevation of surrounding mucosa.

Verrucous
- Older patients.
- Poor-fitting dentures and history of tobacco use.
- More common on buccal mucosa.
- Warty, bulky appearance.
- Grows laterally, pushes but does not invade deeper tissues.
- Sections to be examined carefully for invasive SCC.

Diagnosis
- Incidental finding on oral examination.
- Persistent painful ulcer.
- Physical examination should include bimanual examination to assess depth and fixation and fiberoptic endoscopy to evaluate spread and multifocal lesions.

- CT scan: soft-tissue spread, lymph nodes, particularly good for bony invasion.
- MRI: soft tissue extension and lymph nodes.

Staging
- T1: tumor <2 cm in greatest dimension.
- T2: tumor >2 cm but <4 cm in greatest dimension.
- T3: tumor >4 cm in greatest dimension.
- T4: tumor invading adjacent structures (e.g., cortical bone, extrinsic muscles of tongue, maxillary sinus, skin [skin of neck for lip]).
- N0: no regional lymph node metastasis.
- N1: single ipsilateral node 3 cm or less.
- N2a: Single ipsilateral node >3 cm but <6 cm.
- N2b: Multiple ipsilateral nodes <6 cm.
- N2c: Bilateral or contralateral nodes <6 cm.
- N3: any lymph node >6 cm.
- M0: no distant metastases.
- M1: distant metastases.
- Stage I: T1N0M0.
- Stage II: T2N0M0.
- Stage III: T3N0, T1-T3N1M0.
- Stage IV: everything else.

Treatment
General treatment guidelines
- Most T1 and T2 tumors can be treated equally well with XRT or surgery.
- Most T3 and T4 tumors require multimodality therapy for best results.
- Alternatively, larger tumors may be treated with chemotherapy and XRT organ preservation protocols.

Treatment by site
Lip
- Small lesions may be managed equally well with surgery or XRT.
  - V-shaped or W-shaped excision with primary closure are needed for lesions less than one-third of the lip.
- Larger lesions may require multimodality therapy.
  - For lesions greater than one-third but less than two thirds of the lip, switch flaps (e.g., Abbe, Estlander) are needed for reconstruction.
  - For lesions greater than two-thirds of the lip, Gilles fan flap or Karapandzic flap are needed for reconstruction.
- No consensus has been reached for prophylactic neck dissection.
  - Some would use for lower lip T3 and T4 tumors.
  - Others would base their decision on endophytic/exophytic nature of tumor.
  - Increased rates of metastasis for commissure involvement should be noted.

Anterior two thirds of tongue
- Surgery or XRT for small T1 and T2 lesions.
  - Excision with adequate margins (e.g., partial glossectomy).
  - Transoral or via mandibulotomy.
    - Defect repaired possible by primary closure, skin graft, or tongue flap or allowed to heal by secondary intention.
  - Unilateral neck dissection for lateralized disease, bilateral for midline disease.
  - Elective neck dissection most performed on T2 or higher primary.
  - Depth of invasion >6 mm correlated with increased neck disease.
- Combined therapy for T3 and T4 appears to give better results than single modality.
  - Excision may require mandibulotomy or pull-through for exposure.
  - Gross invasion of the mandible requires mandibulectomy.
  - Reconstruction is best with regional, pedicle, free flap.
  - Unilateral or bilateral neck dissection is often indicated.

Floor of mouth
- Surgery or XRT for T1 and T2 lesions.
  - Excision with adequate margins.
  - Transoral, pull-through, via mandibulotomy.
  - Defect repaired possible by primary closure, skin graft, or allowed to heal by secondary intention.
  - Unilateral neck dissection for lateralized disease, bilateral for midline disease.
  - Elective neck dissection most performed on T2 or higher primary.
- Combined therapy for T3 and T4: better results suggested than with single modality.
  - Excision may require mandibulotomy or pull-through for exposure.
  - Gross invasion of the mandible requires mandibulectomy.
  - Reconstruction is best with regional, pedicle, or free flap.
  - Unilateral or bilateral neck dissection may be indicated.

Alveolar ridge
- Most prefer surgery; secondary to high rate of bone invasion.
- Combined treatment may be indicated for advanced lesions.
- Small lower alveolus lesions may be resected transorally or by pull-through.
- Tumors involving medullary portion of mandible require mandibulectomy.

- Maxillary alveolus lesions frequently require partial or total maxillectomy.
- Reconstruction options include skin graft, local, pedicle, free flaps, and bone plating.
- Prosthetic reconstruction is frequently employed for maxillary defects.
- Cervical metastases from the lower alveolus is more frequently performed than cervical metastases from the upper alveolus.
- Most would perform elective neck dissection on T2 and higher primary.

Buccal mucosa
- Surgery or XRT for T1 and T2 lesions.
- T1 lesions more easily resected.
- Most T2 lesions more easily treated with XRT.
- Larger lesions require multimodality therapy.
- Reconstruction (see Alveolar Ridge).

Hard palate
- XRT may be used to treat small tumors without bone involvement.
- In most cases, surgery is preferred because of bone involvement.
- Small tumors can be resected perorally.
- If the periosteum is involved, a partial-thickness removal of the underlying bone is required.
- Tumor invading bone requires a full-thickness palate resection.
- Larger tumors may require maxillectomy.
- Defects are lined with skin graft and later reconstructed with a prosthesis.
- Patients with larger tumors may benefit from multimodality therapy.
- Most feel elective neck dissection is not indicated.

Retromolar trigone
- Small T1 tumors may be treated equally well with XRT or surgery.
  - Reconstruction is with skin graft.
- Most T2 tumors will require resection of part of the palate that increases morbidity; these are better treated with XRT.
- T1 and T2 tumors invading bone need to be addressed with surgery, including mandibulectomy.
- T3 and T4 tumors require multimodality treatment.
  - Reconstruction requires local, pedicle, and/or free flap, and often a maxillary prosthesis.

Prognosis
Lip
- 5-year survival rates:
  - T1 and T2: 90%+ with XRT or surgery.
  - T3: 75%.
  - T4: 50%.

□ With positive cervical nodes, average 5-year survival rate 55%.

Tongue
- 5-year survival rates:
  □ T1: 80%.
  □ T2: 56%.
  □ T3: 25%.
  □ T4: 10%-20%.
- 3-year survival rates
  □ Stage I: 67%.
  □ Stage II: 48%.
  □ Stage III: 33%.

Floor of mouth
- 5-year survival rates:
  □ Stage I: 68%-90%.
  □ Stage II: 50%-80%.
  □ Stage III: 28%-65%.
  □ Stage IV: 9%-30%.

Buccal mucosa
- 5-year survival rates
  □ Stage I: 75%.
  □ Stage II: 65%.
  □ Stage III: 30%.
  □ Stage IV: 20%.

Alveolus
- 5-year survival rates
  □ Stage I: 78%.
  □ Stage II: 64%.
  □ Stage III: 35%.
  □ Stage IV: 15%.

Retromolar trigone
- 5-year survival rates
  □ Stage I: 90%.
  □ Stage II: 80%.
  □ Stage III: 65%.
  □ Stage IV: 30%.

Other malignant lesions
Lymphoma
- Rare in oral cavity, more common in oropharynx.
- May occur in tongue or submandibular nodes.

Melanoma
- Rare.
- Most lesions pigmented.
- Most frequently in men 50-70 years of age.
- Treatment: wide local excision.
- Prognosis: poor; 5-year survival rate 5%-15%.

Kaposi's sarcoma
- Seen in AIDS patients.

- Treatments: excision, intralesional chemotherapy, laser ablation, cryosurgery, radiation.
- Asymptomatic lesions sometimes observed.

Minor salivary gland malignancies
- Approximately 70% tumors malignant.
- Most common in posterior aspect of hard palate.
- Adenoid cystic most common (30%).
- Mucoepidermoid also approximately 30%-50%; low grade with excellent prognosis.
- Adenocarcinoma (20%).
- Treatment: wide local excision, elective neck dissection not indicated, radiation with positive margins or high-grade malignancies.
- 5-year survival rate 40%.

OROPHARYNX CARCINOMA

Definition
- Oropharynx: anterior boundary from circumvallate papillae (below) and junction of hard and soft palate (above); extends from level of hard palate to pharyngoepiglottic folds.

Incidence and epidemiology
- Oropharyngeal carcinoma relatively uncommon lesion.
- Incidence in the United States (1993): 9200.
- Mortalities: 3800.
- More common in the patients >45 years of age; commonly present with neck mass (>40%).
- Risk factors: alcohol and tobacco use, as well as a history of radiation exposure (>10 years prior to presentation).

Clinical manifestations
- Early: dull pain, otalgia, globus sensation.
- Late: odynophagia, dysphagia, muffled voice, hemoptysis, neck mass, weight loss, trismus (may indicate pterygoid muscle invasion).

Staging (including subsites)
Tumor (T)
- T1: tumor <2 cm in greatest dimension.
- T2: tumor >2 cm but <4 cm.
- T3: tumor >4 cm.
- T4: tumor invasion into adjacent structures (e.g., mandible, hard palate, deep muscles of tongue, larynx, pterygoid muscles).

Regional lymph nodes (N)
- NX: unable to assess regional lymph nodes.
- N0: no regional lymph node metastasis.
- N1: metastasis in single ipsilateral lymph node, <3 cm.

- N2: metastasis in single ipsilateral lymph node, >3 cm but <6 cm or bilateral/contralateral lymph nodes <6 cm.
- N2a: metastasis in single ipsilateral node, <6 cm.
- N2b: metastasis in multiple ipsilateral nodes, <6 cm.
- N2c: metastasis to contralateral node.
- N3: metastasis to neck node, >6 cm.

Tumor subsites
Base of tongue
- Increased rate of cervical metastasis (>60%, 20% bilateral metastasis).
- More aggressive than oral tongue cancer.

Soft palate
- Typically found at earlier stage than other sites given more visible location.
- 20%-45% regional metastasis.

Tonsil/lateral pharyngeal wall
- Most common site of oropharynx carcinoma.
- Regional metastasis (6%-75%).
- Higher instance of lymphoma/lymphoepithelioma.

Posterior pharyngeal wall
- Locally aggressive, but less metastatic potential than base of tongue lesions.
- >90% of oropharyngeal carcinomas SCC.
- Other lesions: malignant melanoma, minor salivary gland tumors, sarcomas, lymphoma, lymphoepithelioma.

Diagnosis
- Examination and biopsy.
- CT scan with contrast/MRI with enhancement: determination of local spread and neck metastases.

Treatment
General considerations
- Possible to manage T1 and T2 with single modality therapy (radiation or surgery).
- Multimodality therapy required for T3 and T4.
- Necessary to address neck with surgery or radiation even if N0.

Subsites
Tonsil
- T1 and T2: radiation first-line therapy with surgical salvage.
- T3 and T4: composite resection with postoperative radiation.

Soft palate
- T1 and T2: radiation with surgical salvage.
- T3 and T4: excision with postoperative radiation.

Base of tongue
- Usually found at advanced stage.
- T1 and T2: radiation with surgical salvage.
- T3 and T4: radiation with surgical salvage or primary surgery with postoperative radiation.

Prognosis
Tonsil (5-year survival rate)
- Radiation alone, N0 neck.
  - T1: 85%.
  - T2: 75%.
  - T3: 45%.
  - T4: 25%.
- Positive neck nodes decrease prognosis by at least one-half.
- Advanced lesions do somewhat better with combined approach therapy.

Soft palate (5-year survival rate)
- Radiation alone:
  - T1: 85%.
  - T2: 75%.
  - T3: 30%.
  - T4: 20%.
- Decreased prognosis by at least one-half with positive neck nodes.
- Advanced lesions do somewhat better with combined-approach therapy at base of tongue.
- Difficult to treat.
- Regardless of modality, 20%-50% 5-year survival rate.

 RECONSTRUCTION OF ORAL CAVITY AND OROPHARYNGEAL DEFECTS

Lip Reconstruction
- The ideal reconstruction should result in a lip that:
  - Is sensate.
  - Has sphincter or muscle function that maintains a watertight, continent seal.
  - Allows sufficient opening for food, dentures, and oral hygiene.
  - Is aesthetically acceptable.
- It is not possible to satisfy all of these criteria in every instance, and careful preoperative evaluation is essential. Appropriate evaluation and planning should include:
  - An estimate of the magnitude and location of the anticipated defect.
  - An assessment of whether the area has been previously irritated.
  - The degree of laxity of the lip and adjacent cheek tissue.
  - Whether the patient wears dentures.
  - Whether palpable lymph nodes may require sacrifice of the facial artery or arteries.

- Surgical procedures to reconstitute the lip may be classified as follows:
  - Those that use remaining lip tissue.
  - Those that borrow tissue from the opposite lip.
  - Those that use adjacent tissue.
  - Those that use distant flaps.

Defects of less than half of the lip

- Vermilion mucosal defects may be reconstructed with *mucosal advancement flaps* from inside the mouth. To prevent the free lip margin from being pulled toward the tongue and to maintain the natural fullness of the lower lip, the undermined mucosa can be made into laterally based bipedicled flaps and advanced anteriorly. The resulting defect in the gingivolabial sulcus is left to granulate and remucosalize.
- When vermilion substance has been lost in addition to mucosa, a muscle-mucosal flap from the ventral surface of the tongue may be used. This flap is based posteriorly with the free edge of the flap attached to the mucocutaneous border. Between 10 and 20 days later, the pedicle is transected at the tongue tip, retaining muscle for bulk and mucosa for vermilion reconstruction. This technique does not limit tongue mobility, although the newly created vermilion has a pebbled surface. To prevent development of a second lip primary tumor, vermilionectomy is performed and repaired with mucosal advancement flaps if leukoplakia, hyperkeratosis, or actinic cheilitis is present in the remaining lip tissue.
- Full thickness defects of up to one-half of the lip width can usually be managed with primary closure, particularly if the perioral tissue is lax and has not been irradiated. Shield or V-excision is usually adequate, whereas W-plasty modification accentuates the mental protuberance. Lateral advancement with incisions placed in the mental crease may be required when the defect base is broad. Every attempt should be made not to extend incisions beyond the mental crease in order to avoid a pointed chin deformity. Primary closure should be in three layers (i.e., mucosa, muscle, and skin) with careful reapproximation of the "white line" at the vermilion border on either side of the defect.
- Primary closure of defects in the midline of the upper lip can be facilitated by excising a crescent of cheek skin in the perialar region. Perialar skin excision allows advancement of the remaining lip segments and lessens the wound tension after primary closure. An Abbe flap may be used in the midline if there is excessive tension on the wound closure.

Defects of one-half to two-thirds of the lip

- The *Karapandzic* labioplasty is the primary choice. The advantages of this orbicularis oris myocutaneous flap are its ease of design and the preservation of motor and sensory innervation of the lip. The main disadvantage is that a relative microstomia can occur, which precludes the use of dentures. In addition, the circumoral scars can be unsightly. The technique begins with circumoral skin incisions within the nasolabial and nasomental creases. The lateral border of the orbicularis oris muscle is mobilized from the other supporting perioral muscles to allow tension-free closure. Blunt dissection of the muscle allows identification and preservation of the superior and inferior labial arteries and the neurovascular pedicles that enter the muscle from its periphery. The underlying oral mucosa usually does not require transection for mobilization.

- *Abbe-Estlander* flaps transfer full-thickness tissue from one lip to the opposite lip and permit close skin texture and color match with the surrounding tissue. The disadvantages are that a second-stage procedure is needed and that the transferred tissue is denervated but may reinnervated over time. Abbe-Estlander flaps should be designed so that the height of the flap equals the height of the tissue excised. The width of the flap should be about half the width of the tissue excised, to maintain appropriate lip proportions. The pedicle should be narrow to facilitate rotation, but the labial artery must be preserved. The secondary defect should be closed in three layers.

- The Abbe flap was originally designed to close medial defects, and it can be based either medially or laterally, depending on the location of the defect. When an Abbe flap is designed from the upper lip, lateral lip tissue should be used. The pedicel crosses the oral stoma and may be severed in 2-3 weeks. The Estlander flap was originally used to reconstruct defects near the corner of the mouth. The superiorly based Estlander flap should be modified so that it lies within the nasolabial fold. The resultant donor-site scar is hidden in the nasolabial crease, and the flap is easily rotated. The blunting of the new oral commissure may be corrected by secondary commissuroplasty when desired.

Defects greater than two-thirds of the lip

- Large defects of the upper lip (*one half to two thirds of the lip*) can be reconstructed as described.
- Midline lower lip defects may be corrected by using any of several modifications of the Bernard repair, which essentially uses full-thickness advancement flaps from adjacent cheek tissue. These techniques have the advantages of using innervated local tissue and one-stage reconstruction and can reconstruct large upper- and lower-lip defects. The Webster

modification of the Bernard cheiloplasty is a reliable technique. The Burrow's triangles are designed so that the medial vertical limb is incorporated into the melolabial fold. The width of the base of the triangle is calculated so that the distance from the oral commissure to the lateral portion of the base equals half of the width of the lip tissue excised. A lateral vertical limb is then drawn to complete the triangle. Burrow's triangles of skin and subcutaneous tissue only are excised. As the transverse incisions are deepened along the base of the triangle, the neurovascular supply to the orbicularis oris and buccinator muscles is identified and preserved. A mucosal flap based on the superior margin of the cheek flap is elevated to create a new vermilion. Usually, incisions through skin and muscle are required around the mental crease, with Burrow's triangles strategically placed in the submental area to allow sufficient advancement of the cheek flaps.

- Full-thickness inferiorly based nasolabial flaps may be used to reconstruct lateral lip defects of up to 75% of the lip height. The disadvantage of this technique is that the flaps are not innervated, and in raising the flaps, the upper lip is usually denervated.
- Repair with distant flaps is required for defects involving the entire lip or adjacent soft tissue of the cheek or chin or when the adjacent cheek tissues are inadequate or contracted. The revascularized radial forearam–free flap is an excellent reconstructive option in this situation. The skin paddle can be centered over the palmaris longus tendon and the skin folded over this tendon to provide internal and external skin lining. The two ends of the palmaris longus tendon can be attached to the remaining orbicularis oris muscle to suspend and support the reconstruction. The vermilion can be secondarily reconstructed with a mucosal flap from the tongue, upper lip, or cheek, or medical tattooing will give an acceptable result. Pectoralis major myocutaneous flap remains another popular, dependable distant flap for transferring muscle and skin for a one-stage lip reconstruction. The flap can be folded on itself to provide intraoral and external coverage, but the flap bulk is variable and the skin is insensate. In addition, oral competence often requires adequate support for the reconstructed lip, which can be achieved. A fascia lata graft can be sutured to sling the lower lip to the remaining upper lip muscle.

Oral Cavity Reconstruction

- Reconstruction of the oral cavity after major ablative surgery poses a major challenge for the head and neck surgeon. Advanced planning is essential in reviewing the several options available. The optimal goal of reconstruction is to achieve maximal restoration of function and cosmesis with minimal morbidity to the patient.
- Free-skin grafts or dermal grafts are useful in closing defects of the tonsil and lateral posterior tongue areas. These are sutured in place and are generally held with a sutured bolster.

Local Flaps

- Moderately sized defects that cannot be closed primarily or by split-thickness skin grafts often can be repaired with local mucosal flaps.

Tongue Flap

- A common local flap used to reconstruct defects of oral cavity.
- Effective method of repairing defects of limited size in floor of mouth and retromolar trigone.
- Potential for defects requiring larger tongue flaps to significantly reduce tongue mobility and create disability for patient.

Skin Flap

- Consists of skin and underlying subcutaneous tissue, which is transferred from one site to another, retaining its vascular attachment to body at all times during transfer.
- Typically used in lip reconstruction. Unilateral or bilateral nasolabial flaps can be used to reconstruct anterior floor of mouth defects.

Regional Flaps

- Surgical defects that result from resection of Stage 3 and 4 tumors of the oral cavity usually require regional and distant flaps for reconstruction of soft tissue defects.
- A regional flap is one that originates in an area close, but not adjacent, to the defect.

Forehead flap
- Based on superficial temporal artery.

Deltopectoral flap
- Based on three or four perforating branches of internal thoracic artery.

Pectoralis myocutaneous flap
- Based on thoracoacromial and occasionally branches of lateral thoracic perforators from internal thoracic.

- Has the advantage of being an axial flap, which may be elevated as a strip of muscle and an attached segment of overlying skin for one-stage reconstruction. A portion of the flap may be turned on itself to provide tissue for the inner and outer aspects of the oral cavity. The flap has sufficient bulk to provide structural support when a mandibulectomy is necessary for tumor exenteration. Pectoralis flaps along with innervated latissimus dorsi flaps retain their bulk and provide excellent closure of tongue-base defects.

Trapezius myocutaneous flap
- Can be based inferiorly on transverse cervical artery and vein or supply on branches of posterior occipital and deep cervical vessels.
- Particularly suited for reconstruction of full-thickness defects in lower portions of oral cavity and may incorporate scapular spine for one-stage mandibular reconstruction.
- Skin grafts often necessary to cover defects.

Sternocleidomastoid flaps
- Useful for small defects of oral cavity.
- Blood supply from branches of thyrocervical trunk, superior thyroid, and occipital arteries.
- Major disadvantage: limited amount of skin that can be harvested; usually flap of only 3 cm or less in width can be used.
- Contraindicated if neck dissection is being performed.

Microvascular Free Flaps

- Advantage: large amount of tissue available and flexibility of usage in difficult oropharyngeal reconstruction.
- Disadvantages.
- Extra time required, which lengthens already long surgical procedure.
- The recipient defect site must have an appropriate artery and vein available, which can pose problems following prior neck dissection and radiation therapy.

Radial Forearm-Free Flap

- Thin pliable skin with capacity for neurosensory restoration.
- Morbidity of skin graft to volar surface of forearm, which can be subsequently removed after adjacent skin expansion.

Greater Omentum-Free Flap

- Excellent for complicated oropharyngeal lesions, such as radiation treatment failures in the tonsillar fossa.

OPTIONS FOR RECONSTRUCTION OF ORAL-MANDIBULAR DEFECTS

Bone Grafting (Iliac Crest, Rib Graft, Tibia)

Indications
- Nonunion of mandibular bone following fracture.
- Loss of significant amount of bone in the absence soft tissue loss.

Contraindications
- Absence of healthy tissue at recipient site (i.e., irradiated tissue, infected site, persistent malignancy).
- Adequate blood supply.
- Lack of remaining mandible to which to secure bone graft.
- Patient not healthy enough to undergo procedure.

Advantages
- Adequate functional results.
- Good cosmetic results.
- Minimal donor site morbidity.

Disadvantages and complications
- Limited application due to requirement of little to no soft tissue loss.
- Graft resorption (rare in setting of healthy recipient tissue).

Rotation Flaps (Pectoralis, Deltopectoral, Bipedicled Scalp Flap)

Indications
- Defects with a large loss of soft tissue requiring skin and/or mucosal replacement.
- Defects with minimal bone loss that does not include symphysis.

Contraindications
- Pectoral agenesis.
- Point not healthy enough to undergo procedure.

Advantages
- Able to provide intraoral or external skin covering.
- Can combine with bone graft, skin graft.
- Good functional result.

Disadvantages and complications
- Donor site morbidity.
- Poor cosmetic result.
- Flap failure with resulting fistula.

Free Flap (Fibular)

Indications

- Defects with large loss of soft tissue requiring skin, mucosal, or bone replacement.

Contraindications

- Point unable to withstand procedure.
- Peripheral vascular disease.

Advantages

- Able to reconstruct large defects.
- Good cosmetic result.
- Good functional result.

Disadvantages and complications

- Donor site morbidity.
- Flap failure.
- Time intensive procedure.

 ## LARYNGEAL CARCINOMA

- 1%-5% of all malignancies diagnosed annually.
- Approximately 11,000 new cases in United States annually, with 3700 deaths annually.
- More common in men than women (8:1), with average age of onset at 60-62 years of age.
- At presentation, confined to larynx (60%), regional mets (25%), distant mets (15%).
- Incidence of multiple synchronous tumors: 0.5%-1%.
- Incidence of metachronous tumors: 5%-10% (lung most common site)

Etiology

- Smoking (6-39 times more likely than nonsmokers; less than 5% of cases have no smoking history).
- Alcohol abuse.
- Smoking and alcohol abuse (the combined risk is 50% greater than the additive risk of each).
- Concurrent pathology: esophageal reflux, radiation to neck, presence of laryngocele, history of juvenile papillomatosis, laryngeal keratosis.
- Occupational exposures: mustard gas, asbestos, wood dust, refinery products.

Pathology
By site

- Supraglottic (from tip of epiglottis to ventricle): 67%.
- Glottic (from ventricle to 1 cm below TVC): 31%.
- Subglottic (from 1 cm below TVC to cricoid): 2%.

By cell type

- SCC (including spindle cell variant): 94%.
- Verrucous carcinoma: 2%-4%.
- Adenocarcinoma: 1%.

- Sarcoma (fibrosarcoma, chondrosarcoma, rhabdomyosarcoma, malignant fibrous histio): 1%.
- Metastatic (melanoma, renal cell, prostate, breast, lung, stomach): <1%.

Patterns of spread

- Local extension and lymphatic spread most common routes.

Barriers to spread

- Quadrangular membrane (above false cords) for supraglottic tumors.
- Conus elasticus (between true cords and cricoid) for glottic and subglottic tumors.

Supraglottis

- Extensive lymphatics feed the preepiglottic space and the neck bilaterally.
- Incidence of nodal metastasis varies from 25%-50% depending on the tumor stage.
- 20%-35% are bilateral.
- Tumors on the epiglottis that invade the preepiglottic space via perforations in the cartilage may enter the paraglottic space, which communicates with the entire larynx in the vertical dimension.

Glottis

- Limited lymphatic drainage.
- Local metastasis less than 10%, partially due to earlier detection (smaller tumor causes more symptoms here).
- Usually slow-growing, well-differentiated tumors that spread in predictable ways.

Subglottis

- Often silent and poorly differentiated
- Often extends into cricoid cartilage to involve paratracheal and cervical lymphatics in large number of cases.

Staging system for carcinoma of the larynx
Tumor stage (T)
Glottis

- T1: tumor limited to vocal cords with normal mobility.
- T1a: tumor limited to one vocal cord.
- T1b: tumor involving both cords.
- T2: tumor extending into supraglottis or subglottis with impaired vocal cord mobility.
- T3: tumor confined to larynx with vocal cord fixation.
- T4: tumor invading through thyroid cartilage, with direct extralaryngeal spread.

Supraglottis

- T1: tumor limited to one subsite with normal vocal cord mobility.

- T2: tumor involving >1 subsite of supraglottis or glottis with impaired vocal cord mobility.
- T3: tumor limited to larynx with vocal cord fixation; may invade medial pyriform sinus, postcricoid area, preepiglottic space
- T4: tumor invading thyroid cartilage, extralaryngeal spread.

Subglottis
- T1: tumor limited to subglottis.
- T2: tumor extending to glottis with or without vocal cord fixation.
- T3: tumor limited to larynx with vocal cord fixation.
- T4: tumor invading cricoid, thyroid cartilage, with extralaryngeal invasion.

Regional lymph nodes (N)
- NX: cannot be assessed.
- N0: no regional lymph node metastases.
- N1: metastasis in single ipsilateral lymph node (LN), <3 cm.
- N2a: metastasis in single ipsilateral LN, >3 cm but <6 cm.
- N2b: metastasis in multiple ipsilateral LNs, <6 cm.
- N2c: metastasis in contralateral or bilateral.

Distant metastases (M)
- MX: cannot be assessed.
- M0: no distant metastases.
- M1: distant metastases.

Stage grouping (Table 5)
Treatment of larynx cancer
Treatment options (glottic carcinoma)
Tis (in situ carcinoma)
- Vocal fold stripping with reoperation as often as required to remove Cis.

T1 and T2 (surgery and radiation equivalent survival)
- Surgical options (based on site and extent of lesion):
  - Endoscopic cordectomy (e.g., CO_2 laser, cold).

TABLE 5. Stage Groupings			
Stage	**Tumor**	**Lymphatic Nodes**	**Distant Metastases**
0	Tis	N0	M0
I	T1	N0	M0
II	T2	N0	M0
III	T3	N0	M0
	T1-T3	N1	M0
IV	T4	N0, N1	M0
	Any T	N2, N3	M0
	Any T	Any N	M1

- Thyrotomy with cordectomy.
- Hemilaryngectomy.
- Supracricoid laryngectomy.
- Endoscopic laser laryngectomy (controversial).
- Radiation therapy advantages:
  - May result in better voice (controversial).
  - Small fields for early larynx carcinoma.
- Surgical advantages:
  - Can use radiotherapy for future primaries.
  - Cheaper.
  - Treatment in single visit (often outpatient surgery).
- Radiation failures: often total laryngectomy for salvage.
- Surgical failures: often second organ-sparing procedure or XRT.

T3 and T4
- Radiotherapy alone: high local failure rate and low survival rate.
- Induction chemotherapy with radiation becoming more popular (organ sparing).
- Total laryngectomy: definitive procedure.

Treatment options (supraglottic)
T1 and T2 (radiation or surgery)
- Surgical options (based on site and extent of lesion):
  - Endoscopic epiglottectomy.
  - Supraglottic laryngectomy.
  - Supracricoid laryngectomy.
  - Endoscopic laser resection (controversial).
- Surgical advantages:
  - Radiotherapy held in reserve for recurrence or second primary.
  - Radiotherapy failures often require total laryngectomy for salvage.
  - Excellent functional results often noted.

T3 and T4 (chemoradiation or surgery)
- Chemoradiation remains experimental.
- Surgical options are total laryngectomy or near-total laryngectomy.
- Selected T3 supraglottic lesions can get supracricoid or extended supraglottic laryngectomy.

Treatment options (subglottic)
- Extremely rare lesion; large controlled studies not available
- Possible to control small lesions with radiotherapy, otherwise need total laryngectomy (no organ preservation procedures).

Regional lymphatics
- Supraglottic region has bilateral draining lymphatics and often needs bilateral neck dissection at time of surgery.

- Role of radiotherapy in control of low-volume neck disease is controversial; many authors recommend neck dissection even in setting of postoperative radiotherapy.
- Early glottic cancers rarely require neck dissection.

- Advanced stage cancers need neck dissection, including paratracheal node dissection

Conservation Laryngectomy

- See Tables 6 and 7.

TABLE 6. Procedures for Glottic Carcinoma

Procedure for Glottic Carcinoma	Components Excised	Indications	Contraindications	Complications
Laryngofissure and cordectomy	Ipsilateral TVC	T1 glottic carcinoma limited to membranous TVC	T1: TVC motion impairment T2: extension onto vocal process of arytenoid or anterior commissure	Seroma, hematoma, infection
Vertical partial laryngectomy	TVC with overlying soft tissue and cartilage; extended procedures may resect arytenoid mucosa, FVC, contralateral TVC	T1-T2 glottic carcinoma	T1: involvement of ant. commissure T2: advanced T2 T3: impaired VC mobility T4: subglottic extension	Seroma, hematoma, infection
Frontolateral partial laryngectomy (extended vertical partial laryngectomy)	Anterior 2/3 ipsilateral TVC and anterior 1/3 contralateral TVC associated thyroid cartilage	T1a and T1b glottic carcinomas that approach or involve only 1-2 mm of contralateral cord	T1: extension onto vocal process of arytenoid T2: vocal cord paralysis secondary to TA muscle invasion T3: subglottic extension	Seroma, hematoma, infection
Anterior frontal vertical partial laryngectomy (extended vertical partial laryngectomy)	Membranous portions of both TVCs underlying soft tissue and midline vertical segment of thyroid cartilage	T2 glottic carcinomas involving membranous portions of both TVCs and extending subglottically beneath anterior commissure	T1: extension onto vocal process of arytenoid T2: >1 cm subglottic extension T3: vocal cord paralysis secondary to TA muscle invasion	Seroma, hematoma, infection
Extended fronto-lateral partial laryngectomy with epiglottic laryngoplasty (extended vertical partial laryngectomy)	Both TVC, both FVC, ipsilateral arytenoid, thyroid ala	T1-T3 glottic carcinoma	T1: involvement of contralateral arytenoid T2: subglottic extension	Delayed decannulation, aspiration, upper airway obstruction
Supracricoid partial laryngectomy with cricohyoido-epiglottopexy	Both TVC, both FVC, entire thyroid cartilage, both paraglottic spaces, ipsilateral arytenoid	Selected T2-T3 glottic carcinomas (particularly T2 glottic carcinomas too extensive for vertical partial laryngectomy)	T1: immobile arytenoid T2: lesions originating in ventricle or anterior commissure T3: subglottic extension >10 mm anterior or >5 mm posteriorly T4: preop respiratory impairment	Dysphagia, infection, aspiration

TABLE 7. Procedures for Supraglottic Carcinoma

Procedure for Supraglottic Carcinoma	Components Excised	Indications	Contraindications	Complications
Supraglottic laryngectomy	Epiglottis, preepiglottic space, hyoid bone, thyrohyoid membrane, upper half of thyroid cartilage, supraglottic mucosa including both AE folds, ventricles, and valleculae (may also be extended to one arytenoid, superiormedial piriform sinus, and base of tongue)	T1 and T2 supraglottic carcinomas (particularly those confined to laryngeal surface of epiglottis and FVCs), highly selected T3 and T4 supraglottic carcinomas	T1: extension to TVCs or anterior commissure T2: vocal cord fixation	Fistula, aspiration, inability to decannulate, TC fistula, dysphagia
Supracricoid laryngectomy with crico-hyoidopexy	Epiglottis, preepiglottic space, entire thyroid cartilage, both AE folds, TVCs, FVCs, ipsilateral arytenoid	T1 and T2 supraglottic carcinomas extending to ventricle, infrahyoid epiglottis, or posterior third of FVC T3 transglottic carcinomas with marked limitation of TVC T1 or T2 supraglottic carcinomas extending to glottis or anterior. commissure with or without impaired cord mobility, selected T4s invading thyroid cartilage	T1: subglottic extension <10 mm anteriorly or a >5 mm posteriorly T2: arytenoid cartilage fixation T3: massive invasion of preepiglottic space T4: extension to pharyngeal wall or intrarytenoid region T5: cricoid cartilage invasion	Fistula, aspiration, inability to decannulate, dysphagia

Total Laryngectomy

Indications
Malignant disease
- Thyroid cartilage invasion.
- Bilateral arytenoid involvement.
- Subglottic extension.
- Thyroid tumors with thyroid cartilage destruction.
- Recurrence after conservation surgery.
- Recurrence, persistence after definitive radiation, chemoradiation.
- Medical/pulmonary disease preventing conservation surgery.

Benign disease
- Radiation necrosis of larynx.
- Chronic, severe, intractable aspiration.

Contraindications
- Inability to undergo general anesthesia.
- Unresectable neck disease.
- Distant metastasis.

Complications
Early
- Hematoma.
- Infection.
- Pharyngocutaneous fistula.
- Wound dehiscence.

Late
- Stomal stenosis.
- Stricture of neopharynx.
- Hypothyroidism (especially post radiation therapy).

Total Laryngopharyngectomy

Indications
- Piriform sinus cancer (with or without laryngeal extension).

- Posterior hypopharyngeal cancer.
- Postcricoid cancer.

Contraindications

- Inability to undergo general anesthesia.
- Involvement of prevertebral musculature.
- Unresectable neck disease.
- Distant metastasis.

Complications

- Same as for total laryngectomy with higher fistula and stenosis rates.
- Reconstructive options: unique complications depending on option selected.

Vocal Rehabilitation after Laryngectomy

- Rapid, effective voice restoration is critical to the successful prevention of psychological, social, and economic consequences.
- Transnasal esophageal insufflation test is designed to see if a patient can sustain vocalization artificially before a procedure is performed (to assess for functionality and rule out cricopharyngeal spasm).

Methods of rehabilitation
Esophageal voice

- Requires no surgery.
- Variable in success rate (depends on such factors as patient motivation, extent of resection, postoperative radiation, development of pharyngeal stenosis, inconvenience of therapeutic sessions).
- Air actively injected or inhaled into cervical esophagus and immediately expelled, causing vibration of opposing mucosal surfaces.

Electronic devices

- Transcervical or transoral devices are available.

Pharyngeal constrictor myotomy

- For cricopharyngeal spasm if transnasal insufflation test reveals spasm or hypertonicity.

Pharyngeal plexus neurectomy

- For cricopharyngeal spasm.

Primary voice restoration

- TEP combined with pharyngeal constrictor myotomy or pharyngeal plexus neurectomy at the time of laryngectomy.

Tracheoesophageal puncture

- Developed first by Singer and Blom (1980).
- Indications
  - Careful counseling is necessary to guide patient expectations.

- Patient should have the ability to maintain the prosthesis.
- COPD with poor airflow would be insufficient to produce vocalization.
- Stoma should be greater than 1.5 cm in diameter, without evidence of pharyngeal stenosis.
- TEP as a secondary procedure has yielded excellent results

- Treatment
  - Patients undergo a rigorous process of fitting and instruction.
  - Fitting begins 3 days following secondary TEP.
  - Placement of the voice prosthesis occurs 8-10 days after barium swallow confirms suture line competence.
    - Voicing is avoided until 12-14 days to prevent fistula formation.
    - Patients are then taught how to occlude the TEP to phonate or are fitted with a tracheostoma valve (Blom-Singer, Provox)
  - Mucosa vibrates in segments of the pharyngoesophagus resulting from airflow, which is under pulmonary control (may change intensity of voice with change in air flow).
- Complications
  - Bleeding.
  - Edema (rare).
  - Infection, abscess formation, mediastinitis.
  - Leakage through prosthesis (valve damage by *Candida,* failure of device, contact against posterior esophageal wall).
  - Leakage around prosthesis (indication of TEP dilation, either from necrosis or positioning of prosthesis).
  - Prosthetic extrusion or aspiration.
  - Microstoma (<2.0 cm requires tracheoplasty or soft silicone laryngectomy tube).
  - Tracheoesophageal-related flatulence (mostly from continuous air being forced across site during inspiration, or in those with hypertonic pharyngeal constrictor or esophageal stricture).
  - Granuloma (if present, must increase length of prosthesis, or if too large, excise granulation tissue).
  - Immediate aphonia and dysphonia (valve stuck in closed position, too much pressure on valve, or pharyngeal constrictor spasm or hypertonicity).
  - Delayed aphonia and dysphonia (stenosis of esophageal end of puncture tract).
  - Insufficient tracheostoma valve seal (functional failure of sealant in system).
  - Fungal infection of prosthesis (*Candida albicans*): interferes with functionality of prosthesis.

HYPOPHARYNGEAL SQUAMOUS CELL CARCINOMA

American Joint Committee on Cancer's Staging of Hypopharyngeal Cancer

- T1: Tumor is limited to one subsite and is less than 2 cm in greatest dimension.
- T2: Tumor involves more than one subsite or measures >2 cm but not >4 cm without fixation of the hemilarynx.
- T3: Tumor measures >4 cm or with fixation of the hemilarynx.
- T4: Tumor invades adjacent structures (e.g., thyroid cartilage, cricoid cartilage, carotid, thyroid, esophagus, soft tissues of the neck, or prevertebral fascia)

Subsites

- Pyriform sinus.
- Posterior wall.
- Postcricoid area.

Regional Disease

- NX: Regional lymph nodes unable to be assessed.
- N0: No regional lymph node metastasis.
- N1: Metastasis in a single ipsilateral lymph node, 3 cm or less in greatest dimension.
- N2: Metastasis in a single ipsilateral lymph node, more than 3 cm but not more than 6 cm in greatest dimension; or in multiple ipsilateral lymph nodes, none more than 6 cm in greatest dimension; or in bilateral or contralateral lymph nodes, none greater than 6 cm in greatest dimension.
- N2a: Metastasis in a single ipsilateral lymph node greater than 3 cm but not more than 6 cm in greatest dimension.
- N2b: Metastasis in multiple ipsilateral lymph nodes, none greater than 6 cm in greatest dimension.
- N2c: Metastasis in bilateral or contralateral lymph nodes, none greater than 6 cm in greatest dimension.
- N3: Metastasis in a lymph node greater than 6 cm in greatest dimension.

Distant Metastasis (M)

- MX: Distant metastasis unable to be assessed.
- M0: No distant metastasis.
- M1: Distant metastasis.

Stages

- I: T1N0M0.
- II: T2N0M0.
- III: T3N0M0, T1N1M0, T2N1M0, T3N1M0.
- IV: T4NxM0, TxN2M0, TxN3M0, TxNxM1.

Primary tumor treatment options

- Surgery.
- Radiation therapy.
- Surgery with preoperative or postoperative radiation therapy.

Surgery

T1-T2

- Treatment options for early hypopharyngeal cancer include partial pharyngectomy with or without partial laryngectomy, or definitive radiotherapy. Failure will likely require a total laryngopharyngectomy.
- Tumors of the hypopharyngeal wall may be resected through a transhyoid or lateral pharyngotomy approach.
- The defect can be reconstructed with a split-thickness skin graft, a pedicled flap, or a free flap.
- Tumors of the medial wall of the pyriform sinus may be treated with a partial laryngopharyngectomy.

T3-T4

- Tumors with vocal fold fixation or large tumor mass undergo multimodality treatment. In most instances, this requires total or near total laryngopharyngectomy, with postoperative radiation therapy.

Radiation Therapy

T1-T2

- These tumors of the pyriform sinus, pharyngeal wall, and postcricoid area may be treated with definitive radiation therapy.

T3-T4

- Radiation therapy is not a definitive treatment for these tumors of the hypopharynx. However, many patients will require postoperative radiation therapy.

Treatment of the Neck

- Risk of occult metastasis may be as high as 60%.
- Bilateral lymph node metastases are common.
- Retropharyngeal lymph node metastases are common.

Surgery

- No neck: ipsilateral and contralateral dissection of stages II-IV, retropharyngeal nodes; and stage IV nodes for those undergoing laryngectomy.

- N1 neck: ipsilateral dissection of stages II-IV or a modified radical neck dissection (IV), contralateral dissection of stages II-IV, retropharyngeal nodes; and stage IV nodes for those undergoing laryngectomy.
- N2-N3 neck: radical neck dissection, modified radical neck dissection, selective neck dissection based on ipsilateral and contralateral disease burden, retropharyngeal nodes; and stage IV nodes for those undergoing laryngectomy.

Radiation therapy

- N0-N1: treatment of ipsilateral and contralateral necks.
- N2-N3: may be used as adjuvant to surgery.

Options for Reconstruction of the Hypopharynx and Cervical Esophagus

Split thickness skin graft

Indications
- Small posterior hypopharyngeal wall defects.

Contraindications
- Cannot be used in larger defects.

Advantages
- Fast.
- Simple.
- Minimal bulk (useful when larynx has been preserved).

Disadvantages and complications
- Limited applicability.
- High rate of stenosis.
- High rate of fistula.

Regional myocutaneous flap (e.g., deltopectoral, pectoral)

Indications
- Noncircumferential hypopharyngeal and/or cervical esophageal defect.
- Only used in the case of total laryngectomy.

Contraindications
- Laryngeal preservation.
- Pectoral agenesis.

Advantages
- Decreased operative time.
- Avoid intraabdominal procedure.

Disadvantages and complications
- Bulky (can interfere with swallowing).
- High rate of fistula.
- High rate of stenosis.
- Poor speech results.

Gastric pullup

Indications
- Reconstruction of esophageal defect, especially with lesions that extend below sternum.

Contraindications
- Extensive lung disease.
- Liver disease.

Advantages
- Single anastomosis.
- Entire esophagus removed, improving chances for negative surgical margins

Disadvantages and complications
- Morbidity of mediastinal portion of procedure (e.g., pneumothorax, hemothorax, pulmonary contusion)
- Long-term complaints of satiety, emesis, dumping

Free-tissue transfer (jejunal autograft)

Indications
- Reconstruction of esophagus in patients not requiring resection of esophagus caudal to thoracic inlet.

Contraindications
- Extension of tumor into thoracic esophagus.

Advantages
- Low rate of stenosis.
- Low rate of fistula.
- Self-lubricating.

Disadvantages and complications
- Microvascular expertise required.
- Prolonged operating time.
- Laparotomy required.

Selected References from the Recent Literature

1. Adelstein DJ. Oropharyngeal cancer: the role of chemotherapy. [Review] [32 refs]. *Current Treatment Options in Oncology* 2003;4:3-13.
2. Al Sarraf M, Reddy MS. Nasopharyngeal carcinoma. [Review] [38 refs]. *Current Treatment Options in Oncology* 2002;3:21-32.
3. Anderson WF, Hawk E, Berg CD. Secondary chemoprevention of upper aerodigestive tract tumors. [Review] [146 refs]. *Seminars in Oncology* 2001;28:106-120.
4. Bales C, Kotapka M, Loevner LA *et al*. Craniofacial resection of advanced juvenile nasopharyngeal angiofibroma. [Review] [25 refs]. *Archives of Otolaryngology—Head & Neck Surgery* 2002;128:1071-1078.
5. Barnes C, Sexton M, Sizeland A *et al*. Laryngo-pharyngeal carcinoma in childhood. [Review] [15 refs]. *International Journal of Pediatric Otorhinolaryngology* 2001;61:83-86.

6. Browne JD. The midfacial degloving procedure for nasal, sinus, and nasopharyngeal tumors. [Review] [12 refs]. *Otolaryngologic Clinics of North America* 2001;34: 1095-1104.

7. Cavalot AL, Gervasio CF, Nazionale G *et al.* Pharyngocutaneous fistula as a complication of total laryngectomy: review of the literature and analysis of case records. [Review] [21 refs]. *Otolaryngology—Head & Neck Surgery* 2000;123:587-592.

8. Chan AT, Teo PM, Johnson PJ. Nasopharyngeal carcinoma. [Review] [54 refs]. *Annals of Oncology* 2002;13:1007-1015.

9. Chan AT, Teo PM, Johnson PJ. Nasopharyngeal cancer. [Review] [43 refs]. *Cancer Treatment & Research* 2003;114:275-293.

10. Chen YK, Lin LM, Lin CC. Malignant fibrous histiocytoma of the tongue. [Review] [11 refs]. *Journal of Laryngology & Otology* 2001;115:763-765.

11. Coppit GL, III, Perkins JA, Manning SC. Nasopharyngeal teratomas and dermoids: a review of the literature and case series. [Review] [32 refs]. *International Journal of Pediatric Otorhinolaryngology* 2000;52:219-227.

12. Couch ME. Laryngopharyngectomy with reconstruction. [Review] [41 refs]. *Otolaryngologic Clinics of North America* 2002;35:1097-1114.

13. Ferlito A, Rinaldo A. Paraneoplastic syndromes in patients with laryngeal and hypopharyngeal cancers. [Review] [80 refs]. *Annals of Otology, Rhinology & Laryngology* 2000;109:109-117.

14. Ferlito A, Buckley JG, Shaha AR *et al.* Rationale for selective neck dissection in tumors of the upper aerodigestive tract. [Review] [73 refs]. *Acta Oto-Laryngologica* 2001;121: 548-555.

15. Ferlito A, Shaha AR, Buckley JG *et al.* Selective neck dissection for hypopharyngeal cancer in the clinically negative neck: should it be bilateral?. [Review] [48 refs]. *Acta Oto-Laryngologica* 2001;121:329-335.

16. Ferlito A, Shaha AR, Rinaldo A. Prognostic value of Delphian lymph node metastasis from laryngeal and hypopharyngeal cancer. [Review] [9 refs]. *Acta Oto-Laryngologica* 2002;122:456-457.

17. Ferlito A, Shaha AR, Lefebvre JL *et al.* Organ and voice preservation in advanced laryngeal cancer. [Review] [34 refs]. *Acta Oto-Laryngologica* 2002;122:438-442.

18. Flint PW. Minimally invasive techniques for management of early glottic cancer. [Review] [46 refs]. *Otolaryngologic Clinics of North America* 2002;35:1055-1066.

19. Garden AS. Organ preservation for carcinoma of the larynx and hypopharynx. [Review] [81 refs]. *Hematology—Oncology Clinics of North America* 2001;15:243-260.

20. Genden EM, Ferlito A, Scully C *et al.* Current management of tonsillar cancer. [Review] [49 refs]. *Oral Oncology* 2003;39:337-342.

21. Gilbert J, Forastiere AA. Organ preservation trials for laryngeal cancer. [Review] [81 refs]. *Otolaryngologic Clinics of North America* 2002;35:1035-1054.

22. Goodwin WJ. Distant metastases from oropharyngeal cancer. [Review] [8 refs]. Orl; *Journal of Oto-Rhino-Laryngology & Its Related Specialties* 2001;63:222-223.

23. Greenman J, Homer JJ, Stafford ND. Markers in cancer of the larynx and pharynx. [Review] [98 refs]. *Clinical Otolaryngology & Allied Sciences* 2000; 25(1):9-18.

24. Ha PK, Califano JA, III. The molecular biology of laryngeal cancer. [Review] [100 refs]. *Otolaryngologic Clinics of North America* 2002;35:993-1012.

25. Harrison LB, Ferlito A, Shaha AR *et al.* Current philosophy on the management of cancer of the base of the tongue. [Review] [31 refs]. *Oral Oncology* 2003;39:101-105.

26. Helliwell TR. Best Practice No 169. Evidence-based pathology: squamous carcinoma of the hypopharynx. [Review] [52 refs]. *Journal of Clinical Pathology* 2003;56: 81-85.

27. Herrmann K, Niedobitek G. Epstein-Barr virus-associated carcinomas: facts and fiction. [Review] [62 refs]. *Journal of Pathology* 2003;199:140-145.

28. Hinerman RW, Amdur RJ, Mendenhall WM *et al.* Hypopharyngeal carcinoma. [Review] [37 refs]. *Current Treatment Options in Oncology* 2002;3:41-49.

29. Horn C, Thaker HM, Tampakopoulou DA *et al.* Tongue lesions in the pediatric population. [Review] [19 refs]. *Otolaryngology—Head & Neck Surgery* 2001;124:164-169.

30. Jorissen M, Eloy P, Rombaux P *et al.* Endoscopic sinus surgery for juvenile nasopharyngeal angiofibroma. [Review] [48 refs]. *Acta Oto-Rhino-Laryngologica Belgica* 2000;54: 201-219.

31. Klaassen I, Braakhuis BJ. Anticancer activity and mechanism of action of retinoids in oral and pharyngeal cancer. [Review] [107 refs]. *Oral Oncology* 2002;38:532-542.

32. Koch WM. Total laryngectomy with tracheoesophageal conduit. [Review] [27 refs]. *Otolaryngologic Clinics of North America* 2002;35:1081-1096.

33. Koren R, Kristt D, Shvero J *et al.* The spectrum of laryngeal neoplasia: the pathologist's view. [Review] [40 refs]. *Pathology, Research & Practice* 2002;198:709-715.

34. Laramore GE, Coltrera MD. Organ preservation strategies in the treatment of laryngeal cancer. [Review] [37 refs]. *Current Treatment Options in Oncology* 2003;4:15-25.

35. Lee DJ. Definitive radiotherapy for squamous carcinoma of the larynx. [Review] [60 refs]. *Otolaryngologic Clinics of North America* 2002;35:1013-1033.

36. Lee JH, Machtay M, McKenna MG *et al.* Radiotherapy with 6-megavolt photons for early glottic carcinoma: potential impact of extension to the posterior vocal cord. [Review] [47 refs]. *American Journal of Otolaryngology* 2001;22:43-54.

37. Lee JT, Chen P, Safa A *et al.* The role of radiation in the treatment of advanced juvenile angiofibroma. [Review] [43 refs]. *Laryngoscope* 2002;112:1213-1220.

38. Lee SP. Nasopharyngeal carcinoma and the EBV-specific T cell response: prospects for immunotherapy. [Review] [64 refs]. *Seminars in Cancer Biology* 2002;12:463-471.

39. Licitra L, Bernier J, Grandi C *et al.* Cancer of the oropharynx. [Review] [95 refs]. *Critical Reviews in Oncology-Hematology* 2002;41:107-122.

40. Liu FF. Novel gene therapy approach for nasopharyngeal carcinoma. [Review] [108 refs]. *Seminars in Cancer Biology* 2002;12:505-515.

41. Lo KW, Huang DP. Genetic and epigenetic changes in nasopharyngeal carcinoma. [Review] [95 refs]. *Seminars in Cancer Biology* 2002;12:451-462.

42. Lu B, Yalcin S. Squamous cell carcinoma of the tongue in a patient with Fanconi's anemia: a case report and review of the literature. [Review] [41 refs]. *Annals of Hematology* 2002;81:294-298.

43. Mignogna MD, Fedele S, Lo RL *et al.* Costs and effectiveness in the care of patients with oral and pharyngeal cancer: analysis of a paradox. [Review] [12 refs]. *European Journal of Cancer Prevention* 2002;11:205-208.

44. Nadal A, Cardesa A. Molecular biology of laryngeal squamous cell carcinoma. [Review] [71 refs]. *Virchows Arch* 2003;442:1-7.

45. Nunes FD, Loducca SV, de Oliveira EM *et al.* Well-differentiated liposarcoma of the tongue. [Review] [13 refs]. *Oral Oncology* 2002;38:117-119.

46. Ozturk O, Ozek H, Cansiz H *et al.* Primary malignant melanoma of the pharynx. [Review] [18 refs]. *Journal of Laryngology & Otology* 2001;115:931-934.

47. Raab-Traub N. Epstein-Barr virus in the pathogenesis of NPC. [Review] [102 refs]. *Seminars in Cancer Biology* 2002;12:431-441.

48. Raaijmakers E, Engelen AM. Is sensorineural hearing loss a possible side effect of nasopharyngeal and parotid irradiation? A systematic review of the literature. [Review] [29 refs]. *Radiotherapy & Oncology* 2002;65:1-7.

49. Rafferty MA, Fenton JE, Jones AS. The history, aetiology and epidemiology of laryngeal carcinoma. [Review] [41 refs]. *Clinical Otolaryngology & Allied Sciences* 2001;26:442-446.

50. Remijn EE, Marres HA, van den Hoogen FJ. Endoscopic laser treatment in premalignant and malignant vocal fold epithelial lesions. [Review] [28 refs]. *Journal of Laryngology & Otology* 2002;116:1019-1024.

51. Rice DH. Endonasal approaches for sinonasal and nasopharyngeal tumors. [Review] [17 refs]. *Otolaryngologic Clinics of North America* 2001;34:1087-1093.

52. Rinaldo A, Howard DJ, Ferlito A. Laryngeal chondrosarcoma: a 24-year experience at the Royal National Throat, Nose and Ear Hospital. [Review] [54 refs]. *Acta Oto-Laryngologica* 2000;120:680-688.

53. Rudat V, Wannenmacher M. Role of multimodal treatment in oropharynx, larynx, and hypopharynx cancer. [Review] [65 refs]. *Seminars in Surgical Oncology* 2001;20:66-74.

54. Samlan RA, Webster KT. Swallowing and speech therapy after definitive treatment for laryngeal cancer. [Review] [104 refs]. *Otolaryngologic Clinics of North America* 2002;35:1115-1133.

55. Scully C. Oral squamous cell carcinoma: from an hypothesis about a virus, to concern about possible sexual transmission. [Review] [113 refs]. *Oral Oncology* 2002;38:227-234.

56. Strome SE, Weinman EC. Advanced larynx cancer. [Review] [37 refs]. *Current Treatment Options in Oncology* 2002;3:11-20.

57. Teknos TN, Hogikyan ND, Wolf GT. Conservation laryngeal surgery for malignant tumors of the larynx and pyriform sinus. [Review] [56 refs]. *Hematology–Oncology Clinics of North America* 2001;15:261-276.

58. Thekdi AA, Ferris RL. Diagnostic assessment of laryngeal cancer. [Review] [15 refs]. *Otolaryngologic Clinics of North America* 2002;35:953-969.

59. Thompson LD, Gannon FH. Chondrosarcoma of the larynx: a clinicopathologic study of 111 cases with a review of the literature. [Review] [58 refs]. *American Journal of Surgical Pathology* 2002;26:836-851.

60. Tufano RP. Organ preservation surgery for laryngeal cancer. [Review] [49 refs]. *Otolaryngologic Clinics of North America* 2002;35:1067-1080.

61. Weinstein GS. Surgical approach to organ preservation in the treatment of cancer of the larynx. [Review] [92 refs]. *Oncology (Huntington)* 2001;15:785-796.

62. Zeitels SM, Casiano RR, Gardner GM *et al.* Management of common voice problems: committee report.[comment]. [Review] [85 refs]. *Otolaryngology—Head & Neck Surgery* 2002;126:333-348.

63. Zinreich SJ. Imaging in laryngeal cancer: computed tomography, magnetic resonance imaging, positron emission tomography. [Review] [49 refs]. *Otolaryngologic Clinics of North America* 2002;35:971-991.

BENIGN DISEASES OF THE THYROID

Graves' Disease

Etiology and pathogenesis
- Autoimmune hyperthyroidism is caused by circulating thyroid-stimulating antibodies that bind to and activate thyroid-stimulating hormone (TSH) receptors.
- Different autoantibodies (e.g., ocular muscle cells and fibroblasts) seem to be involved in mediating the infiltrative ophthalmopathy (50% of patients) associated with this disease.

Epidemiology
- Most common in women in their third to fourth decades of life.

Pathology
- Hypervascular thyroid gland with cellular hypertrophy and hyperplasia.

Signs and symptoms
- As per hyperthyroidism:
  - Tachycardia.
  - Anxiety, irritability.
  - Heat intolerance.
  - Proximal muscle weakness, atrophy.
  - Warm, smooth skin.
  - Weight loss.
  - Amenorrhea.
- Ocular symptoms.
  - Exophthalmos.
  - Proptosis.
  - Lid retraction, lid lag.
  - Diplopia.
- Pretibial myxedema.

Investigations
- Decreased TSH.
- Increased T4 and T3.
- Increased radioactive iodine uptake on scan.

Treatment
Radioactive iodine (I^{131})
- Treatment of choice in nonpregnant adults.
- Contraindicated in pregnancy.
- High incidence of posttreatment hypothyroidism.

Medications
- Propylthiouracil (PTU).
  - Blocks organification of iodine, resulting in decreased thyroid hormone production.
  - Blocks conversion of peripheral T4 to T3.
- Methimazole.
  - Blocks organification of iodine, resulting in decreased thyroid hormone production.
  - Medications continued for 6-12 months after euthyroid state achieved; significant relapse rate when therapy discontinued.

Indications for surgery
- Failed or refused medical treatment.
- Pregnant patient who cannot be controlled on low dose PTU.
- Question of malignancy.
- Obstructive goiter.

Ophthalmopathy
- May be worse after radioactive iodine treatment; treated with prednisone 0.5 mg/kg.
- Surgical decompression (see chapter in Rhinology section).

Toxic Multinodular Goitre

- Presents in older females with more insidious onset than Graves' disease.
- Treated with I^{131} after initiation of beta-blockers.

Toxic Adenoma

- Presents as nodule with symptoms of hyperthyroidism.
- "Hot nodule" on thyroid scan.
- Treatment: excision, especially in younger patient; I^{131} as alternative.

Thyroid Storm

- Acute exacerbation of thyrotoxicosis.

Etiology
- Major stress (e.g., sepsis, myocardial infarction, surgery, diabetic ketoacidosis) in patient with unrecognized hyperthyroidism.
- Inadequate therapy in hyperthyroid patient.

Clinical presentation
History
- Fever.
- Anxiety, psychosis.
- Hyperhidrosis, heat intolerance.
- Muscle weakness.
- Diarrhea, nausea, vomiting.
- Tachycardia, arrhythmias

Physical examination
- Tremor.
- Fever.
- Tachycardia.

- Warm, moist skin.
- Altered mental status.
- Goiter, lid lag.

Investigations
- Thyroid function tests.
- Cultures: blood and urine.
- Electrolytes, BUN, creatine, glucose.
- ECG.
- CXR (pneumonia, congestive heart failure [CHF]).

Treatment
- PTU 400 q8h.
- Sodium iodide 250 mg IV q6h *or* potassium iodide (SSKI) 5 gttes po q8h *or* Lugol's solution 10 gttes q8h.
- Note: PTU must be given 1 hour prior to iodide to prevent the iodide from *increasing* thyroid storm.
- Dexamethasone 2 mg IV q6h or hydrocortisone 100 mg IV q6h (prevents thyroid hormone release and conversion of T4 to T3).
- Beta-blockers (e.g., propranolol, atenolol).
- Acetaminophen for fever.
- Aggressive hydration with glucose containing solution.

Thyroiditis

Definitions
- Acute: may be bacterial, viral, fungal, rarely parasitic.
- Subacute: granulomatous or de Quervain's
- Chronic:
  - Reidel's (struma): rare, inflammatory (autoimmune); typically affects woman.
  - Hashimoto's: autoimmune disorder, primarily affects middle-aged women.

Pathology
- Acute: infiltration with polymorphonuclear neutrophil leukocytes (PMNs).
- Subacute (de Quervain's): mixed inflammatory infiltrate with giant cell granulomas.
- Chronic:
  - Riedel's: mixed inflammatory infiltrate (primarily lymphocytic) with extensive fibrosis.
  - Hashimoto's: extensive lymphocytic infiltrate with lymphoid follicles; atrophic thyroid follicles lined by Hurthle cells (follicular cells with brightly eosinophilic granular cytoplasm).

Clinical presentation
- Suppurative thyroiditis: present with fever, severe neck pain, focal tenderness, erythema of overlying skin.

- Subacute: pain, fever, enlarged thyroid, initial signs of hyperthyroidism; development of hypothyroidism subsequent to resolution of inflammation in some patients.
- Riedel's: painless, slowly enlarging, hard thyroid mass; may be mistaken for thyroid carcinoma potential for development of hypothyroidism.
- Hashimoto's: enlarged thyroid gland associated with hyperthyroidism in early stages of disease; decrease in gland size as hypothyroidism ensues.

Investigations
- TSH, free T4.
- White blood cell count (WBC) with differential.
- Blood cultures in suppurative.
- Antimicrosomal antibodies (in >90% of patients with Hashimoto's).
- Serum thyroglobulin (elevated in subacute—useful in monitoring course of disease).
- CT or MRI if abscess suspected.

Treatment
- If hyperthyroid, treat symptoms with beta-blockers.
- Control pain with NSAIDs and, if severe, prednisone.
- If hypothyroid, start levothyroxine 25-50 μg/day and monitor TSH q 6-8 weeks.
- Start IV antibiotics with or without incision and drainage of neck abscess in suppurative labyrinthitis.
- Note that Hashimoto's associated with increased risk of papillary carcinoma and lymphoma.

Goiter

Diffuse nontoxic (colloid)
- Endemic (low iodine).
- Sporadic (idiopathic).
- Treat with potassium iodide if endemic, otherwise no treatment unless obstructive (surgery).

Nodular
- Seen in up to 5% of population.
- Etiology unknown.
- No treatment unless obstructive or if one nodule shows risk of malignancy (see following section).

Evaluation of Thyroid Nodule
- Seen 0.8% of men and 5.0% of woman.
- Risks for malignancy include:
  - History of radiation to head and neck.
  - Family history of pheochromocytoma, cancer of thyroid, hyperparathyroidism (multiple endocrine neoplasia [MEN] II).
  - Dysphagia or hoarseness.
  - Nodule >2 cm.

- ▫ Regional lymphadenopathy.
- ▫ Fixation to adjacent tissues.
- ▫ <40 years of age, male.

Evaluation
Fine needle aspiration (FNA)
- Test of first choice
- If FNA shows cancer, surgery is recommended.
- If FNA shows a cystic lesion, then the patient is followed. If the cyst does not recur, the patient is then followed. If the cyst recurs, it is reaspirated, at which point the cyst may be followed but is typically removed because FNAs are less accurate when evaluating cystic lesions.
- If FNA reveals benign cells in a solid lesion, then a radionucleide is performed.
  - ▫ If the scan reveals increased uptake ("hot"), then the lesion is removed (or treated with I^{131}) if:
    - T4 is elevated.
    - If the lesion is large.
      - ○ A small hot nodule may be followed.
  - ▫ If the scan shows no increased uptake, then:
    - The lesion can be followed (some will institute levo thyroxine suppressive treatment: 100-200 μg qd).
    - If the lesion does not regress, a repeat FNA is performed and the lesion may then be followed or may be resected.

DISEASES OF THE PARATHYROID GLANDS

Hyperparathyroidism

Primary hyperparathyroidism
- 0.1% of adults.
- More frequent in patients >50 years of age.
- Caused by increased secretion of PTH.
- Results in hypercalcemia, hypercalcuria, hypophosphatemia.
- Adenoma.
- Single adenoma in 80% of cases.
- Double adenoma in 5% of cases.
- Hyperplasia 15% of cases.
- Carcinoma 2% of cases.

THYROID CANCER

- 1% of all new cancers.
- Approximately 12,000 cases per year.
- Incidence: 4 per 100,000.

Papillary thyroid cancer
Incidence and epidemiology
- 80% of all thyroid carcinomas.
- Radiation major risk factor.
- Found in 10% of all autopsies (male = female).

- 30-40 years of age.
- Female:male = 3:1.

Pathology
- Papillary and follicular components.
- Large pink cell.
- Granular cytoplasm. "Orphan Annie eyes" (i.e., clear nuclei with marginated chromatin).
- Psammoma bodies: calcified basophilic spheres in stroma; pathognomonic for papillary carcinoma.
- Squamous metaplasia.
- Lymphocytic infiltrate.
- 10% encapsulated.
- Hürthle cell variant (aggressive).
- Follicular variant.
- 10% invade locally.
- 36% of adults nodal metastases.
- 80% of children nodal metastases.
- Correlation of frequency of nodal metastases with increasing primary tumor size central and lateral nodal drainage.
- Mediastinal and bilateral cervical nodal involvement in large tumors → mortality 3 times greater.
- <1% present with distant metastases.
- 5%-10% develop distant metastases → lung, bone.

Evaluation
- Thyroid mass or nodule on physical examination.
- FNA (cornerstone of diagnosis).
- Ultrasound (may localize other sites within thyroid).
- CT scan to evaluate nodal metastases.
- Thyroglobulin staining.

Treatment
- Surgery: decreased recurrence with total thyroidectomy vs. lobectomy.
- Neck dissection for patients with locally invasive disease and nodal metastases.
- I^{131} postoperatively lowers risk of distant metastases.
- External beam radiation for tumors that do not concentrate iodine.

Prognosis
- 30-year mortality rate 6%.
- 30-year recurrence rate 31%.
- Poorer prognosis indicated by the following factors:
  - ▫ Age: high recurrence at extremes of age.
  - ▫ Gender: higher mortality rate in men.
  - ▫ Graves' disease: more invasive tumors.
  - ▫ Tumor size.
  - ▫ Invasion.
  - ▫ Distant metastases.

Follicular thyroid cancer
Incidence and epidemiology
- 10% of thyroid cancers.

- Older age group.
- Uncommon in children.
- Females>males.
- Not typical in autopsy specimens.

Pathology
- Encapsulated.
- Benign on frozen section and FNA.
- Capsular and angioinvasion.
- Microfollicles and solid cell masses histologically.
- Some capsular and angioinvasion in minimally invasive type.
- Satellite nodules in highly invasive type.
- 20% distant metastases → bone, brain, lung.
- Potential for small tumors to metastasize distantly.

Evaluation
- As per papillary carcinoma.

Treatment
- Surgery-decreased recurrence with total thyroidectomy vs. lobectomy.
- Neck dissection for patients with locally invasive disease and nodal metastases.
- I^{131} post-operatively lowers risk of distant metastases.
- External beam radiation for tumors that do not concentrate iodine.

Prognosis
- 30-year mortality rate 15%.
- 30-year recurrence rate 24%.
- Age: high recurrence at extremes of age.
- Gender: men have higher mortality than women.
- Graves' disease: more invasive tumors.
- Increased tumor size = poorer prognosis.
- Invasion of surrounding structures = poorer prognosis.
- Distant metastases.

Anaplastic thyroid cancer
Incidence and epidemiology
- Usually arises from differentiated thyroid cancer.
- May develop after radiation for Hodgkin's lymphoma.
- Low iodine intake.
- Age > 60.
- Female:male = 2:1.

Pathology
- Infiltrative.
- Hemorrhage and necrosis.
- Well-differentiated thyroid carcinoma foci in one-third of patients.
- Must be differentiated from lymphoma.
- Thyroglobulin positive.

- May contain sarcomatous and epithelial elements.
- Rapidly growing.
- Regional metastases.
- Tracheal invasion in 25% of patients.
- Distant metastases to lung in 50% of patients.

Evaluation
- History and physical examination: rapidly growing, hard, fixed neck mass; may have rapidly progressive airway compromise.
- FNA.
- CT scan of chest to evaluate distant metastases, local invasion.
- Immunohistochemical staining crucial to differentiate from lymphoma and medullary thyroid carcinoma.

Treatment
- Surgery: thyroidectomy.
- External beam radiation.
- Chemotherapy.

Prognosis
- Very poor.
- Mortality within 6-8 months.

Medullary carcinoma of the thyroid gland (MTC)
Incidence and epidemiology
- 5%-10% of all thyroid malignancies.
- 13.4% of all deaths related to thyroid carcinomas.
- Average age at diagnosis approximately 40 years of age; patients with sporadic disease present later.

Genetics
- Sporadic (75%).
  - Unilateral.
  - No familial pattern.
  - No associated abnormalities.
- Familial (25%).
  - Bilateral.
  - Autosomal dominant with nearly complete penetrance, but variable expressivity.
  - Syndromes.
  - MEN-IIA: MTC, pheochromocytoma, parathyroid hyperplasia.
  - MEN-IIB: MTC, pheochromocytoma, neural hypertrothy.
  - FMTC (familial medullary thyroid carcinoma).
  - Missense mutations in RET protooncogene.

Pathology and patterns of spread
- Develops in C cells, which are located in superior portion of thyroid lobe.
- Macroscopically, has solid appearance; cut surface = white and gritty.
- Tumors: histologically, spindle cell appearance.

- On special staining, has properties characteristic of amyloid; however, material not amyloid but prohormone calcitonin (i.e., polypeptide hormone secreted by C cells).
- C cells: great biosynthetic activity, secretion of several hormones and biogenic amines, including calcitonin (important clinically), adrenocorticotropic hormone (ACTH), histaminase carcinoembryogenic antigen, vasoactive peptide.
- C cell hyperplasia: histologic abnormality that precedes development of MTC.
- MTC: slow growth and metastasis to regional lymph nodes.
- Most common sites of distant metastasis: liver, lung, bone, brain.

Physical examination
- Thyroid nodule with or without enlarged lymph nodes, multicentric in familial syndromes.
- Tachycardia/hypertension for pheochromocytoma to evaluate for MEN syndromes.

Investigations
- Biochemical examination.
  - Measurement of plasma calcitonin level following intravenous administration of calcium and pentagastrin.
  - 24-hour urinary excretion rates of catecholamines and metabolites to exclude presence of pheochromocytoma.
  - Serum calcium and parathyroid hormone to exclude hyperparathyroidism.
- Genetic testing for familial forms of MTC.

Treatment
- Surgery
  - In primary MTC:
    - Total thyroidectomy and resection of lymph nodes in central zone of the neck should be performed.
    - If enlarged lymph nodes are found in central zone or the lateral neck, a modified neck dissection is performed.
    - If pheochromocytoma is identified, it should be removed prior to performing the thyroidectomy.
    - Measuring stimulated plasma calcitonin levels following thyroidectomy is a valuable means of determining persistent or recurrent disease.
    - If postoperative plasma calcitonin is not elevated above the basal level, patients should be followed annually for 5 years.
  - In MTC associated with genetic syndrome:
    - *Prophylactic* early thyroidectomy is often curative in family members of kindred with RET protooncogene mutations.

- In MEN-IIA and FMTC, surgery should be performed around 5 years of age.
- In MEN-IIB, surgery should be performed during the first year of life
  - In persistent or recurrent MTC.
    - Total thyroidectomy and meticulous resection of central and lateral lymph nodes in the neck may be curative in some patients.
    - Chemotherapy and radiotherapy are generally ineffective.

Prognosis
- MTC is a slow-growing tumor, and patients may live for years with evidence of distant metastatic disease.
- Only age and stage of the disease are independent predictors of survival in multivariate analysis.
- Patients who are younger than 45 years of age, are female, and have MTC confined to thyroid have the best overall prognosis.

Selected References from the Recent Literature

1. Cohen EG, Tuttle RM, Kraus DH. Postoperative management of differentiated thyroid cancer. [Review] [123 refs]. *Otolaryngologic Clinics of North America* 2003;36:129-157.
2. Bentley AA, Gillespie C, Malis D. Evaluation and management of a solitary thyroid nodule in a child. [Review] [63 refs]. *Otolaryngologic Clinics of North America* 2003;36:117-128.
3. Sniezek JC, Holtel M. Rare tumors of the thyroid gland. [Review] [44 refs]. *Otolaryngologic Clinics of North America* 2003;36:107-115.
4. Clayman GL, el Baradie TS. Medullary thyroid cancer. [Review] [81 refs]. *Otolaryngologic Clinics of North America* 2003;36:91-105.
5. Boone RT, Fan CY, Hanna EY. Well-differentiated carcinoma of the thyroid. [Review] [91 refs]. Otolaryngologic *Clinics of North America* 2003;36:73-90.
6. Kim N, Lavertu P. Evaluation of a thyroid nodule. [Review] [58 refs]. *Otolaryngologic Clinics of North America* 2003;36:17-33.
7. Castro P, Fonseca E, Magalhaes J et al. Follicular, papillary, and "hybrid" carcinomas of the thyroid. [Review] [45 refs]. *Endocrine Pathology* 2002;13:313-320.
8. Tallini G. Molecular pathobiology of thyroid neoplasms. [Review] [104 refs]. *Endocrine Pathology* 2002;13:271-288.
9. Bojunga J, Kusterer K, Schumm-Draeger PM et al. Polymerase chain reaction in the detection of tumor cells: new approaches in diagnosis and follow-up of patients with thyroid cancer. [Review] [88 refs]. *Thyroid* 2002;12:1097-1107.
10. Anderson CE, McLaren KM. Best practice in thyroid pathology. [Review] [30 refs]. *Journal of Clinical Pathology* 2003;56:401-405.
11. Pasieka JL. Anaplastic thyroid cancer. [Review] [56 refs]. *Current Opinion in Oncology* 2003;15:78-83.

12. Kinder BK. Well-differentiated thyroid cancer. [Review] [42 refs]. *Current Opinion in Oncology* 2003;15:71-77.

13. Roman SA. Endocrine tumors: evaluation of the thyroid nodule. [Review] [41 refs]. *Current Opinion in Oncology* 2003;15:66-70.

14. Hammoud ZT, Mathisen DJ. Surgical management of thyroid carcinoma invading the trachea. [Review] [21 refs]. *Chest Surgery Clinics of North America* 2003;13:359-367.

15. Mazzaferri EL, Robbins RJ, Spencer CA et al. A consensus report of the role of serum thyroglobulin as a monitoring method for low-risk patients with papillary thyroid carcinoma. [Review] [49 refs]. *Journal of Clinical Endocrinology & Metabolism* 2003;88:1433-1441.

16. Nagataki S, Nystrom E. Epidemiology and primary prevention of thyroid cancer. [Review] [74 refs]. *Thyroid* 2002;12:889-896.

17. Knudsen N, Laurberg P, Perrild H et al. Risk factors for goiter and thyroid nodules. [Review] [85 refs]. *Thyroid* 2002;12:879-888.

18. Sherman SI. Thyroid carcinoma. [Review] [168 refs]. *Lancet* 2003;361:501-511.

19. Parthasarathy KL, Crawford ES. Treatment of thyroid carcinoma: emphasis on high-dose ^{131}I outpatient therapy. [Review] [38 refs]. *Journal of Nuclear Medicine Technology* 2002;30:165-171.

20. Hung W, Sarlis NJ. Current controversies in the management of pediatric patients with well-differentiated nonmedullary thyroid cancer: a review. [Review] [198 refs]. *Thyroid* 2002;12:683-702.

21. Larson SM, Robbins R. Positron emission tomography in thyroid cancer management. [Review] [12 refs]. *Seminars in Roentgenology* 2002;37:169-174.

22. Harris PE. The management of thyroid cancer in adults: a review of new guidelines. [Review] [7 refs]. *Clinical Medicine* 2002;2:144-146.

23. Haigh PI. Follicular thyroid carcinoma. [Review] [32 refs]. *Current Treatment Options in Oncology* 2002;3:349-354.

24. Sarlis NJ. Metastatic thyroid cancer unresponsive to conventional therapies: novel management approaches through translational clinical research. [Review] [168 refs]. *Current Drug Targets—Immune Endocrine & Metabolic Disorders* 2001;1:103-115.

25. Puxeddu E, Fagin JA. Genetic markers in thyroid neoplasia. [Review] [143 refs]. *Endocrinology & Metabolism Clinics of North America* 2001;30:493-513.

26. Gimm O. Multiple endocrine neoplasia type 2: clinical aspects. [Review] [115 refs]. *Frontiers of Hormone Research* 2001;28:103-130.

27. Lips CJ, Hoppener JW, Thijssen JH. Medullary thyroid carcinoma: role of genetic testing and calcitonin measurement. [Review] [79 refs]. *Annals of Clinical Biochemistry* 2001;38: 168-179.

28. Modigliani E, Franc B, Niccoli-sire P. Diagnosis and treatment of medullary thyroid cancer. [Review] [73 refs]. *Best Practice & Research Clinical Endocrinology & Metabolism* 2000;14:631-649.

29. Hansford JR, Mulligan LM. Multiple endocrine neoplasia type 2 and RET: from neoplasia to neurogenesis. [Review] [129 refs]. *Journal of Medical Genetics* 2000;37:817-827.

30. Le HN, Norton JA. Perspective on RET proto-oncogene and thyroid cancer. [Review] [80 refs]. *Cancer Journal* 2000;6:50-57.

32. Van Nostrand D, Atkins F, Yeganeh F et al. Dosimetrically determined doses of radioiodine for the treatment of metastatic thyroid carcinoma. [Review] [63 refs]. *Thyroid* 2002;12:121-134.

33. Malchoff CD, Malchoff DM. The genetics of hereditary nonmedullary thyroid carcinoma. [Review] [41 refs]. *Journal of Clinical Endocrinology & Metabolism* 2002;8: 2455-2459.

34. Lane H, Jones MK. Management of nodular thyroid disease. [Review] [15 refs]. *Practitioner* 2002;246:266-269.

35. Weiss RE, Lado-Abeal J. Thyroid nodules: diagnosis and therapy. [Review] [55 refs]. *Current Opinion in Oncology* 2002;14:46-52.

36. Massine RE, Durning SJ, Koroscil TM. Lingual thyroid carcinoma: a case report and review of the literature. [Review] [50 refs]. *Thyroid* 2001;11:1191-1196.

37. Baloch ZW, LiVolsi VA. Neuroendocrine tumors of the thyroid gland. [Review] [172 refs]. *American Journal of Clinical Pathology* 2001;115 Suppl:S56-S67.

38. Baloch ZW, LiVolsi VA. Prognostic factors in well-differentiated follicular-derived carcinoma and medullary thyroid carcinoma. [Review] [128 refs]. *Thyroid* 2001;11:637-645.

39. Puxeddu E, Fagin JA. Genetic markers in thyroid neoplasia. [Review] [143 refs]. *Endocrinology & Metabolism Clinics of North America* 2001;30:493-513.

NECK DISSECTION

Definition

- Surgical procedure performed to remove the fibrofatty contents of specific areas of the neck; designed to remove metastatic disease to cervical lymph nodes.

Indications

- Identified metastatic disease to cervical lymph nodes from upper aerodigestive tract, salivary gland, skin, and other malignancies of the head and neck.
- Neck dissection is indicated in cases of primary malignancies with high risk for nodal metastases.

Contraindications

- Unresectable disease (e.g., carotid artery involvement).

Classification

Triangles of the neck

- Anterior triangle: bordered by the SCM muscle posteriorly, the mandible superiorly, the clavicle inferiorly, and the midline medially.
  - The anterior triangle is further divided into smaller triangles by the digastric and omohyoid muscles.
  - The submandibular triangle lies between the digastric muscle inferiorly and the mandible superiorly.
  - The superior and inferior carotid triangles lie inferior to the digastric and are separated by the omohyoid muscle.
- The posterior triangle is formed by the SCM anteriorly, the trapezius posteriorly, the clavicle inferiorly, and the mastoid tip superiorly.
  - It is further divided into the occipital triangle (superior) and the subclavian (inferior) triangles by the omohyoid muscle.

Levels of cervical lymph nodes

- The head and neck contains over 300 lymph nodes, generally following venous structures.
- Based on patterns of metastatic spread, the cervical lymph nodes have been classified based on the following levels:
  - Levels I-IV are located in the anterior triangle, Level V in the posterior triangle
  - Level I: found in the submandibular triangle:
    - Level Ia: submental nodes.
    - Level Ib: submandibular nodes.
  - Level II: located along the upper third of the internal jugular vein (above the carotid bifurcation/hyoid bone).
  - Level III: located along the middle third of the jugular vein, between the carotid bifurcation and the omohyoid.
  - Level IV: lower third of the jugular vein, between the omohyoid and the clavicle.
  - Level V: posterior triangle.
  - Level VI: "anterior compartment" of the neck, between the common carotid arteries, inferior to the hyoid bone; contains the paratracheal, pretracheal, perithyroidal, and precricoid (Delphian) nodes.

Staging of lymph node metastases

- Nx: nodes cannot be assessed.
- N0: No nodal metastases.
- N1: Single ipsilateral node, <3 cm in diameter.
- N2a: Single ipsilateral node: diameter >3 cm, but ≤6 cm
- N2b: Multiple ipsilateral nodes, no single node >6 cm.
- N2c: Bilateral or contralateral nodes, none >6 cm.
- N3: Massive adenopathy, >6 cm.

Types of Neck Dissections

Radical neck dissection

- En bloc resection of fibrofatty tissue from one side of the neck (Levels I-V).
- Includes resection of the internal jugular vein (IJV), CN XI, and SCM.
- Does not include the following regions:
  - Postauricular.
  - Suboccipital.
  - Perifascial.
  - Buccinator.
  - Retropharyngeal.
  - Central compartment (level VI).
- Indicated for patients with advanced neck disease with gross involvement of the IJV, CN XI, and SCM.

Modified radical neck dissection

- Level I-V dissection.
- Preservation of one or more of the IJV, CN XI, and/or SCM.

Selective neck dissection

- Preservation of one or more of the lymphatic groups that are removed in radical or modified radical neck dissections.

Supraomohyoid neck dissection

- Removal of fibrofatty tissues and lymph nodes contained in Levels I-III.
- Indicated as a prophylactic treatment in oral cavities carcinomas with no identifiable cervical metastases.

Lateral neck dissection

- Removal of fibrofatty tissues and lymph nodes contained in levels II, III, and IV.

- Indicated as a prophylactic treatment in laryngeal, hypopharyngeal, and oropharyngeal carcinomas with no identifiable cervical metastases.

Anterior neck dissection
- Removal of fibrofatty tissues and lymph nodes contained in level VI.
- Indicated in cancers of the thyroid, hypopharynx, cervical esophagus, cervical trachea, and subglottic larynx.
- Hypoparathyroidism a major complication of this procedure.

Posterolateral neck dissection
- En bloc resection of nodes in the following regions:
  - Suboccipital, postauricular, levels I-III, level V superior to the XIth nerve
- Indicated in cutaneous malignancies of scalp, postauricular, and suboccipital regions.

Extended neck dissection
- For patients with advanced disease, includes a radical neck dissection supplemented by removal of one or more of the following lymphatic and nonlymphatic structures:
  - Parapharyngeal nodes.
  - Retropharyngeal nodes.
  - Superior mediastinal nodes.
  - Paratracheal nodes.
  - Hypoglossal nerve.
  - Vagus nerve.
  - Paraspinal muscles.
  - Carotid artery.

Complications
Infection
- Use prophylactic antibiotics.

Hematoma
- Use suction drains.
- Early surgical intervention to ligate bleeding vessel.

Chylous fistula

Thoracic duct anatomy
- Length: 37-45 cm (abdomen to neck).
- Starts at **cisterna chyli** (level of L2) and drains into **left subclavian vein**
- Thoracic duct drains all but right side of head and neck, right upper extremity, right lung, right side heart (drained by right lymphatic duct).
- Goes posterior to median arcuate ligament between azygous vein and the aorta.
- Crosses to the left side at T4-T6.

- Forms an arch anterior to scalenus anterior muscle, then descends to junction of left subclavian vein and IJV. Located medial and posterior to left common carotid artery, vagus, and IJV.
- Duct anterior to the thyrocervical trunk and the transverse cervical artery.
- In 7%, duct has two terminal ends; in 4%, duct has three terminal ends.
- May receive additional tributaries:
  - Jugular trunk: drains deep cervical lymph nodes.
  - Subclavian trunk: axillary lymph nodes.
  - Left bronchomediastinal trunk = left chest and mediastinum.
  - Eight to ten unidirectional valves, with terminal valve at junction of SCV.
  - Three layers: the middle muscular layer propels chyle.

Physiology
- Transports 4 L/day in healthy adult (range 10-100 ml/kg).
- Cholinergic stimulation increases the tone of the wall.
- Respiration increases flow.
- 95% of transported fluid from GI tract and liver; 5% from skeletal muscle
- Chyle includes: lymphocytes; immunoglobulins; enzymes; Vitamins D, E, A, K; and triglycerides.
(Note: Triglycerides in chyle > triglycerides in plasma.)
- Normal protein concentration = 20-30 g/L (4% protein, mostly albumin).

Effects of loss
- Hypovolemia, hyponatremia, hypoproteinemia, acidosis, and hypocalcemia.
- Immune compromise if long standing.
- Mortality of postesophagectomy chylothorax is up to 50% because of bacterial and fungal infections if not corrected.

Etiology
- Esophageal surgery.
- Neck dissection: 2% with 90% associated with surgery of the left side.
- On the right side, fistula is caused by injury to the lymphatic channel.
- Thyroid surgery: 0.2% to 0.5%.
- Trauma: penetrating injury, hyperextension of spine, blunt abdomen trauma, violent coughing episodes, tumors (especially lymphoma).

Detection
- Hard to detect intraoperatively because patient is NPO, so fluid tends to be clear.
- Chyloma, persistent chyle leak, or pleural effusion (chylothorax) visible.

- Fluid sampling of drain fluid may reveal levels of triglycerides and lymphocytes greater than that in serum.
- Chyle contains fat from the intestinal lacteal system, giving it the characteristic whitish color. Infusing a dose of cream or other high-fat liquid per NGT causes sudden change in color (whitish)
- Lymphangiography can assist in identification of the site of leak in chest.
- Intraoperatively, placing the patient in Trendelenburg position and having anesthesiologist hyperinflate lungs will increase intrathoracic pressure and force chyle into wound.
- Meticulous isolation and double ligation of the thoracic duct.
- Early postoperative period, may see sudden increase in drainage.
- Laboratory examination will be positive for chylomicrons.

Treatment
- Conservative if drainage is less than 1200 ml/day; successful in 75%
- NPO may be sufficient to stop leak.
- TPN (but can eventually result in a deficiency of linoleic acid [found only on long-chain triglycerides]).
- Dietary oral fat intake, except medium-chain triglycerides, withheld.
- Pressure dressing over the lower neck.
- Continued suction drainage.
- Electrolyte repletion.
- Surgery is indicated if >1200 ml/day or if pleural drainage >1 L/day for 5 days.
- Can irrigate the site, then oversew with cellulose or fibrin glue.
- Transthoracic approach:
  ▫ Open or abdominal ligation (success >95%).
  ▫ Thoracoscopic technique has recently gained wider recognition and acceptance.
- Other modalities:
  ▫ Fibrin glue
  ▫ Pleurodesis with talc or tetracycline
  ▫ Pleuroperitoneal shunts (limited success)
  ▫ Abx.
  ▫ Continuous somatostatin infusion to decrease GI production of chyle.
  ▫ Pectoralis muscle flaps.
- If chylous fistula results from neck dissection for malignancy, need to consider early surgery in order to insure XRT can begin within 6 weeks.

Vascular
- Bilateral internal jugular vein occlusion (e.g., resection on one side and thrombosis on the other).
  ▫ Complications include facial and cerebral edema.
  ▫ Blindness.

- IJV rupture: very rare.
- Carotid artery:
  ▫ Hypotension and bradycardia secondary to manipulation.
  ▫ Intraoperative trauma: repair at the time of surgery with primary closure.
  ▫ Rupture: "blow-out."
    - Incidence: 5%; mortality: 50%.
    - Rupture can result from wound breakdown, infection, salivary fistula. Preoperative radiation is an additional risk factor.
    - May be heralded by a sentinel bleed.
    - If a rupture is pending, elective ligation is associated with a significant decrease in morbidity and mortality.
    - In an acute rupture, apply direct pressure, transfuse, and ligate at a site proximal to the open wound.

Nerve
- Trigeminal nerve
  ▫ Branches at risk are the inferior alveolar nerve and the lingual nerve.
- Facial nerve
  ▫ Cervical branch supplies the platysma, so sacrifice is immaterial.
  ▫ Marginal mandibular branch at risk.
  ▫ Main trunk at risk with parotid involvement.
- Vagus nerve
  ▫ Superior laryngeal nerve trauma may result in aspiration.
  ▫ Recurrent laryngeal nerve.
  ▫ Main trunk may be violated during dissection, especially with ligation of the IJV at the skull base. If violation of the main trunk is observed, a primary repair should be performed.
- Spinal accessory nerve
  ▫ Transection of the XIth nerve results in a syndrome characterized by shoulder pain, stiffness, drooping, limited abduction and flexion, and aberrant scapular rotation.
- Hypoglossal nerve
  ▫ At risk in laryngectomy.
- Sympathetic trunk
  ▫ Runs deep to the carotid sheath along the prevertebral fascia.
  ▫ Violation of the cervical trunk results in an ipsilateral Horner's syndrome.
- Phrenic nerve
  ▫ Receives contributions from roots of C3, C4, and C5.
  ▫ Only nerve to run medial to lateral in the neck.
  ▫ Runs deep to the fascia overlying the scalene muscles, therefore preservation of the phrenic nerve requires dissecting superficial to this plane.

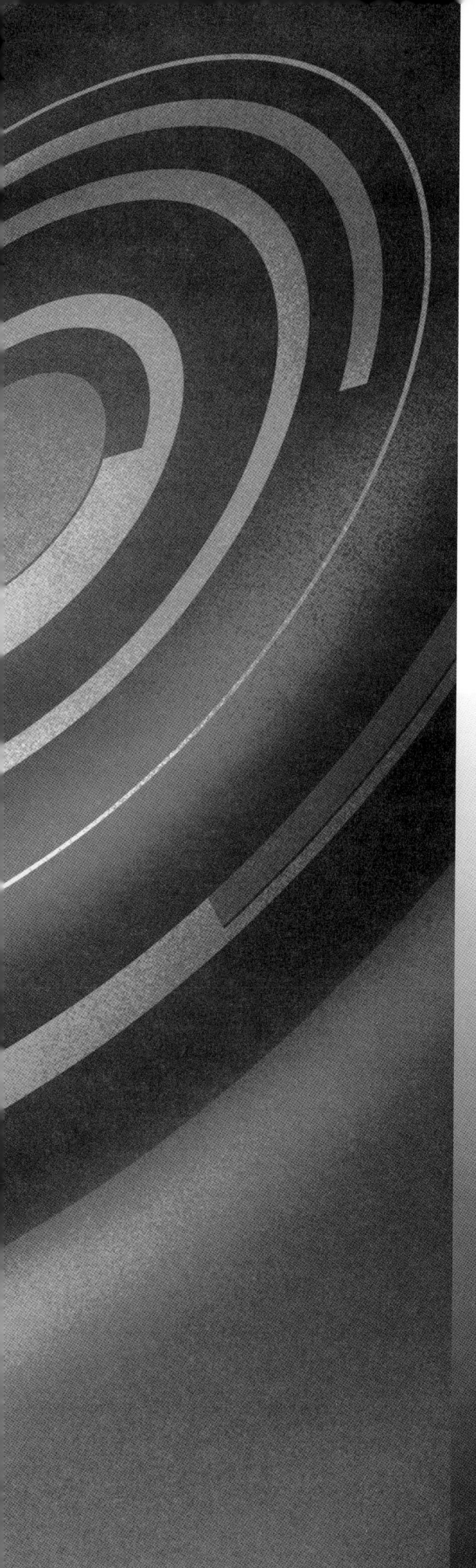

Trauma of the Head and Neck

FRONTAL SINUS FRACTURES

Anatomy
- Reaches adult size by 15 years old.
- Pyramidal structure in frontal bone with base (floor) created by orbital roof.
- Drains into anterior portion of middle meatus (50%) or anterior infundibulum (50%).
- Arterial supply: supraorbital and supratrochlear arteries (via ophthalmic).
- Venous drainage: facial vein, ophthalmic vein (to cavernous sinus), foramina of Breschet (to subarachnoid space).
- Anterior table thick.
- Posterior table thin.

Etiology and mechanism of injury
- Fracture of frontal bone requires high force, usually (75%) associated with other facial fractures.
- Motor vehicle accident (MVA) (50%).
- Assault: gunshot, baseball bat.

Clinical manifestations
Symptoms/signs
- Pain.
- Numbness.
- Epistaxis.
- Frontal swelling.
- Diplopia.
- CSF rhinorrhea.

Physical examination
- Depressed fragments of skull.
- Brain/cerebrospinal fluid (CSF)/dura in wound.
- Epistaxis.

Investigations
- Computed tomography (CT) scan: axial and coronal thin cuts.
- Nasal endoscopy (if frontal recess is involved).

Treatment
Anterior table fracture
- Nondisplaced: observe.
- Displaced: explore.
  - Frontonasal orifice not involved: reduce and microplate.
  - Frontonasal orifice involved: reduce and obliterate sinus or perform endoscopic frontal sinusotomy.

Anterior and posterior tables involved
- Nondisplaced (less than width of bone):
  - If pneumocephalus/CSF leak, observe 4-7 days. If no resolution, explore, reduce, repair, and obliterate, cranialize, or preserve/restore sinus function.

- If no leak, no treatment.
- Noncomminuted but displaced: explore, repair, reduce, and possibly obliterate, cranialize, or preserve/restore sinus function.
- Comminuted.
  - Frontonasal orifice comminuted: cranialization.
  - If floor not involved: reduce and obliterate.

Surgical approach
- Through lacerations: avoid extending lacerations.
- Bicoronal flap: note male pattern baldness.
- Gull wing or butterfly incision: not cosmetically desirable.

Complications (may be late)
- Meningitis.
- CSF leak.
- Intracranial abscess.
- Pneumocephalus.
- Cavernous sinus thrombosis.
- Chronic sinusitis.
- Mucocele/mucopyocele.
- Osteomyelitis of frontal bone.

ORBITAL FRACTURES

- Between 25% and 50% of patients with orbital fractures also suffer ocular injury (scleral or corneal laceration, dislocation or tear of the lens, retinal detachment, vitreous hemorrhage, hyphema, extraocular muscle laceration, cranial nerve damage, optic nerve transection).
- All fractures of the middle third of the face must be evaluated as potential orbitozygomaticomaxillary injuries; ultimate goal must be exact anatomic restoration of midfacial skeleton, not simply repositioning of component parts.
- Diplopia and restricted movement are not definitively diagnostic of orbital fracture, because swelling and bleeding can cause same findings.

Etiology of orbital blow-out fractures
- Produced by impact of a blunt force to front of orbit, sudden rise of intraorbital pressure → posterior displacement of orbital contents.
- Force is thus transmitted to orbital walls; floor and medial wall (lamina papyracea) are paths of least resistance; can have herniation of contents through inferior defect with incarceration of orbital contents.

Anatomy
- Vertical buttresses: paired nasomaxillary, zygomaticomaxillary and pterygomaxillary struts arise in alveolar process and project superiorly to skull base.
- Horizontal buttresses: frontal bar, inferior orbital rims, maxillary alveolus and palate, zygomatic process

(temporal), and serrated edge of the greater wing of the sphenoid bone.

- Buttress system exists to resist vertical forces of mastication; middle third of face provides excellent stability for this function. Horizontal forces are more weakly reinforced, and disruption of single buttress can cause collapse of entire system.

- Two critical external arcs of contour are horizontal and vertical.
  - Vertical arc is traced out by zygomatic process of frontal bone, over zygoma and to the zygomaticomaxillary buttress area of lateral antral wall of the maxilla.
  - Horizontal arc runs from maxilla near lacrimal fossa, across zygoma to the zygomatic process of the temporal bone.
  - Point of intersection of these external arcs defines the malar prominence.
- Orbital floor is concave, lying 3 mm below inferior orbital rim; bone may be <0.5 mm thick; globe rests in this concavity.
  - Posteriorly, floor is convex, sloping upwards as it goes posteromedially into medial orbital wall.
  - Posterolaterally, floor is separated from greater wing of sphenoid bone by inferior orbital fissure.

Orbital forces

- Forces are transmitted through zygoma via sphenoidal and orbital processes.
- Concave central portion of orbital floor often suffers comminuted injury, severity depends on strength of impact.
- Forces can be transmitted to convex portion of orbital floor and medial wall.
- Forces to high lateral orbital rim result in fracture dislocations of lateral orbital wall; orbital plate of sphenoid bone may be impacted into orbital apex or middle cranial fossa.
- Recessed or depressed globe results from one or more orbital wall pushing outward and damaging suspensory ligaments of the globe; orbit becomes more spherical, less conical in shape.

Patient evaluation

- CT scan.
- Coronal cuts necessary to evaluate orbital floor.
- Practitioners must evaluate floor and medial wall, particularly convex posterior floor and gentle slope of floor onto medial wall.
- Orbital injuries that are likely to produce enophthalmos:
  - >2 cm^2 area of floor disruption.
  - Volume change >1.5 mL (5% of orbit volume).
  - 3 mm displacement of inferior or medial wall = 7%-12% change in volume.

Clinical
Enophthalmos

- Globe position affected by integrity of orbital walls and suspensory ligaments of globe.
- Enophthalmos may not appear immediately.
- Intact, dislocated zygoma may be displaced medially and may mask volume changes from blow-out fractures of other orbital walls; until it is replaced, globe may appear to have normal projection.
- Common cause of posttraumatic enophthalmos is incomplete repair of posterior (convex) portion of orbital floor or medial orbital wall.

Ophthalmologic examination

Must assess:

- Visual acuity (subjective and objective in both eyes).
- Pupillary function.
- Ocular mobility.
- Anterior chamber: rule out hyphema.
- Fundus: rule out gross disruptions.

Treatment
General

- Ideal to wait at least 7 days before surgery so that edema is minimized; preoperative steroids may help.
- Orbital wall reconstruction can only begin after repair of the zygoma and the buttress system is complete.
- Extended access technique for greater exposure creates more accurate reduction of fractures; coronal, sublabial, and transconjunctival approaches can all be used.
- Vertical buttress can be exposed inferiorly through extended sublabial incisions that deglove maxilla.

Zygoma

- Lateral wall portion is reconnected to greater wing of sphenoid.
- If sphenoid wing is fractured, lateral component of zygoma can be used as landmark for replacing orbital floor component of sphenoid.
- If orbital contents herniate into temporal and infratemporal fossa, split calvarial graft is ideal for reconstructing lateral orbital wall because calvarium is already in surgical field with lateral approach; graft can be stabilized to frontal bone or zygoma with plate and screws.

Orbital wall reconstruction

- Must occur after zygoma and buttress system, including frontal bar, are stabilized.
- Lateral, medial, and inferior walls should be replaced in exact pretrauma position.
- Roof should be placed higher than normal, because convexity is hard to duplicate; bone is attached to the

reconstructed frontal bar at higher level than pretrauma state, thus avoiding inferior displacement of globe.

Orbital floor
- Medial floor (maxilla) can be reconstructed with intact portions as template.
- Small defect in anterior concave segment can be repaired with alloplastic implant (e.g., polypropylene mesh); entire defect must be exposed to allow fixation of graft.
- If posterior convex floor is involved, implant must be more rigid than polypropylene mesh, because there is often no residual floor posterior or medial to defect to attach this implant. More rigid alloplastic material (e.g., porous high-density polyethylene) is better suited and does not require 360-degree support.
- If lamina papyracea is involved, more rigid graft needed (outer table calvarial bone graft); it allows rigidity, needs less surface for attachment, can be fixed to zygoma or reconstructed orbital rim, and requires adequate floor dissection.
- Care must be taken to avoid impingement on orbital apex from posterior end of bone graft for posterior floor defects.

Complex
- Involvement of concave anterior floor, convex posterior floor, and medial orbital wall. Must completely expose medial orbital wall; best done with coronal incision.
- Bone cannot be shaped to fit all defects but can be patched and fixed with metal plates that serve as a cradle for grafted bone.
- Plates offer flexibility and can serve as a cradle for grafted bone, but present problems with chronic infections given the proximity of metal to the ethmoid and maxillary sinuses.

Complications
Lid damage
- Ectropion and increased scleral show can be reduced with a transconjunctival incision.
- Orbicularis muscle must be spared.
- Periosteum over inferior orbital rim should be incised 2-3 mm anterior to the crest on the downward slope of the rim.

Visual loss
- Orbit may not be able to be reconstructed if manipulation of globe during surgical procedure will worsen ocular injury or cause total vision loss.
- If injured orbit contains only seeing eye, goal is aimed at returning globe to functional position and not at total reconstruction of orbital volume and shape.

- Intraoperative tonometry and funduscopy should be considered, especially when large posterior implants are used (may cause increased intraocular pressure).

Implant visibility
- Plate over inferior rim can create irregular contour because of thin overlying skin; therefore avoid plating this region unless absolutely necessary.
- Use screws with <1.3 -mm diameter to minimize detection.

FRACTURES OF THE NASOETHMOID (NOE) COMPLEX

Anatomy
- The nasoethmoid (NOE) complex comprises the nasal, frontal, ethmoid, maxillary, and lacrimal bones. Fracture of the complex may result in telescoping and splaying of these structures.
- The vertical buttress of the NOE is the frontal process of the maxilla. The horizontal buttresses are the superior and inferior orbital rims.
- Medial canthal tendon (MCT) attaches in a tripartite configuration around the lacrimal sac. MCT anchors the eyelid structures to the medial orbital wall and maintains the palpebral configuration, the lid-to-globe contact, and the lacrimal pump system.
- In normal state, the three components of the MCT attach to the medial orbital wall in three different vectors. Disruption of each vector adds a different feature to the resultant dysfunction of the MCT, particularly in its aesthetic role.

Etiology and mechanism of injury
- Unilateral or bilateral impaction of the frontal processes of the maxilla and the nasal bones into the orbital space may occur, with secondary communition of the ethmoid air cells and out-fracturing of the medial orbital wall.
- NOE fractures may be associated with panfacial injuries (caused by broad-surfaced impact force) that separate the middle third of the face from the skull base.
- Fractures are classified based on severity of injury. Impact velocity is the major determinant of the severity of the NOE injury.
  - Type I: *Low-velocity* injuries are often unilateral and create a minimally to moderately displaced large fragment composed of the frontal process of the maxilla, lacrimal bone, and anterior-most portion of the lamina papyracea. The attachment of the three components of the MCT is usually intact, and repair consists of realignment of the bony fragments.

❑ Type II: *Medium-velocity* injuries may be unilateral, but more often they are bilateral and create a moderately displaced large fragment in the MCT area. The site of attachment of the posterior horizontal component of the MCT is destroyed. Anterior-horizontal and vertical components of MCT usually remain attached to the frontal process of maxilla.

❑ Type III: *High-velocity* injuries produces severe comminution of the entire NOE complex with bilateral detachment of the all three components of each MCT.

Clinical manifestations

- The nasal dorsum is flattened.
- The attachment of the three components of the MCT may be partially or totally disrupted. Widening of the intercanthal distance increases as the number of disrupted components of the MCT increases.
- Symptoms of MCT disruption include diplopia and epiphora. Signs include telecanthus, dystopia (malposition), narrowing of the palpebral fissure, crepitus over the nasal bones and medial orbital rim, and CSF leak.

Investigations

- Diagnosis of NOE fractures can be made on physical examination alone if gross telescoping of the nasal bones has occurred and the intercanthal distance is greater than one half of the interpupillary distance.
- Bimanual examination is performed by placing an elevator or clamp intranasally beneath the frontal process of the maxilla and a finger directly over the MCT insertion. Any movement of the frontal process differentiates the injury from a simple comminuted nasal fracture.
- Edema may obscure posterior telescoping and intercanthal widening.
- Both diagnosis and accurate portrayal of the extent of bone fragmentation are readily detectable with the CT scan. MCT disruption cannot be seen on CT; however, indirect evidence exists if the bone in the area is found fragmented.

Treatment

- Reduction of associated facial fractures prior to repair of NOE fractures realigns buttresses. Reconstruction of the medial orbital rim and nasal dorsum allow for redraping of the overlying soft tissues and reattachment of the MCT.
- A combination of subciliary or subconjuctival, sublabial, and coronal incisions may be necessary. Use of associated lacerations is usually inadequate.
- Fixation may be accomplished with fine-gauge, stainless-steel wire or a microplating system.

- The posterior horizontal components are stabilized via a transnasal 28-gauge wire that is initially passed around the anterior horizontal component (just medial to the lacrimal sac) of the tendon. The vector of the wire is in a superiomedial aspect of the contralateral orbit. Bilateral injuries are treated in the same fashion, with the transnasal wire from each side being anchored independently in the contralateral orbit.
- Lacrimal system injury can be diagnosed by instilling fluorescein in the eye; it can be detected on pledgets in the inferior meatus. Lacrimal system injury repair may be delayed in favor of the optimum MCT repair. An attempt at simultaneous lacrimal system repair often leads to a compromised MCT repair.
- Split calvarial bone is a superior choice in reconstruction of the dorsonasal area. It offers few long-term complications, good resistance to bone resorption, excellent postoperative contour, and a natural feel of the nasal complex.

Complications

- Injury to frontal recess and cribriform plate.
- Pseudohypertelorism deformity from detachment or misalignment of MCT.
- CSF rhinorrhea.
- Anosmia.
- Ocular injury.
- Lacrimal system interruption.
- Brain injury.

 NASAL FRACTURES

Anatomy

- Nasal skin thin and loose over the upper two thirds of the nose and thicker and adherent over the lower third.
- Excellent blood supply; heals rapidly with minimal scarring.
- Sensory innervation via supratrochlear, infratrochlear, anterior ethmoidal, and infraorbital nerves.
- Nasal pyramid: involves two rectangular nasal bones articulating with frontal process of maxilla.
- Cartilages of the external nose: consist of paired upper lateral cartilages, lower lateral cartilages, and sesamoid cartilages.
- Septum consists of the vomer posteriorly and inferiorly, the perpendicular plate of the ethmoid bone posteriorly, and the quadrangular cartilage anteriorly.

Etiology and mechanism of injury

- In urban areas, fractures are usually secondary to fights, auto accidents, or sports; in rural areas, fractures are due to work accidents, sports, or leisure activities.

- The pattern of nasal fractures varies with the direction of applied forces: either frontal, lateral, or superiorly directed (from below).
- Frontal forces cause injuries varying from minor injury to the lower margin of nasal bones to marked flattening of the external skeleton.
- Lateral forces typically cause a depressed fracture of the ipsilateral nasal bone, but if strong enough, they can also fracture the contralateral nasal bone.
- Superiorly directed forces are most likely to produce septal fractures and dislocations (dislocation of the quadrangular cartilage from maxillary crest).

Clinical manifestations

- Signs and symptoms:
  - Altered appearance.
  - Epistaxis.
  - Nasal airway obstruction.
  - Lacerations.
  - Mucosal tears.
  - Ecchymosis/edema.
  - Hematoma, including septal hematoma.
  - Subcutaneous emphysema: secondary to attempts to blow clots from nose.
  - Associated ocular injury: subconjunctival hemorrhage, periorbital ecchymosis, scleral chemosis, and lid edema.

Investigations

- Plain radiographic studies usually unnecessary (50% of nasal fractures will not appear).
- Photographs for documentation of deformity.

Treatment

- Optimum management occurs during first 3 hours after injury.
- If reduction not performed within 3 hours, reductions should be performed in 3-7 days.
- Indications for closed reduction include:
  - Unilateral or bilateral fracture of the nasal bones
  - Fracture of the nasal-septal complex with nasal deviation less than one half the width of the nasal bridge
- Indications for open reduction:
  - Deviation of nasal pyramid greater than half the width of nasal bridge.
  - Extensive fracture-dislocation of the nasal bones and septum.
  - Open septal fractures.
  - Fracture-dislocation of the caudal septum.
  - Unsatisfactory results after closed reduction.

Complications

- Septal hematoma: associated with persistent pain, swelling, and obstruction:
  - Superinfection and abscess can cause cartilage erosion and subsequent saddle nose deformity.
  - Treatment includes drainage, imbrication of the mucosa, and packing.
- Epistaxis:
  - Usually resolves spontaneously but can require control by nasal packing, cautery, or vessel ligation.
  - Profuse bleeding may indicate involvement of the anterior or posterior ethmoidal arteries, or sphenopalatine branch of the internal maxillary artery.
- Late complications:
  - Airway obstruction.
  - Fibrosis and scar contracture.
  - Septal perforation.
  - Saddle nose deformity.

ZYGOMA FRACTURES

Anatomy

- Zygoma articulates with the frontal, maxillary, sphenoid, and temporal bones.
- *The zygoma forms the following:*
- Lateral cheek (malar) prominence.
- External arcs of contour (intersection defines position of malar prominence).
- *Horizontal arc:* maxilla (near lacrimal fossa), zygoma, zygomatic process of temporal bone.
- *Vertical arc:* zygomatic process of frontal bone, zygoma, lateral antral wall.
- Lateral orbital wall.
- Orbital floor/maxillary sinus roof.
- Attachment for the lateral canthal ligament and masseter muscle.
- Zygoma forms *buttress system* in the middle third of the face; mechanical adaptation to masticatory forces.
  - *Vertical struts (buttresses):*
    - Nasomaxillary.
    - Zygomaticomaxillary.
    - Pterygomaxillary.
  - *Horizontal struts (buttresses)*
    - Frontal bar.
    - Inferior orbital rims.
    - Maxillary alveolus and palate.
    - Zygomatic process (temporal).
    - Serrated edge of the greater wing of the sphenoid bone.

Types of fractures

- Simple
  - Blows directed just anterior to the ear may result in isolated depressed fracture of the zygomatic arch.
- Complex
  - Multiple components (zygomaticomaxillary complex [ZMC]), usually displacement of the

orbital floor, the anterior and lateral walls of the maxillary sinus, separation of the zygomaticofrontal (ZF) or zygomaticosphenoid suture lines.

"Tetrapod" fracture
- ZF suture.
- Zygomatic arch.
- Infraorbital rim.
- Lateral orbital wall.

Clinical manifestations
- Point tenderness over fracture.
- Flattening of upper cheek (masked by edema/hematoma), lowering of the lateral canthal ligament attachment.
- Subconjunctival hemorrhage.
- Trismus: impingement on temporalis and/or coronoid process of mandible.
- Subcutaneous emphysema.
- Epistaxis.
- Limited ocular mobility/diplopia.
- Hypesthesia over V_2 distribution: injury to infraorbital nerve quite common.

Physical examination
- Observation: asymmetry, depressed malar eminence.
- Palpation of the orbital rims and zygomatic arch for significantly displaced fractures (may be obscured by edema/hematoma).
- Extraocular muscle function (limited gaze or diplopia).
- Visual acuity: ophthalmology consultation to document visual acuity should always be obtained when injuries occur to the middle third of face.

Investigations
- Radiologic studies: CT scan fine cuts of orbits/sinuses demonstrate degree of displacement and comminution. Useful in planning the repair of complex midface injuries.

Treatment
- Attempt to repair either before onset of swelling or after swelling has subsided (3-5 days after injury).
- Repair of the zygoma to focus on reestablishing the external arcs of contour, which serve as the framework for the repair of any associated orbital wall fractures.
- Complex fractures: zygomatic arch may serve as a useful point of alignment for repositioning the arcs of contour.
- Release of the masseter muscle from the zygoma will ease the mobilization of the zygoma.

Zygomatic fracture without comminution of inferior orbital rim and/or lateral antral wall
- No displacement of zygoma: no treatment.
- Displacement of zygoma:
  - If displaced at inferior orbital rim and lateral antral wall:
    - Closed = Gillies approach: incision behind the hairline, anterosuperior to the helix of the ear, through the temporalis fascia (avoiding the superficial temporal artery and frontal branch of facial nerve).
    - If this fails, open approach with fixation at lateral antral wall (intraoral incision: extended Caldwell-Luc incision) with or without fixation at inferior orbital rim through transconjunctival incision.
  - If displaced at inferior orbital rim, lateral antral wall, and ZF suture, open approach with fixation at ZF suture (access via a brow incision) and lateral antral wall with or without fixation at inferior orbital rim through transconjunctival incision.

Zygomatic fracture with comminution of inferior rim and/or lateral antral wall
- No comminution of zygomatic arch with loss of continuity of fragments: arch exposed via intraoral approach with fixation at ZF suture and lateral antral wall with or without fixation at inferior orbital rim through transconjunctival incision.
- Comminution of zygomatic arch with loss of continuity of fragment: zygomatic arch fixation via temporal approach. Stabilization of zygoma as above.

Complications
- Flattened cheek secondary to inadequate reduction/fixation.
- Enophthalmos: unrecognized significant orbital floor defect.
- Temporary or permanent infraorbital anesthesia.
- Blindness: packing floor or orbit fractures into the globe by antral approach or excessive orbital traction at surgery.
- Lower lid ectropion.
- Depressed scar over the infraorbital rim caused by direct rim approach.

 LE FORT'S (ORBITOZYGOMATICOMAXILLARY) FRACTURES

Anatomy
Buttress system
- The bony architecture of the midface is arranged in a lattice work of vertical buttresses and horizontal beams.

- ❑ Vertical buttresses
  - Zygomaticomaxillary: lateral (bears greatest load of masticatory forces).
  - Nasomaxillary: medial.
  - Pterygomaxillary: posterior.
- ❑ Horizontal beams
  - Alveolus.
  - Orbital floor.
  - Orbital rims.
  - Supraorbital bar.

Le Fort fractures I, II, and III

Pure Le Fort's fractures are rare. The whole face must be examined and orbitozygomaticomaxillary injuries described using the system of vertical buttresses and horizontal beams.

- *Le Fort I:* low horizontal fracture between maxilla and palate/alveolar arch complex
  - ❑ Includes fractures of the paired nasomaxillary and zygomaticomaxillary vertical buttresses.
  - ❑ May continue posteriorly through the pterygoid plates or between palate and maxilla.
  - ❑ Also involves nasal floor, septum, piriform aperture, and anterolateral maxilla
- *Le Fort II:* pyramidal
  - ❑ Starts at the nasal bones and crosses the frontal process of the maxilla and lacrimal bones.
  - ❑ Changing direction, fracture then descends through the floor of the orbit, infraorbital rim, and lateral maxillary sinus wall.
  - ❑ Often extends through the pterygoid plates.
- *Le Fort III:* Craniofacial dysjunction
  - Fracture extends from nasofrontal suture lines, frontal process of the maxilla, lacrimal bones, ethmoid sinus, lamina papyracea before crossing the orbital floor to the inferior orbital
  - Across the lateral orbital wall through the zygomaticofrontal suture.
  - Through the zygomatic arch.
  - Through the pterygoid plates.

Clinical manifestations

- Airway obstruction (more common with Le Fort II and III).
- Variable degrees of maxillary retrusion and rotation.
- Palatal edema.
- Midface elongation.
- Severe midface edema and ecchymosis.
- Epistaxis (internal maxillary artery).
- Gaze restriction (entrapment of orbital muscles).
- Enophthalmos.
- Blindness.
- Epiphora.
- Tooth avulsion.
- Hypesthesia (V_2).

Clinical evaluation

- Airway, breathing, circulation (ABC).
- Bleeding control.
- Physical examination:
- Visual inspection.
- Palpation.
- Occlusal evaluation.
- Assessment of mobility of maxilla.
- Ophthalmologic evaluation.
- Neurologic evaluation.
- Radiologic evaluation: CT scan: 2-3–mm slices in axial and coronal planes with an appropriate bone widow.

Treatment

Goal:
- To restore the projection and height of the face.
- To recreate pretraumatic occlusion.

Timing:
- Early intervention with open reduction and direct rigid fixation.
- Can be successfully completed up to 3 weeks after injury.

Exposure:
- Le Fort I: sublabial incision.
- Le Fort II: periorbital incision and sublabial approach.
- Le Fort III: bicoronal incision.
- Reduction with digital or hook traction (Rowe forceps).
- Fixation: rigid with plates.
- Postreduction imaging with CT scans.

Management of specific fractures

Le Fort I fractures

- Minimally displaced Le Fort I fractures can be reduced and stabilized with intermaxillary fixation.
- If displacement or mobility of maxilla is present, open approach is necessary.
- Ivy loops or arch bars are placed to set occlusion (IMF alone is inadequate because mandibular muscle pull will distract; thus fixation is required).
- Medial and lateral buttresses are then repaired using 1.2- to 1.7-mm monocortical miniplates.
- Arch bars are left and patient followed closely for 8-12 weeks to identify and correct occlusal problems.

Le Fort II fractures

- Often impacted into superior portion of midface, thus first require disimpaction.
- Occlusion then established with Ivy loops or arch bars.
- Plates at lateral maxillary wall, infraorbital rim, or nasomaxillary junction.
- Postoperative IMF guidelines similar to Le Fort I.

Le Fort III fractures: "craniofacial dysjunction"

- Occlusion established with Ivy loops or arch bars.

- 1.0- to 1.5-mm plates are used at zygomaticofrontal suture, frontonasal area, and zygomaticotemporal area.
- CSF leak commonly seen, often associated with intracranial injury, which requires stabilization first.
- External fixation with a head frame rarely used
  - Offers advantages in unstable fractures, severely retrodisplaced or comminuted fractures, or in those with significant bone loss.

Complications
Early
- Hemorrhage
  - Treat with pressure, ligation.
  - May cause swelling and airway compromise, although uncommon.
- Infection
  - Usually related to contaminated, open wounds.
  - Irrigation, debridement, antibiotics.
  - Gross contamination: possibly best managed by packing, healing by secondary intention, and later revision.
- CSF leaks
  - Related to fractures that cross the cribriform plate.
  - Early diagnosis necessary because contamination, packing may lead to meningitis.
  - Most leaks stop with conservative management, fracture reduction.
  - Spinal drainage and mannitol possibly required by larger leaks.
  - Persistent leakage may require extradural repair or craniotomy.
- Blindness
  - Rare.
  - May result from fracture through orbital apex, or retro-orbital hematoma.
  - Visual evaluation mandatory.
- Ectropion
  - Most common complication seen after subciliary or rim incision.
  - Resolves with conservative measures such as massage, steroid injection if scars.
- Diplopia and enophthalmos
  - Should be noted and corrected at surgery.

Late
Complications may be seen weeks to months after injury and repair.
- Nonunion
  - When bone is devitalized, improperly reduced or immobilized, or infected.
  - Underlying cause to be treated.
  - May require grafts, prolonged fixation.
- Malunion
  - May result from unstable fixation, misdiagnosis, or improper establishment of occlusion.

- Treatment may require exploration, refracture, and fixation or grafting.
- Diplopia
  - Results from extraocular muscle imbalance caused by entrapment, scarring, motor nerve injury.
  - Treatment may require reexploration, release of scar, or muscle surgery.
- Epiphora
  - Results from damage to canalicular system.
  - May respond to conservative treatment of dilation and irrigation. Dacryocystorhinostomy often needed.
- Chronic sinusitis
  - Pain/sensation.
  - Some patients may feel plates, necessitating removal.

 MANDIBLE FRACTURES

Epidemiology
- Second most common facial fracture; nasal bone most common.
- Most common sites of fracture:
  - Condyle: 36%.
  - Body: 21%.
  - Angle: 20%.
  - Parasymphysial: 14%.
  - Alveolar: 3%.
  - Ascending ramus: 3%.
  - Coronoid: 2%.
  - Midline (symphyseal): <1%.
- Women have less cortical bone, therefore fracture occurs with less applied force.
- 60%-90% of fractures occur in men.
- 20-30–year age group most commonly involved.
- Most common cause: blunt trauma (MVA, assaults, falls).
- In children, cranial injuries much more common than mandibular injuries.

Anatomy
- Mandible is composed of two cortical plates with intervening medullary bone.
- Inferior alveolar artery (branch of internal maxillary artery) enters mandible on its lingual aspect, high on ascending ramus, through mandibular foramen.
- Inferior alveolar nerve (branch of mandibular nerve) courses parallel to artery.
- Symphysis is the chin prominence at midline of mandible.
- Parasymphysis is lateral to symphysis (i.e., area at the canine tooth).
- Mental foramen is located along vertical line between first and second premolar.
- Body is the horizontal area from parasymphysis to angle.
- Body and ascending ramus meet at the angle.

- Retromolar trigone is the area posterior to last molar.
- Ramus splits superiorly to form the coronoid process (anteriorly) and condyle (posteriorly).
- Area between coronoid process and condyle is called the *sigmoid notch.*
- Condyle articulates with glenoid fossa of temporal bone via temporomandibular joint (TMJ).

TMJ
- Synovial, diarthrodial joint.
- Capable of hinge, gliding, and rotational movement.
- Articulating surfaces covered with fibrocartilage, not hyaline cartilage.

Areas of inherent bone weakness: common areas of fracture
- Condylar area (thin bone, third molar).
- Parasymphysis (canine tooth root).
- Depressors of mandible: suprahyoid muscles (anterior belly of digastric, mylohyoid, geniohyoid, genioglossus) and lateral pterygoid muscle.
- Elevators of mandible: temporalis, masseter, medial pterygoid muscles.
- Lateral pterygoid muscle is the only protruser.

Dentition
- 20 primary teeth; 32 permanent teeth (8 in each quadrant: 2 incisors, 1 bicuspid, 2 premolars, 3 molars).
- Numbering begins at maxillary *right* third molar (#1) to maxillary *left* third molar (#16) to mandibular left third molar (#17) to mandibular right third molar (#32).

Fracture classification
- Fractures that extend through periodontal membrane surrounding tooth root and communicate with oral cavity are *open fractures.*
- Favorable vs unfavorable fractures (based on muscle forces acting on fractured fragments).
  - Horizontally favorable: fracture line is directed inferiorly and anteriorly.
  - Horizontally unfavorable: fracture line is directed inferiorly and posteriorly.
  - Vertically favorable: fracture line passes from outer surface of mandible posteriorly and medially (as in sagittal split osteotomy).
  - Vertically unfavorable: fracture line is directed from posterior to anterior (muscles pull mandible fragment medially).
- *Greenstick fracture:* only one cortex is fractured.
- *Compound fracture:* associated with external wound; all fractures through tooth roots are compound.
- Fractures that involve only alveolar bone and associated teeth are called *dentoalveolar fractures;* all of these are considered open fractures.

Signs and symptoms
- Intraoral bleeding.
- Tenderness.
- Edema.
- Trismus (normal opening: 40-50 mm).
- Malocclusion.
- Deviation of jaw on opening.
- Palpable stepoffs.
- Hypesthesia/anesthesia of lower lip/chin.
- Loose/damaged teeth.
- Intraoral/facial lacerations.
- Floor of mouth hematoma.
- Open bite deformity: bilateral subcondylar fractures.
- Unilateral subcondylar fracture: occlusion of side of fracture and open bite on nonfractured side.

Imaging
- Panorex: most information for least cost. Detects 92% of fractures. Good for lateral fractures, TMJ, tooth root involvement. Midline structures not well visualized. Need cooperative patient.
- Mandibular series: lateral, oblique, posterior-anterior, and Towne's view (for condylar regions). Only detects 66% of fractures but can be used in uncooperative or obtunded patients.
- CT: detailed images of bone and soft tissue. More information on condylar region and lingual aspect of mandible. Plain films not needed if CT planned or already done.

Treatment
General
- ABCs.
- Other injuries stabilized.
- Open fractures: antibiotics (e.g., clindamycin), tetanus toxoid.
- Repair by 7-10 days (the earlier the repair, the better the outcome).
- Analgesics and Barton's bandage provide pain relief until definitive treatment.

Teeth involved in line of fracture
- Teeth fractured through root or pulp chamber, teeth with significant decay, loose teeth with severe periodontal disease should be extracted.
- Loose but healthy tooth (root intact): stabilize to attempt salvage.
- Third molar management in angle fractures.
  - Left in (vs extraction) to provide more stability.
  - Removal if fracture reduction prohibited.
  - Rate of infection higher if teeth remain.

Fixation techniques
Semirigid fixation
- Maxillomandibular fixation (MMF): arch bars with interdental wiring, four-screw intermaxillary fixation, ivy loops.
- External fixation devices: Joe Hall Morris appliance.

- Good for minimally displaced, favorable fractures with easily reducible occlusion.
- Interdental fixation maintained 2-6 weeks (younger, healthier patients need less time).
- Advantages: simple, no soft tissue dissection.
- Disadvantages: weight loss, tooth decay, gingivitis, immobile TMJ.
- Contraindications: patient unwilling or unable to cooperate (elderly, obtunded, mentally retarded, alcoholics, drug addicts, those predisposed to vomiting/aspirating).

Rigid fixation
- Plates and screws.
- Most plates made of titanium (inert, biocompatible, resistant to corrosion).
- Need to use sharp drill bit at low speeds (<1000 rpm) with constant irrigation in order not to overheat the bone.
- Overheating leads to bone necrosis and causes loosening of screws.
- Loose screws will cause fixation failure; they should be removed.
- Plate should be passively adapted to underlying bone with slight overbend over the fracture site.

Tension band principles
- When a fracture occurs in the horizontal segment of the mandible, the tensile forces (i.e., the pull of the muscles) act to displace the fracture at the alveolar border and compress the fracture at the inferior border.
- Fixation systems should be placed at the superior border of the mandible to overcome the distraction forces.
- The fixation system on superior border functions as a tension band.
- The inferior border remains closed because of the natural compressive forces.
- Methods of establishing tension band:
  - Bridging teeth across fracture line with arch bar or ivy loops.
  - Placement of monocortical miniplate across fracture line.

Compression plating
- Prevents interfragmentary motion of the mandible fracture.
- Two methods:
- Dynamic compression plates
  - Two oval holes on either side of the fracture line are placed eccentrically.
  - Compression created by screws placed within oval holes is greater than pressures created during mandibular function, thus creating a stable fracture line.
  - Holes have an inclined and horizontal beveled surface that allows the screw to glide toward the medial aspect of the plate as it is being threaded.
  - Bone moves medially towards opposite fracture fragment as screw is tightened.
  - Useful only in noncomminuted, transverse fractures.
- Lag screws (static compression)
  - Gliding hole is overdrilled in outer cortex; screw passes without engaging bone.
  - Second threaded hole (size of screw) placed in the far cortex.
  - As screw engages the threaded hole, the two bone fragments are forced together.
  - Useful for long or oblique fracture lines (i.e., symphyseal fractures, oblique fractures of the body, angle, and subcondylar regions that have significant overlapping segments).

Neutralization plates (a.k.a. reconstruction plates)
- Used in comminuted fracture with or without bone loss.
- May be used with bone grafts.
- Larger and stronger than compression plates.
- Minimum two screws on either side of fracture.

Soft tissue approaches to the mandible
- Intraoral incisions should be used whenever possible.
  - Incision in vestibule with 5-10 mm cuff of mucosa gives exposure from symphysis to angle and ascending ramus.
  - Disadvantages: limited visibility of the inferior border of the mandible, no visualization of lingual cortex.
- Extraoral approaches are variations of standard facelift and parotidectomy incisions.
  - Cervical "smile" incision used for severely comminuted and bilateral fractures.
  - Edentulous patients with atrophic mandibles need extraoral approaches.

Treatment options
- None: isolated coronoid fractures.
- Soft/liquid diet: unilateral subcondylar fracture with normal occlusion/minimal displacement.
- MMF alone: most stable fractures with adequate dentition.
- Open reduction with internal fixation (ORIF) with or without MMF: everything else.
- Body and angle fractures approached transorally.
- Ramus and condyle fractures require percutaneous or open approach.

Duration of MMF
- Young healthy patient with subcondylar fracture: 3-4 weeks.
- Young healthy patient with other fracture: 6 weeks .
- Elderly/sick patient: 6-8 weeks.

Factors that favor ORIF
- Unstable fractures.
- Multiple fractures.

- Associated midface fractures.
- Poor dentition.
- Very young/very old patient who would not tolerate MMF and would become nutritionally compromised.
- Severe chronic obstructive pulmonary disease (COPD) to facilitate clearing of secretions.
- Poorly controlled epileptic.
- Alcoholic, psychotic, intellectually challenged.

Special situations:
- Edentulous patient: use dentures or Gunning's splint for MMF with or without ORIF and plate/wire fixation.
- Condylar head fractures: most can be managed by MMF. Major ORIF indication:dislocation.
- Bilateral subcondylar fractures: need to perform ORIF on one of them.
- Pediatric fractures: most require circummandibular wiring, piriform aperture/zygomatic arch suspension to stabilize arch bars.

Management of specific fractures
- General principles same for all fractures.
- Anatomic reduction of fracture segments.
- Stabilization of reduced fragments.

Symphysis
- Fractures possibly hard to detect, especially if nondisplaced.
- May only present with sublingual hematoma or chin laceration.
- Rule out associated subcondylar fractures.
- Treatment
  - Arch bars or equivalent used as tension bands to restore occlusion.
  - Exposure: intraoral approach or via laceration of chin, if present.
  - Plate placed at midportion of symphysis (below tooth roots).
  - If associated subcondylar fx present, longer/stronger plate to be considered.
  - Alternatively, minimum of two lag screws perpendicular to the fracture line and parallel to each other may be used.

Parasymphysis
- Similar approach to symphyseal fractures.
- Intraoral approach.
- Mental nerve to be bluntly dissected and retracted; found close to mucosal surface near canine and first bicuspid.

Body
- Intraoral approach
  - Reset occlusion.
  - Place monocortical tension band.

  - Place mandibular plate at inferior border.
  - Avoid inferior alveolar neurovascular bundle
- Sagittal or oblique fractures of body and parasymphysis can also be fixated with lag screws.

Angle
- Difficult to achieve accurate reduction and fixation.
- Intraoral incision with wide stripping of periosteum:
  - Reduce fracture.
  - MMF.
- Place L-shaped plate at inferior border, avoiding inferior alveolar nerve.
  - Monocortical 2-0 miniplate placed at superior border as tension band.
- Percutaneous fixation (at least two screws on either side of fracture) if poor exposure intraorally.

Condylar and subcondylar fractures
By location:
- Intracapsular (fracture of head within ligamentous capsule).
- High subcondylar.
- Low subcondylar (at level of sigmoid notch).
- All involve TMJ, so early mobilization needed to prevent complications.
- Normal occlusion + nondisplaced/minimally displaced fracture: conservative management with soft diet.
- Abnormal occlusion + minimally displaced fracture: short-term MMF (heavy elastics 2 weeks, then lighter elastics and physical therapy).
- Indications for open reduction:
  - Proximal segment >30 degrees displaced off the ascending ramus.
  - Shortening of ascending ramus with telescoping of fragments and open bite deformity.
  - Condylar head displaced out of condylar fossa.
  - Inability to restore normal occlusion with closed reduction.
  - Bilateral neck fracture with loss of vertical height.
  - Foreign body in condylar neck (e.g., gunshot wound).
- Techniques: plate/screw fixation, direct wiring, removal of proximal fragment + plate fixation to distal fragment, replacement of condyle with rib graft.
- Fracture below midneck: intraoral alignment/reduction, stabilization with bone-holding clamps, MMF, percutaneous placement of passively adapted 2.4-mm plate/screws, release of MMF.
- Endoscopic approaches to condyle recently described.
- All approaches involve areas where facial nerve susceptible to injury.

Comminuted fractures
- Usually from high-energy injuries.
- Useful to get preoperative study models and acrylic splints.
- Removal of all nonviable/devascularized bone prior to fixation.
  - Stepwise reduction of small fragments with monocortical miniplates.
  - MMF.
  - Large reconstruction plate to span all fracture segments (at least three screws on each side).

Dentoalveolar injuries
- 80% of all traumas to oral cavity occur in the area of the four anterior maxillary teeth.
- All teeth to be counted after injury; missing teeth should be noted and retrieved if possible.
- Rule out airway teeth with chest and neck radiographs.
- Treatment as open fractures: tetanus prophylaxis, antibiotics, reduction/fixation.
- Several types:
- Tooth fractures:
- Ellis classification:
  - Class I: fracture of tooth enamel only; painless, not emergency, refer to dentist.
  - Class II: fracture of dentin; painful, need medicated paste to cover exposed dentin.
  - Class III: involves pulp or neurovascular bundle: extremely painful, urgent dental consult.
- Tooth luxation:
  - Malposition of tooth in socket, indicates periodontal ligament and neurovascular bundle damage.
  - Treatment: gentle manipulation of tooth into position + dental referral for splinting.
- Tooth avulsion
  - Dental emergency, tooth should be reimplanted in socket immediately.
  - Practitioner to irrigate with normal saline, place in buccal vestibule, call dentist.
  - If patient at risk for aspirating tooth, tooth placed in cold milk or sterile saline and dentist called.
  - Dentist reimplants tooth and splints it to surrounding teeth.
  - Soft diet and antibiotics to follow; endodontic treatment needed for ultimate salvage.

Complications
General factors that predispose to complications include:

1. Systemic factors
- Age.
- Nutritional status.
- Systemic disease: diabetes mellitus (DM), vasculitides, compromised immune function.

2. Local factors
- Poor oral hygiene.
- Nonvital or abscessed tooth in fragment line.
- Hematoma.
- Foreign bodies:
- Status of dentition:
  - Edentulous.
  - Impacted dentition.

3. Treatment
- Delayed
  - Complication rate three times higher after delay of 10 days.
  - Optimal results if reduced within a few days of injury.
  - Good results obtained if done within 2 weeks.
  - Children and condyle fractures should be repaired earlier, because rapid healing by fibrosis will impair proper reduction.
- Inadequate
  - Improper or inadequate fixation allows mobility and associated complications

Postoperative care
- Oral hygiene.
- Antibiotics.

Patient compliance
- Minimizing load

Specific complications
Respiratory complications
Airway obstruction
- Hemorrhage, edema, teeth, dentures, retrodisplacement of tongue.
- Bilateral parasymphysial or condylar fractures, allowing free-floating central segment to be pulled posteriorly by muscle attachments, causing obstruction.
  - Acutely pull segment forward.
  - Usually needs tracheostomy.
  - Needs early reduction and fixation.

Aspiration
- Dentures, teeth.
- Secretions, emesis with MMF.
  - Wire cutters at bedside.
  - Antiemetics.
  - Delay MMF after arch bars placed until recovery of anesthesia.

Poor pulmonary toilet with MMF
Vascular complications
Hemorrhage
- Usually serious only with gunshot, major soft tissue injury.
- Treat with pressure, ligation.

AV fistula

- Rare.
- Treat with embolization.

Internal carotid artery (ICA) thrombosis

- Rare, mandibular fragments cause ICA trauma, thrombosis.

Neurologic complications
Inferior alveolar anesthesia

- Most common complication of body fractures.
- Dependent on degree of nerve injury.
- Minimize fracture manipulation.
- Approximate cut ends.
- Some return of sensation provided by accessory innervation from C2-C3.

Infectious complications

- From nonvital/damaged/infected tooth in fracture line, foreign body (FB) in wound, poor hygiene, inadequate reduction and fixation.
- Remove source of infection, drain abscess, antibiotics, maintain immobilization.
- If bony infection proceeds to sequestrum formation, sequestrectomy and bone graft required.

Bony complications

- Bone union occurs in 4-8 weeks: 4 in children, 6 in adults, 8 in the elderly.

Delayed union

- When union does not occur in the above timeframe.
- Ultimately will progress to union with additional immobility, treatment (removal of infected tooth, sequestrum).

Nonunion

- When fracture persists indefinitely without evidence of healing.
- Fibrous pseudoarthrosis at fracture with instability that does not resolve.
- Most frequent cause of delayed union and nonunion: inadequate reduction or immobilization.
- Factors: delayed treatment, postoperative trauma, poor blood supply, infection, inadequate reduction.
- Not factors: sex, age, cause of fracture, site of injury, periosteal stripping, general health.
- If mobility persists upon release of fixation after 6-8 weeks, reimmobilized for 2-12 more weeks, factors like loose teeth, foreign bodies corrected.
- Surgery required to treat nonunion.
  - Site exposed extraorally.
  - Interposed fibrous tissue, foreign bodies, sequestra removed.
  - Bone ends should be freshened, reapproximated, plated.
  - Large bone gaps require bone graft, fixation.
  - 6-8 additional weeks of fixation required

Malunion

- When bone heals under poor anatomic reduction.
- Functional and cosmetic difficulties such as malocclusion, pain, asymmetry.
- Slight occlusal discrepancies treatable with orthodontics, extractions.
- Significant discrepancies require osteotomy, reestablishment of normal occlusion.

TMJ complications
Joint stiffness

- From atrophy of masticator muscles, fibrous adhesions caused by hematoma organization in condylar fractures.
- Therapy: Jaw exercises, serial advancement of tongue depressors, and dietary advancement usually provide resolution.

Bite deviation

- Because of forces applied by pterygoids, external pterygoid shortened after healing on fractured side, thus deviation seen toward fracture side with mouth opening
- Deviation is common.
- Little functional significance because occlusion is correct.

Ankylosis
Growth Disturbance

- Occurs in children.
- Most commonly unilateral underdevelopment, with deviation to injured side.
- Treated with osteotomy, bone grafting.

Aseptic osteomyelitis and necrosis of condylar head

- Blood supply via neck to fractured articular portion disrupted, resulting in pain, limitation of movement; treatment by surgical removal of necrotic condyle.

 LARYNGEAL TRAUMA

Etiology and epidemiology

- Second most common cause of death in head and neck trauma (no. 1: intracranial).
- Three fourths caused by blunt trauma; one fourth caused by penetrating trauma.
- Airway obstruction resulting from soft tissue, cartilage, or blood.
- Mechanism of injury in blunt trauma: direct, blunt injury to the anterior neck and forceful impact of larynx against cervical spine.

- Mechanisms of penetrating trauma: penetrating knife wound leaves even wound edges. Projectile injury results in soft tissue loss.
- Associated soft tissue injury to great vessels and esophagus (Levels I, II, and III).

Classification
- By anatomic divisions:
  - Supraglottic.
  - Glottic.
  - Subglottic (most cases of pediatric trauma).

Clinical manifestations
Soft tissue
- Hematoma extension to the subglottis limited by conus elasticus.
- Hematoma spreads from ipsilateral paraglottic space to preepiglottic space to contralateral paraglottic space.
- Direct injury to the cricothyroid muscle mimics superior laryngeal nerve injury.

Bone injury
- Hyoid fracture: painful dysphagia with crepitus at fracture site.
- No respiratory distress.

Cartilage injury
Thyroid Cartilage: Age-Dependent Injury
- In children: cartilage forced against cervical spine. See linear fracture down thyroid prominence and vocal cord avulsion.
- In adults: multiple stellate fractures; breach of internal perichondrium; shortened AP diameter of larynx; epiglottis avulsion and prolapse into lumen possible concerns.

Cricoid Cartilage: Complete ring
- Usually seen with fractured thyroid cartilage.
- Fractures in two or more sites.
- High frequency of associated recurrent laryngeal nerve (RLN) injury.

Tracheal Cartilage
- Avulsion through cricotracheal membrane (cricotracheal separation).
- Severe respiratory obstruction and subcutaneous emphysema.
- Usually death at scene.

Symptoms
- Voice change:
  - Hematoma causes hoarseness.
  - Avulsed cord causes air wasting and weak voice.
- Pain:
  - Aggravated by coughing or swallowing.
- Dyspnea:
  - Frequent, slowly developing stridor.
- Odynophagia
- Cough:
  - Hemoptysis

Signs
- Bruising.
- Laceration.
- Subcutaneous emphysema.
- Flattened thyroid prominence.

Investigations
- AP and soft tissue lateral films may demonstrate endolaryngeal edema and fractures.
- CT (plain or spiral) scan preferred for cross-sectional imaging, ability to define calcified cartilage vs soft tissue injury, and airway compromise.
- CT allows evaluation in patients with supraglottic edema that precludes adequate laryngoscopic evaluation.
- CT can identify transverse or vertical fractures of thyroid or cricoid cartilages, arytenoid dislocation at cricoarytenoid joint, or disruption of cricothyroid joint.
- Fiberoptic laryngoscopy assesses larynx anatomy, arytenoid position, vocal cord position and motion, and edema.
- Chest x-ray evaluates for pneumothorax or pneumomediastinum
- Cervical spine films.

Treatments
- Follow ABCs: secure airway; assess for emergent tracheostomy; avoid cricothyroidotomy (may not bypass level of obstruction). At times, tracheostomy tube can be placed through open wound. Nasotracheal and orotracheal intubation should be avoided.
- For mild cases of hematomas, lacerations, or edema without framework fracture, patient can be observed.
  - Observation for 24 hours to rule out progression of symptoms.
  - Voice rest.
  - Humidified air.
  - Racemic epinephrine.
  - Systemic corticosteroids.
  - Systemic antibiotics with mucosal lacerations.
  - Clear fluid diet.
- Indications for surgical exploration: should be performed as soon as possible:
  - Severe upper airway obstruction.
  - Displaced fracture of the laryngeal skeleton.
  - Increasing subcutaneous emphysema.
  - Hemorrhage.

- Fracture of hyoid:
  - If causing severe pain (odynophagia), fractured segment can be excised.
- Fracture of thyroid:
  - Displaced, linear fracture without internal disruption: wire or suture.
  - If internal derangement (avulsed cord or displaced epiglottis), exploration of laryngeal lumen by midline laryngofissure required. Mucosa repaired with absorbable suture. If extensive mucosa loss, buccal mucosa graft used.
  - Silicon keel: can remain in place for 3-4 weeks.
  - Stent only in cases of extensive comminution or mucosal grafting; soft stent to be used and left in place for 7 days (mucosa) to 3 months (comminution).
  - Thyroid cartilage pieces wired together. Small fragments discarded.
  - External perichondrium reapproximated.
  - Arytenoid repositioned if necessary.
- Fracture of cricoid cartilage:
  - If nondisplaced, can be secured with suture or wire.
  - If crushed, can use costal cartilage graft or hyoid transposition.
  - Exploration to assess integrity of RLN is risky.
- Cricotracheal separation:
  - Tracheostomy.
  - If cricoid intact, mucosal repair performed with absorbable sutures and nonabsorbable sutures placed between superior aspect of cricoid and inferior aspect of second tracheal ring to minimize tension on closure.
  - If cricoid fractured, reconstruction attempted with internal fixation and local soft tissue (strap muscles), closure of separation, and stent.
  - Cricoid resection and thyrotracheal anastomosis only used if other repairs fail.
  - High incidence of RLN paralysis; repair can be attempted but results are poor.
  - High incidence of subglottic stenosis. Meticulous mucosal coverage and stabilization of fracture attempted.
- Results and complications
  - Results depend on degree of injury. Excellent results when no fracture has occurred.

Complications
Granulation tissue
- Develops in presence of bare cartilage.
- May lead to fibrosis and scarring.
- Best treated with prevention at time of repair by ensuring mucosal coverage of cartilage and by limiting duration of stent placement.

- Systemic and local corticosteroids, low-dose radiation not effective.

Stenosis
- Supraglottic: excision of scar and local advancement flap, dermal or mucosal graft. May require excision of significant supraglottic tissue (e.g., epiglottis).
- Glottic and subglottic stenosis: see sections on these disorders.

Vocal cord paralysis
- Must be differentiated from arytenoid fixation. Can be differentiated using direct observation, palpation of the arytenoid, and laryngeal EMG. For management, see section on this topic.

Selected References from the Recent Literature

1. Alexander AEJ, Lyons GD, Fazekas-May MA, *et al:* Utility of helical computed tomography in the study of arytenoid dislocation and arytenoid subluxation. *Annals of Otology, Rhinology & Laryngology* 1997;106:1020-1023.
2. Back MR, Baumgartner FJ, Klein SR: Detection and evaluation of aerodigestive tract injuries caused by cervical and transmediastinal gunshot wounds. *Journal of Trauma-Injury Infection & Critical Care* 1997;42:680-686.
3. Brosch S, Johannsen HS: Clinical course of acute laryngeal trauma and associated effects on phonation. *Journal of Laryngology & Otology* 1999;113:58-61.
4. Deeb ZE, Williams JB, Campbell TE: Early diagnosis and treatment of laryngeal injuries from prolonged intubation in adults. *Otolaryngology–Head & Neck Surgery* 1999; 120:25-29.
5. Gold SM, Gerber ME, Shott SR, *et al:* Blunt laryngotracheal trauma in children. *Archives of Otolaryngology–Head & Neck Surgery* 1997;123:83-87.
6. Jewett BS, Shockley WW, Rutledge R: External laryngeal trauma analysis of 392 patients. *Archives of Otolaryngology–Head & Neck Surgery* 1999;125:877-880.
7. Lykins CL, Pinczower EF: The comparative strength of laryngeal fracture fixation. *American Journal of Otolaryngology* 1998;19:158-162.
8. Merritt RM, Bent JP, Porubsky ES: Acute laryngeal trauma in the pediatric patient. *Annals of Otology, Rhinology & Laryngology* 1998;107:104-106.
9. Offiah CJ, Endres D: Isolated laryngotracheal separation following blunt trauma to the neck. [Review] [14 refs]. *Journal of Laryngology & Otology* 1997;111:1079-1081.
10. Plant RL, Pinczower EF: Pullout strength of adaption screws in thyroid cartilage. *American Journal of Otolaryngology* 1998;19:154-157.
11. Pou AM, Shoemaker DL, Carrau RL, et al: Repair of laryngeal fractures using adaptation plates. *Head & Neck* 1998; 20:707-713.
12. Schoem SR, Choi SS, Zalzal GH: Pneumomediastinum and pneumothorax from blunt cervical trauma in children. *Laryngoscope* 1997;107:351-356.

PENETRATING NECK TRAUMA

- Penetrating neck trauma accounts for 5%-10% of all trauma and has 3%-6% mortality.
- The amount of tissue damage is related to $KE = 1/2\ mV^2$; the higher the velocity, the greater the damage.
- It is also related to the type of weapon, characteristics of the missile, and distance from the victim.

Etiology

- Can be divided into high- and low-velocity weapons (which again determines energy transfer):
- Missiles cause:
  - Direct tissue injury.
  - Temporary cavitation.
  - Distal shock waves.
  - Secondary fragment formation.
- Handguns and shotguns are usually low-velocity weapons, but the amount of damage is related to the distance of the weapon from the victim.
- Tumbling missiles (such as in an M16) cause more radial tissue damage, as do expanding missiles (hunting rifles). Missiles with copper jackets (rifles) travel longer distances with a smoother path.
- High-velocity weapons often result in death because of the previously mentioned properties.
- Other low-velocity weapons include knives, ice picks, razors, and glass, to name a few.

Classification

- Based on stability of patient, and anatomical location of wound(s).
- Unstable patients display massive bleeding, expanding hematomas, hemodynamic instability, hemomediastinum, hemothorax, or hypovolemic shock and require immediate surgical exploration.
- Stable patients must be evaluated for anatomic location of injury and symptomatology to determine treatment.

Anatomic zones of injury

- Zone I: Between sternum and clavicle inferiorly and cricoid superiorly. Bony structures are helpful in protecting structures but make surgical exploration difficult after vascular injury, which accounts for high mortality (12%).
  - Contents: Lung, esophagus, carotid arteries, internal jugular veins, subclavian veins, innominate vessels, brachial plexus, spinal cord.
- Zone II: most common (60%-75%): above cricoid, below mandible. Examination is facilitated by lack of obstructing bony structures present in other zones.
  - Contents: Larynx, trachea, esophagus, carotids, internal jugular, vertebral arteries, spinal cord, phrenic, vagus, and hypoglossal nerves.

- Zone III: Above angle of mandible, which protects region but makes exploration difficult.
  - Contents: Carotids, pharynx, internal jugular vein, vertebral artery, cranial nerves, and spinal cord.

Clinical evaluation

- Always begins with advanced trauma life support (ATLS) protocol:
1. Airway: compromised in 10%; intubation is often required, or tracheostomy (as in the case of massive oral hemorrhage).
2. Breathing: auscultate chest; check for hemothorax, pneumothorax.
3. Circulation: Check peripheral pulses, hemodynamics, secure two large-bore IVs, apply direct pressure to bleeding site. Hypotension without tachycardia suggests spinal cord injury.
4. Protect C-spine until proper clearing is achieved.
5. Full head and neck examination: pay close attention to neurologic status and nature and depth of wound. Avoid blind probing of the wound at all times.

Laryngotracheal injury

- Suggested by:
  - Subcutaneous air.
  - Airway obstruction.
  - Sucking wounds.
  - Hemoptysis.
  - Dyspnea.
  - Stridor.
  - Hoarseness.

Vascular injury

- Suggested by:
  - Shock.
  - Hematoma.
  - Absent pulses.
  - Neurologic deficits.
  - Bruits.
  - Thrills.

Injury to the pharynx or esophagus

- Suggested by:
  - Subcutaneous air.
  - Hematemesis.
  - Dysphagia.
  - Odynophagia.

Algorithm for investigation and exploration
Unstable

- Immediate surgical exploration.

Stable (controversial)

- *Symptomatic:* angiography for injuries to zones I and III, then surgical exploration or embolization.

- *Asymptomatic:* controversial with more recent studies leaning toward a conservative approach.
  - Angiography for zones I, III.
  - Contrast esophagography, esophagoscopy, laryngoscopy for zone I. Between 80% and 90% sensitivity with either swallow study or endoscopy; higher sensitivity if used in combination.
- Zone II directed by clinical examination.
  - Injury identified: proceed with exploration.
  - No injury identified: observation.

Management
Vascular injuries
- Zone I
  - High mortality rate of 12% because of potential for injury to great vessels and esophagus.
  - Signs of significant injury may be hidden from inspection in the mediastinum and chest.
  - One third of patients with a clinically significant injury may be asymptomatic.
  - Sternum and clavicle create significant obstacles to surgical exploration.
  - Vascular perforation requires thoracic surgery to obtain control via a thoracotomy or sternotomy.
  - Mandatory exploration is usually not recommended.
  - Most trauma centers advocate routine angiography of aortic arch and great vessels whether or not the patient is symptomatic.
  - Angiography can identify patients that need a sternotomy or thoracotomy for vascular control.
  - Asymptomatic patients with negative angiograms can be observed safely with good outcomes.
- Zone II
  - Injuries are seldom occult, and physical examination is a good predictor of severity of injury.
  - Symptomatic patients should undergo neck exploration without further studies.
  - If asymptomatic, consider angiography, esophagoscopy/esophagography, and laryngoscopy.
- Zone III
  - Potential for injury to vessels at or near the skull base.
  - One fourth of patients with arterial injuries may be asymptomatic at presentation.
  - Injuries at the skull base can be temporized with pressure, but once delineated, they may require a mandibulotomy in the midline similar to the exposure for a parapharyngeal space tumor or a craniotomy.
  - Routine angiography advocated in all stable patients with Zone III injury.

- Many vascular injuries are amenable to embolization and thus may not require exploration.

Arterial Injuries
- Major arteries should be repaired when possible, except the vertebral, which can be ligated.
- Primary repair of the carotid is performed when possible.
- Injuries not amenable to primary closure may require end-to-end anastomosis, a patch, or grafting with autogenous vein or Gore-Tex.
- Internal carotid injury may also be repaired by transposition of the external carotid artery to the internal carotid artery.
- When the internal carotid artery is injured at the skull base, the distal vessel may not be accessible for circumferential control. A no. 4 Fogarty catheter may be passed beyond the injury; inflation of the balloon will occlude the lumen and control bleeding while the repair is performed. Alternatively, a shunt may be passed over the catheter.
- Injuries to the external carotid branches can be safely suture ligated, because the collateral circulation to the areas supplied by these vessels is good.
- The internal carotid should only be ligated when damage is irreparable, access for repair is impossible, or the patient has suffered profound neurologic damage.
- Carotid repair in the setting of neurologic impairment has been controversial in the past, as the possibility of converting an ischemic infarction into a more severe hemorrhagic infarction has been raised. Recent studies have disputed this concept and support efforts to reestablish blood flow in patients with neurologic impairment.

Venous injuries
- All injured veins in the neck can be safely ligated to control hemorrhage.
- If both internal jugular veins are damaged, an attempt should be made to repair one or both of them to avoid complications arising from venous outflow obstruction.

Subclavian vessel injuries
- Mortality from subclavian injury is high, and the prognosis for subclavian vein injury is worse than that for subclavian artery injury because of the potential for fatal air embolism.
- A median sternotomy or thoracotomy is usually needed for repair.
- Ligation of the subclavian artery should be avoided because of the risks of upper-extremity claudication, ischemia, and subclavian steal syndrome.

Vertebral artery injuries

- Most vertebral artery injuries are amenable to embolization. Surgery is reserved for extremely distal injuries not amenable to embolization.

Digestive tract injuries

- Esophageal injury is the most commonly missed injury with an increase in mortality from 11%-17% with a 12-hour delay in diagnosis.
- Physicians should maintain a high level of suspicion for digestive tract injuries in level I. These injuries may remain clinically silent until the development of serious complications such as mediastinitis and sepsis.
- For suspected injuries, a Gastrografin swallow is recommended, followed by a barium swallow if equivocal.
- Rigid esophagoscopy generally is the diagnostic procedure of choice if the barium swallow is equivocal, or if the patient is intubated or in the OR.
- Sensitivity of contrast esophagography and esophagoscopy are both about 80%-90%.
- Using both esophagoscopy and esophagography together increases sensitivity to 100%.
- Injuries to the nasopharynx or oropharynx are not subjected to dependent drainage of saliva and generally do not require closure.
- Hypopharyngeal or esophageal injury requires early operation, closure, and drainage.
- Injuries should be closed primarily with a two-layer watertight closure and a muscle flap based on the sternoclydomastoid or strap muscles for reinforcement.

Selected References from the Recent Literature

1. Asteri T, Missias G, Tsagaropoulou I, *et al:* Multivascular trauma on an adolescent. Perioperative management. *Journal of Cardiovascular Surgery* 1999;40:425-427.
2. Atta HM, Weaver WL: Re: Penetrating injuries of the neck: selective management evolving [letter; comment]. *American Surgeon* 1998;64:803-804.
3. Atta HM, Walker ML: Penetrating neck trauma: lack of universal reporting guidelines. *American Surgeon* 1998;64:222-225.
4. Back MR, Baumgartner FJ, Klein SR: Detection and evaluation of aerodigestive tract injuries caused by cervical and transmediastinal gunshot wounds. *Journal of Trauma-Injury Infection & Critical Care* 1997;42:680-686.
5. Benson BW, Mohtadi NG, Rose MS, *et al:* Head and neck injuries among ice hockey players wearing full face shields vs half face shields. *JAMA* 1999;282:2328-2332.
6. Biffl WL, Moore EE, Rehse DH, *et al:* Selective management of penetrating neck trauma based on cervical level of injury. *American Journal of Surgery* 1997;174:678-682.
7. Catala J, Puig J, Munoz JM, *et al:* Perforation of the pharynx caused by blunt external neck trauma. *European Radiology* 1998;8:137-140.
8. Demetriades D, Theodorou D, Cornwell E, *et al:* Evaluation of penetrating injuries of the neck: prospective study of 223 patients [see comments]. *World Journal of Surgery* 1997;21:41-47.
9. Eachempati SR, Vaslef SN, Sebastian MW, *et al:* Blunt vascular injuries of the head and neck: is heparinization necessary? *Journal of Trauma-Injury Infection & Critical Care* 1998;45:997-1004.
10. Eddy VA: Is routine arteriography mandatory for penetrating injury to zone 1 of the neck? Zone 1 Penetrating Neck Injury Study Group. *Journal of Trauma-Injury Infection & Critical Care* 2000;48:208-213.
11. Gouny P, Nowak C, Smarrito S, *et al:* Bilateral thrombosis of the internal carotid arteries after a closed trauma. Advantages of magnetic resonance imaging and review of the literature. [Review] [23 refs]. *Journal of Cardiovascular Surgery* 1998;39:417-424.
12. Jacobs I, Niknejad G, Kelly K, *et al:* Hypopharyngeal perforation after blunt neck trauma: case report and review of the literature. [Review] [4 refs]. *Journal of Trauma-Injury Infection & Critical Care* 1999;46:957-958.
13. Kendall JL, Anglin D, Demetriades D: Penetrating neck trauma. [Review] [63 refs]. *Emergency Medicine Clinics of North America* 1998;16:85-105.
14. Nunez DJ, Rivas L, McKenney K, *et al:* Helical CT of traumatic arterial injuries. *American Journal of Roentgenology.* 1998;170:1621-1626.
15. Offiah CJ, Endres D: Isolated laryngotracheal separation following blunt trauma to the neck. [Review] [14 refs]. *Journal of Laryngology & Otology* 1997;111:1079-1081.
16. Park SS: Blunt trauma to the face & neck: initial management. [Review] [4 refs]. *Comprehensive Therapy* 1997;23:730-735.
17. Patton JH, Kralovich KA, Cuschieri J, *et al:* Clearing the cervical spine in victims of blunt assault to the head and neck: what is necessary? *American Surgeon* 2000;66:326-330.
18. Schoem SR, Choi SS, Zalzal GH: Pneumomediastinum and pneumothorax from blunt cervical trauma in children. *Laryngoscope* 1997;107:351-356.
19. Yetiser S, Kahramanyol M: High-velocity gunshot wounds to the head and neck: a review of wound ballistics. *Military Medicine* 1998;163:346-351.

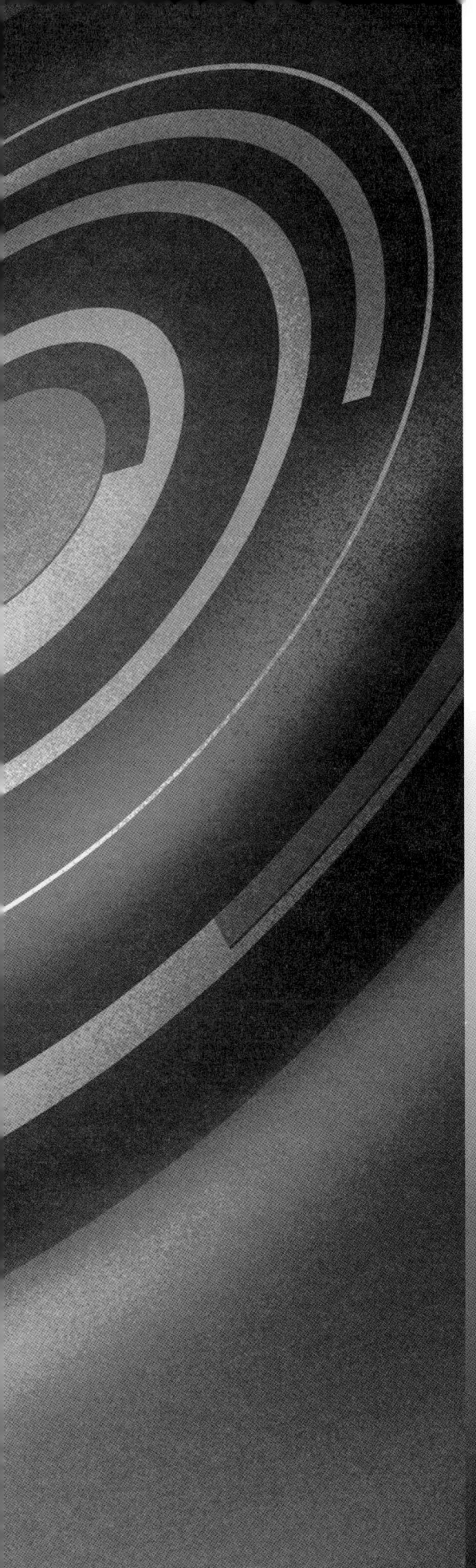

Facial Plastic Surgery

AESTHETIC FACIAL PROPORTIONS

When asked to evaluate a patient who wishes to change his or her facial appearance, it is important for the otolaryngologist to have a solid understanding of the landmarks and standard proportions used in facial analysis. Although the concept of beauty has changed somewhat over time and varies according to culture, certain reference points and favored proportions are consistently useful. Once an initial facial analysis based on standardized landmarks and proportions has been performed, it is important to take into account factors such as body habitus, age, and ethnicity that will affect overall facial harmony and surgical planning.

A general medical history is important for defining patient expectations as well as for determining comorbidities and social history (e.g., cigarette smoking) that may affect surgical risk and wound healing. In addition to addressing facial features and proportions, the physical exam should take into account skin type, degree of laxity, pigmentation, elements of asymmetry, and whether scars from previous procedures have healed well. Photographs taken from specific perspectives (e.g., frontal, lateral, oblique, and basal view) are helpful for surgical planning and postoperative assessment.

Reference Points

A number of landmarks are used to help standardize the approach to facial analysis. The first step in maintaining consistency in facial analysis is placing each patient in the same position. This is done by keeping the *Frankfort horizontal*, a plane defined by the superior external auditory canals and the inferior aspect of the inferior orbital rims, parallel to the floor. A plane perpendicular to the Frankfort horizontal and running through the nasion (Box 1) may be used as a reference for measuring the relative projection of the different regions of the face.

Box 1. Reference Point Definitions

Trichion: midpoint of current or former anterior hairline (approximated by superior limit of action of frontalis muscle)

Glabella: most prominent midline point of the forehead (generally in line with supraorbital rim)

Nasion: deepest/posterior-most midline point between the nose and forehead

Rhinion: meeting of bony and cartilaginous nasal dorsum

Tip: anterior-most point of the nose

Subnasale: meeting of the columella and the upper lip

Pogonion: anterior-most projection of the chin

Menton: inferior-most point of the chin

Facial proportions, anterior view

- One of the classic concepts is to divide the vertical height of the face into equal thirds: hairline to glabella, glabella to subnasale, and subnasale to menton.
- Alternately, measurements can exclude the forehead and primarily take into account the middle and lower face, in which case nasion-to-subnasale should equal 43% of the total distance between nasion and menton. Focusing on the middle and lower face in this way is meaningful for modern applications because the relative proportions of these areas are more easily influenced by aesthetic surgery than the upper face.
- The width of one eye should equal both the intercanthal distance and one fifth the width of the face between the outer aspects of the pinnae.
- The interalar distance should also equal the intercanthal distance, although this feature varies significantly with ethnic background.
- The neck should equal three fifths the width of the face (i.e., three times the width of one eye or the total space between the two outer canthi).
- Symmetry—or the location of the midline of the forehead, nose, lips, and chin along the midsagittal plane—is also an important feature.

Facial proportions, lateral view

In 1984, Powell and Humphreys described the complex relationship of facial features to each other based on an "aesthetic triangle" and five related angles seen in profile. These lines and angles demonstrate that individual features—the forehead, nose, lips, chin, and neck—cannot be altered without affecting each other and the overall balance of the face.

- *Nasofrontal angle (ideally 115-135 degrees):*
  - Angle between the nasal dorsum and a tangent connecting the glabella and nasion.
  - A shallow (more obtuse) nasofrontal angle gives the illusion of nasal lengthening, whereas a deep (more acute) nasofrontal angle is perceived as a shorter nose.
- *Nasofacial angle (ideally 30-40 degrees):*
  - Angle between the dorsum of the nose and the plane of the face (which connects the glabella and the pogonion).
  - An increased nasofacial angle corresponds with greater nasal projection.
- *Nasolabial angle (ideally 90-95 degrees in men and 95-105 degrees in women):*
  - Angle between the columella (line connecting subnasale and the anterior-most point on the columella) and a tangent connecting the subnasale to the mucocutaneous border of the upper lip.

- ▫ Tip rotation is directly related to the nasolabial angle.
- ■ *Nasomental angle (ideally 120-132 degrees):*
  - ▫ Angle between nasal dorsum and nasomental (tip to menton) line.
- ■ *Mentocervical angle (ideally 80-95 degrees):*
  - ▫ Angle between the plane running through glabella and pogonion and a line between the menton and the deepest point between the neck and the submental region.
  - ▫ An increased mentocervical angle may be secondary to prolapse of submental fat, diminished platysma tone, retrognathia, microgenia, or a low hyoid bone.

Facial Features

Forehead and eyes

- ■ The medial aspect of the eyebrow should start approximately 1 cm above the medial canthus and directly superior to the lateral edge of the ala nasi. In women, the eyebrow should arch laterally just above the level of the supraorbital rim. The lateral edge of the brow generally ends at its intersection, with the oblique line extending through the lateral canthus and the alar base. The lateral end of the brow should be at or slightly superior to the level of the medial end of the brow. In men, the arch is less pronounced and more closely follows the level of the supraorbital rim.
- ■ The supratarsal crease lies 7-10 mm above the inferior border of the upper lid margin. The upper lid covers 2-3 mm of the superior edge of the iris, whereas the lower lid covers only about 1 mm of its inferior edge. Lower lid laxity or normal anatomic variation may result in scleral show, meaning sclera is visible between the iris and the lower eyelid.
- ■ Again, the intercanthal distance should be equal to the width of one eye. Ideally, the lateral canthi should be level with or slightly higher than the medial canthi. The distance from the nasion to the vermillion border of the upper lip should be equal to the interpupil distance.
- ■ Brow ptosis and facial lines from repeated use of underlying facial muscles are the two primary age-related changes of the forehead and brow, and they may be improved by a brow lift. Excess skin of the upper lids (dermatochalasis) and fat herniation may be remedied by blepharoplasty. Lower lid laxity may require a shortening procedure to be corrected.

Nose

- ■ The nose is particularly important for overall facial aesthetics because of its central location and the ease with which its irregularities can be seen. The interalar distance should be equal to the intercanthal distance. From the basal view, the tip should be approximately one third of the height of the base, with the nares making up the remaining two thirds. The nares should be wider at the base and taper anteriorly. The width of the tip should be approximately 75% the total width of the base. In profile, 2-4 mL of columella should be visible below the level of the ala. The ala and the tip lobule should be similar in length.
- ■ As described previously, nasal projection can be described in terms of the nasofacial angle.
- ■ Goode described projection as the distance from the nasal tip to a line connecting the nasion to the alar groove. The ratio of projection to the nasal length (nasion to tip) should be 0.55-0.60:1.
- ■ Rotation may be described by the nasolabial angle or as a change in nasal tip location maintaining equidistance from the external auditory canal. Greater tip rotation has a more normal appearance on shorter people.
- ■ The nose can be divided into several aesthetic subunits: the unpaired dorsum and tip and the paired sides, ala, and soft triangles. Incisions placed at the junctions of these aesthetic subunits are less noticeable than ones placed within a subunit.

Lips

- ■ Lower lip height (menton to lower lip vermillion) should be roughly double that of the upper lip (subnasale to upper lip vermillion). The horizontal position of the lips may be evaluated in comparison to the nasomental line, which should be 4 mm anterior to the upper lip and 2 mm anterior to the lower lip. The oral commissure should be in line with the medial limbus.

Chin and neck

- ■ The mentocervical angle is useful for analyzing the chin and neck. Chin augmentation, rhytidectomy, liposuction, and platysmaplasty are methods used to correct a shallow mentocervical angle.

Ears

- ■ The ears are generally even with the supraorbital rim superiorly and the alar facial junction inferiorly. The ratio of width to length should be 0.55-0.60:1. The superior portion of the pinna should not be more than 18-20 mm from the temporal bone (which corresponds to a 20-degree angle between the mastoid and the auricle). Otoplasty may be used to correct underdeveloped antihelices or overdeveloped conchal bowls.

Summary

In order to adequately assess a patient interested in facial aesthetic surgery, it is important to understand the basics of facial analysis. Although ideal proportions vary somewhat according to age, gender, ethnicity, body habitus, and multiple other factors, standardized concepts of facial analysis provide a framework on which to build a coherent evaluation. As demonstrated by Powell and Humphreys' aesthetic triangle, facial features have a complex relationship to one another, so any alteration can affect the harmony of the entire face. Careful documentation, photography, and pre-operative analysis can help to maximize the outcome of aesthetic surgery.

 THE AGING FACE

Pathology

Anatomy of the skin
- The skin is divided into three layers: the epidermis, the dermis, and the superficial fascia.

Epidermis
- This is the most superficial layer of the skin. Epidermal replacement is decreased by 30%-50% in the elderly (longer healing time).
- The epidermis comprises four cell types: keratinocytes (80%), melanocytes, Langerhans' cells, and Merkel cells (function unknown).

Keratinocytes
- Aggregation of keratin filaments (catalyzed by filaggrin) forms macrofibrils, providing a cytoskeleton to the cell, as well as function in intracellular communication from the surface to the nucleus.

Langerhans' cells
- Dendritic cells that most likely mediate immunologic responses within the skin.
- The number of Langerhans' cell decrease with aging or UV exposure.

Melanocytes
- They produce melanin pigment.
- With aging the melanocyte density decreases with each decade by 6%-8%.
- The melanocytic enzyme tyrosinase decreases with age; therefore the elderly do not tan as easily as the young. Melanocytes in older skin are somewhat pleomorphic.
- The rate of epidermal replacement is decreased with aging, by up to 50%.
- There is a loss of polarity of the epidermal layers with blurring of the progression from basal cell layer to granular cell layer.

Dermal-epidermal junction
Basement membrane (BM)
- Attaches the epidermis to the dermis.
- Provides mechanical support.

- Provides a barrier to chemicals or cells.
  Anchoring fibrils in the BM help to anchor the epidermis and the epidermal-dermal junction to the dermis. They are absent in early scars and are lower in number in sun-exposed areas. They are susceptible to degradation by collagenase (which may be inhibited by topical tretinoin).

Rete Ridges
- With aging there is a decrease in the length of the dermal papillae and rete pegs, and the derma-epidermal junctions appear flattened (absent in scars).
- This relative decrease in interface is associated with:
  - Easier dermal-epidermal separation leading to a propensity for torn skin after minor trauma.
  - A decrease in the quantity of available keratinized cells caused by a decrease in the number of basal cells per unit area. This leads to dry skin.
  - A decrease in nutrient transfer.

Hair Shafts
- Extension of the epidermis, which has oncologic implications.

The Dermis
- The papillary dermis is composed of loose collagen, fibrocytes, and blood vessels.
- The reticular dermis is composed of compact collagen and a few fibrocytes.
- The main structural components of the dermis include collagen, reticulin, and elastic fibers embedded in a matrix of ground substance.
- Aging:
  - Skin collagen decreases by 1% per year as a result of decreased production.
  - Organization of collagen changes from small bundles parallel to the skin (infants) to randomly arranged papillary and tight reticular bundles (young adult) to compact bundles either in thick bundles or in loose-woven straight fibers.

Reticulin and elastic fibers
- Elastic fibers are thick and abundant in the papillary dermis in sun-damaged skin.
- Aging: increase in reticular dermis (thick, branched, and random) with decrease in the papillary dermis.

Fibrocytes
- Mostly in the papillary dermis. Can become collagen-producing in wound healing as well as contractile during wound contraction. Makes ground substance (fluid material consisting of glycoproteins and glycosaminoglycans).
- Aging: Fibrocytes decrease with age.

Superficial fascia
- Below dermis; has a fat component and a fibrous component.

Vascular network
- Superficial and deep network of capillaries and arteries. With aging the pericytes surrounding the vessels decrease in number and synthetic activity (increased bruising).

Nerves
- Afferent sensory and efferent autonomic.
  - Eccrine glands: sweat producers; decrease in number and function with aging.

The Aging Face

Etiology
- Secondary to combination of intrinsic and extrinsic factors. Intrinsic aging is characterized by fine wrinkling on pale surface, whereas extrinsic aging is characterized by coarse wrinkles on rough surface.
- Endogenous skin changes with aging:
  - Fine wrinkling.
  - Dermal atrophy.
  - Decrease in subdermal adipose tissue.
  - Loss of elastic fibers (resulting in skin laxity).
  - Decrease in vascular supply (pale appearance).
  - Decrease in melanocyte number (uneven pigmentation).
  - Decrease in intracellular water content results in dry and rough appearance.
  - Decrease in Langerhans' cells leads to increased risk of carcinogenesis or infection.
  - Adipose atrophy.
- Exogenous skin changes with aging:
- Results from chronic sun exposure (photoaging) and smoking.
  - Build-up of elastotic material in papillary dermis (elastosis).
  - Collagen and elastin fiber changes resulting from UV radiation–induced production of matrix-degrading proteinases (MDPs).
  - Decreased vascular supply as a result of cigarette smoking, nevi, hyperpigmentation, and cutaneous lesions.

Medical therapy
- Indications are for cosmetic considerations alone.
- No contraindications exist.
- Drug treatment includes sunscreens, alpha-hydroxy acids, and topical retinoids.
  - Effective sunscreens must block both UVA and UVB rays.

- Tretinoin reduces fine wrinkles, skin discoloration, and skin roughness. Mechanism of action is via increased vascularity as well as increased activity of fibroblasts and keratinocytes. Tretinoin was proven to inhibit the activity of MDP implicated in photodamage. Side effect is termed *retinoid dermatitis*, manifested by redness, dryness, and scaling. Treatment involves dose reduction and steroids.
  - Alpha-hydroxy acids promote epidermal desquamation and are effective at photodamage reduction.

Surgical therapy
- The basic tenet is that epidermal removal at various levels stimulates epidermal regrowth as well as inflammation, which induces reformation of collagen and ground substance. This can be done by a number of methods, including chemical peels, dermabrasion, and laser resurfacing.

Chemical Peel
- Application of an exfoliant stimulates epidermal growth by removing layers of skin. A light peel removes the stratum corneum and thickens the epidermis. A full superficial peel destroys the epidermis, and further destruction induces an inflammatory change in the papillary dermis (medium peel). A deep peel causes an inflammatory response in the deep reticular dermis with new collagen production.

Indications
- To provide cosmetic improvement or to eliminate solar-damaged skin.
- Can improve or minimize facial wrinkles, keratoses, age spots, freckles, and some scars.
- Fitzpatrick classification of sun reactive skin types (Table 1). Types I-III have best potential for favorable outcome, minimal risk.
  - Cosmetic patient selection: skin laxity = lift; fine rhytides = peel.

TABLE 1. Fitzpatrick Classification of Sun-Reactive Skin Types			
Unexposed Skin	**Skin Type**	**Sunburn**	**Tan**
White	I	Yes	No
	II	Yes	Minimal
	III	Yes	Yes
	IV	No	Yes
Brown	V	No	Yes
Black	VI	No	Yes

- Solar damage patient selection: epidermal lesions (actinic, seborrheic changes) = peel; dermal lesions = excision.

Contraindications
Absolute
- Hepatorenal disease (phenol).
- Cardiac disease (phenol).
- Unstable psychiatric disease.
- Allergy.
- Active herpes simplex.

Relative
- Physical restriction (postoperative care).
- Facial radiotherapy.
- Keloid former.
- Fitzpatrick types IV-VI.
- Latent herpes simplex.
- Telangiectasias.
- Medications (e.g., warfarin, estrogens).
- Pregnancy <6 months (pigmentary changes).
- Immunodeficiency (CD4 < 500).
- Male gender (thicker skin, postoperative makeup).

Agents
- Historic: carbolic acid, resorcinol, salicylic acid, naphthol.
- Current: retinoids, alpha-hydroxy acids, trichloroacetic acid (TCA), and phenol.
- Depth of skin pathology determines proper agent:
  - *Superficial:* fine rhytides, some keratoses (maximum every 1-6 weeks).
  - *Medium:* moderate rhytides, actinic keratoses, dyschromias of epidermis/upper dermis (maximum every 3-4 months).
  - *Deep:* heavy rhytides, solar lentigines, superficial premalignant keratoses, acne, melasma.

Superficial
- Jessner's solution.
- 10%-25% TCA.
- Alpha-hydroxy acid.
- Tretinoin.

Medium
- Jessner's TCA.
- 35% TCA.
- CO_2 and 35% TCA.

Deep
- Baker's phenol.
- 45%-50% TCA.

Technique
Preoperative
- Avoidance of sun.

- Retinoids (e.g., tretinoin, retinoic acid, Retin-A):
  - Thin stratum corneum, thicken epidermis, reverse keratinocyte atypia.
  - Redistribute melanin in epidermis, stimulate dermal collagen and glycosaminoglycan deposition.
  - Applied 2 weeks before peel; allows better absorption of agent, promotes healing.
- Alpha-hydroxy acids e.g., glycolic acid):
  - Concentrations 5%-20%: thin stratum corneum; control dry skin, ichthyosis, follicular hyperkeratosis
  - Concentration 50%-70%: full-face chemical peel.
  - Concentration >70%: epidermolysis below stratum corneum; spot treatment for seborrheic keratosis, actinic keratosis, verruca vulgaris.
  - Low concentration; daily use 1-6 weeks before deep peel.
  - Safe in Asians, Blacks, Hispanics without risk of scar formation.
- Prophylactic antivirals (acyclovir, valacyclovir) .
- No makeup for 24 hours.
- Cleansing of skin; removal of surface oils (Septisol/acetone, alcohol/10% glycolic acid, soap/ether).
- Elevation of head to minimize edema; IV hydration (phenol), individualizes analgesia.

Operative
TCA
- A chemical cauterant (coagulates protein in skin); neutralized by dermal serum.
- Stable for up to 6 months.
- Deep peel = concentrations >50%; more scarring, but no hypopigmentation nor cardiac or systemic toxicity.
- Applied evenly to aesthetic units of face with gauze or cotton swab; segments should not overlap.
- Feathered into hairline, vermilion, mandibular margin.

Phenol
- Deep peels for coarse facial rhytides (perioral, periorbital), spotty hyperpigmentation, actinic keratoses, superficial acne scars.
- Effect concentration dependent: <50% -keratolytic -> 50% - deeper penetration; >80% keratocoagulant-protein precipitation prevents extension to deeper tissues.
- Unstable, must mix fresh each time.
- Hemodynamic and cardiac monitoring.
- Applied to aesthetic units one at a time; 15-20 mm between for clearance (60-90 mm total). Feathered into hairline; applied just over vermilion, to within 2 mm of lid margin.

Postoperative

- Occlusion (decreases depth in TCA; increases depth in phenol).
- Face washed five to six times/day with warm water, cleanser; moisturizing ointment applied.
- Patients to avoid picking crusts, which can cause scarring.
- Makeup okay after 7-10 days; return to work okay after 2 weeks.
- Avoidance of sun for 6 months to minimize hyperpigmentation.

Complications
- Cardiac toxicity
  - Phenol can lead to arrhythmias (PAC, PVC, bigeminy, trigeminy).
  - Can occur within minutes, but typically after 30 minutes.
- Bacterial infection
- Uncommon (agents are bactericidal); ointments to treat folliculitis.
- Milia (small epidermal inclusions)
  - Ointment occlusion of pilosebaceous units.
- Herpes simplex reactivation
  - Prophylaxis with acyclovir at 200 mg t.i.d.
  - Increase dose if reactivation occurs.
  - Scarring rare after infection.
- Pigmentary changes
  - Superficial, medium peels: hyperpigmentation; deep peels: hypopigmentation.
  - More common in Fitzpatrick types IV-VI (may require 1-2 years to return to normal).
  - Other risk factors: sun exposure, pregnancy, oral estrogens.
  - Hyperpigmentation treatable with skin lightening quinolones.
- Persistence of erythema
  - Usually lasts 7-14 days, may last 3 months.
  - Avoidance of sun exposure, use of sunscreen at all times, concealing with makeup.
  - Preoperative tretinoin: may reduce postoperative erythema.
  - 1% Hydrocortisone applied for erythema that lasts more than 3 months.
  - Persistence of rhytides (inappropriate choice of agent or inappropriate patient selection).
- Scarring
  - Rare, most common with high TCA concentrations.

LASER SKIN RESURFACING

Indications
- Cosmetic: facial rhytides, rhinophyma.
- Therapeutic: tattoo removal; benign dermal tumors; actinic keratoses.

Main disadvantages
- Delayed wound healing.
- Potential for retinal damage from laser light.
- Expensive, bulky equipment.
- Aerosolization of genetic material.

Laser of choice
- For general laser facial resurfacing, CO_2 laser is current laser of choice: small spot size for excisional work, large spot size for tissue ablation.
- Originally continuous wave lasers only; recent advances include superpulsed and ultrapulsed CO_2 laser for high-energy ablation with less thermal absorption.
- Flash scanner can be used to focus beam more narrowly and move it rapidly over skin.
- Other lasers, although not specifically for resurfacing, include:
  - Q-switched Nd:YAG (pigmented epidermal lesions).
  - Q-switched ruby (tattoo removal).
  - Flash-lamp dye laser (vascular malformations).
  - Copper vapor or continuous wave yellow dye (telangiectasias).

Technique
Preoperative
- Acyclovir treatment started, continued for 7 days postoperatively.
- Topical bleaching agent applied if postoperative hyperpigmentation a preoperative concern.
- Skin rejuvenation: tretinoin and alpha-hydroxy acids.

Operative
- Local anesthesia via appropriate nerve block with 1% lidocaine with 1:100,000 epinephrine; alternately may use EMLA cream.
- Intralesional (within rhytid) injections that distort anatomy to be avoided.
- Smoke evacuator used.
- Work performed within aesthetic units of face.
- Coagulated skin wiped off with saline-soaked gauze after each laser pass.

Postoperative
- Laser-treated areas rinsed with cool water and topical antibiotic ointment applied for 1 week.
- Ice packs and acetaminophen used for 24-48 hours to limit swelling and discomfort.
- Crusts softened with H_2O_2 at 1 week.

Complications
- Bacterial infection:
  - Generally rare with appropriate postoperative care.

- Herpes simplex reactivation, rare if appropriate prophylaxis taken.
- Persistent erythema:
  - Usually lasts 7-14 days, may last 3-4 months.
  - Important to avoid sun exposure and to wear sunscreen during healing period.
  - Preoperative tretinoin may reduce postoperative erythema.
  - 1% hydrocortisone for erythema >3 months.
- Pigmentary changes:
  - Transient hyperpigmentation may occur in up to 30% of patients.
  - More common in patients with Fitzpatrick types IV-VI.
- Scarring (related to excessive thermal damage).
- Retinal damage from laser (operator dependent).

DERMABRASION

Indications
Note: The development of an effective technique that is satisfying for physician and patient generally requires many years.
- Reconstructive: post-acne scars, traumatic scars, surgical scars.
- Cosmetic: tattoo removal, rhytides.
- Therapeutic: actinic keratosis (premalignant), benign tumors (adenoma sebaceum, syringoma, telangiectasia, melasma, rhinophyma).

Contraindications
- Dark-skinned patients: risk of pigmentary change.
- Prior treatment with 13 cis-retinoic acid (Accutane): possible atypical scarring.
- AIDS: aerosolization of blood, tissue products.

Technique
Preoperative
- Acyclovir begun 24 hours preoperatively, continued for 5 days postoperatively.
- Staged analgesia with sedation (e.g., diazepam), regional block including supraorbital, infraorbital and mental foramina blockade.
- Refrigerant provides additional topical analgesia.
- Supplement with nitrous oxide as needed for patient comfort.

Operative
- Natural contour of skin to be maintained; skin frozen with Freon or other refrigerant. (bloodless field; easier to identify papillary dermis [RBC frozen in capillary bed]). Skin should be 0°-30° C (too cold of temperature increases necrosis, scarring).
- Small areas frozen and dermabraded at one time (1-inch squares); frozen skin stabilized with free hand

- Two main types of instruments exist: diamond fraise and wire brush:
  - Diamond fraise:
    - Multiple sizes, shapes, abrasiveness.
    - Flat surface, which allows easy identification of capillary loops and sebaceous glands to gauge depth.
    - Little tendency to grab skin, skip, or ricochet.
    - Can abrade in clockwise or counterclockwise rotation.
    - Balances easily, can be driven at high speeds.
  - Wire brush:
    - One basic shape, one size wire (1/3000 inch).
    - Irregular surface, which makes identification of capillary loops and sebaceous glands difficult.
    - Difficult to balance.
    - Rotational speeds limited to 30,000 rpm (2 mm width), 20,000 rpm (12 mm width).
    - Can only be used in clockwise rotational direction (wires at angle).
- Proceed no deeper than papillary dermis identified by punctate bleeding from capillaries as tissue thaws.
- Procedure generally begins beside nose and works outward. Lip fixed by countertraction to prevent getting caught in dermabrader.

Postoperative
- Topical thrombin for hemostasis.
- Occlusive dressings.
- Prednisone 40 mg × 4 days to control edema.
- Reepithelialization typically in 5-7 days.

Complications
- *Hypertrophic scarring*: occurs when dermabrasion proceeds too deep into papillary dermis. Certain areas more prone to hypertrophic scarring after dermabrasion:
  - Mandibular ramus.
  - Zygomatic arch.
  - Malar eminence.
  - Bossing of chin.
  - Bossing of forehead.
- *Infection*: most common: *Staphylococcus aureus*, herpes simplex virus, *Candida albicans*.
- *Acne flare*: treated with tetracycline.
- *Milia*: Dermal inclusions appearing 3-4 weeks postoperatively. Rare with postoperative tretinoin.
- *Persistent erythema*: treated with topical steroids if persists > 4 weeks; daily use of sunscreens for several months after reepithelialization.
- *Pigmentary abnormalities*: topical hydroquinone with tretinoin for hyperpigmentation.

Selected References from the Recent Literature

1. Baker TM: Dermabrasion. As a complement to aesthetic surgery. *Clinics in Plastic Surgery* 1998; 25:81-88.

2. Demas PN, Bridenstine JB: Diagnosis and treatment of postoperative complications after skin resurfacing. *Journal of Oral & Maxillofacial Surgery* 1999; 57:837-841.

3. Heinz GW, Kikkawa DO: The aging upper and middle face: an overview for the aesthetic surgeon. *International Ophthalmology Clinics* 1997; 37:1-10.

4. Khan JA: Millisecond CO_2 laser skin resurfacing. *International Ophthalmology Clinics* 1997; 37:29-68.

5. Lawrence N: New and emerging treatments for photoaging. *Dermatologic Clinics* 2000; 18:99-112.

6. Manaloto RM, Alster TS: Periorbital rejuvenation: a review of dermatologic treatments. *Dermatologic Surgery* 1999; 25:1-9.

7. Matarasso SL, Hanke CW, Alster TS: Cutaneous resurfacing. *Dermatologic Clinics* 1997; 15:569-582.

8. Orentreich N, Orentreich DS: Dermabrasion. As a complement to dermatology. *Clinics in Plastic Surgery* 1998; 25:63-80.

9. Patel BC: The krypton yellow-green laser for the treatment of facial vascular and pigmented lesions. *Seminars in Ophthalmology* 1998; 13:158-170.

10. Pitanguy I, Radwanski HN: Rejuvenation of the brow. *Dermatologic Clinics* 1997; 15:623-634.

11. Sherris DA, Otley CC, Bartley GB: Comprehensive treatment of the aging face–cutaneous and structural rejuvenation. *Mayo Clinic Proceedings* 1998; 73:139-146.

12. Solish N, Raman M, Pollack SV: Approaches to acne scarring: a review. [Review] [74 refs]. *Journal of Cutaneous Medicine & Surgery* 1998; 2 Suppl 3:24-32.

13. Tarbet KJ, Lemke BN: Clinical anatomy of the upper face. [Review] [33 refs]. *International Ophthalmology Clinics* 1997; 37:11-28.

14. Weinstein C: Carbon dioxide laser resurfacing. Long-term follow-up in 2123 patients. *Clinics in Plastic Surgery* 1998; 25:109-130.

BLEPHAROPLASTY

Indications

- Desire for improved cosmesis.
- Abnormalities corrected by blepharoplasty:
  - *Blepharochalasis:* redundancy and draping of eyelid (particularly upper eyelid) skin. Can even create visual field defects in superior and superior-lateral gaze if skin hangs eyelashes.
  - *Dermatochalasis:* hereditary hypertrophy of skin and orbicularis muscle, unrelated to aging. Occurs in young individuals. Gives a hooded appearance to the upper lid.
  - *Pseudoherniation of fat:* lids with puffy, baggy appearance. Results from weakness in the orbital septum.
  - *Orbicularis muscle hypertrophy:* occurs in the lower lid. Worsening puffiness caused by fat pseudoherniation.

Contraindications

- Any medical condition precluding elective surgery.
- Dry-eye syndrome: excessive tearing, gritty or burning sensation, mucus production, eyelid crusting, frequent blinking.
- Lagophthalmos: preoperative evaluation of brow/lid complex.
- Normal female upper brow: positioned centrally and medially at orbital rim or slightly above, laterally above rim. Otherwise, brow lift should be considered.
- Redundant skin and/or pseudoherniated fat.
- Asymmetries and/or lagophthalmos.
- Preexisting ectropion, entropion, exophthalmos, enophthalmos.

Upper Lid Blepharoplasty

- Elliptical excision of excess skin from the upper eyelid.
- Usually performed under local anesthesia with 1% lidocaine with 1:100,000 epinephrine.
- Lower incision placed horizontally in the upper lid crease, at least 5 mm above the upper lid margin.
- Medial border of the incision should end 1-2 mm medial to the upper lid puncta to avoid webbing.
- Lateral border runs to the sulcus between the lateral orbital rim and lid; can be extended laterally and upward if there is redundant tissue.
- Amount of skin excised estimated by grabbing excess skin with a forceps; must allow for adequate tension as well as eye closure.
- No. 15 blade used to excise skin off muscle; muscle taken only if redundant tissue exists or if the lid crease requires enhancement.

- Pseudoherniated fat excised (if necessary) by opening the orbital septum and dissecting the central and medial fat pads, with care taken not to clamp the superior oblique muscle.
- Only fat that comes into wound should be excised; too much fat removal may lead to lid retraction and overhang of orbital rim.

Lower Lid Blepharoplasty

- Techniques: skin-muscle flap, skin flap, and transconjunctival techniques.
- Skin-muscle flap technique:
  - Subciliary incision made 2-3 mm below the lower lashes extending laterally in a natural skin crease over the orbital rim. Initially incision carried through skin only until pretarsal portion of orbicularis muscle is met, and then skin-muscle flap is elevated and extended to the inferior orbital rim. Method of choice when fat pseudoherniation exists with minimal excess skin.
  - Advantage: safety of submuscular plane.
  - Disadvantage: scar, limited access to medial fat pad.
- Skin flap technique:
  - Oldest and least used approach. Incision similar to that described for skin-muscle flap, but plane of dissection is between skin and muscle all the way to inferior orbital rim. Useful for patient with redundant skin or when muscle resection desired.
  - Advantage: skin and muscle separated makes separate excision easier.
  - Disadvantage: more tedious dissection.
- Transconjunctival approach:
  - Conjunctival incision made on the inner aspect of the lower lid, used when fat is excised. Approach is in preseptal plane between orbicularis oculi and orbital septum.
  - Advantage: no external scar.
  - Disadvantage: skin excision must be accomplished separately.

Major complications of blepharoplasty
Bleeding and hematoma formation
Etiology

- Cut orbicularis muscle.
- Coughing spasm, retching, vomiting.
- Excessive traction of orbital fat.
- Retraction of open vessel.

Clinical manifestations

- Severe pain.
- Vision loss secondary to optic nerve or vascular compression.
- Blindness 1:25,000 (only seen with resection of lower lid fat).

Management

- Hematoma aspiration.
- Reexploration for evacuation of clot and control of hemorrhage.
- With loss of vision: IV mannitol/steroids, lateral canthotomy, lysis of lateral canthal tendon.
- Bony decompression of orbit.

Keratoconjunctivitis Sicca (Dry Eye Syndrome)
Etiology

- Preexisting marginal lacrimal function.
- Prolonged corneal or conjunctival exposure intra-operatively.
- Systemic diseases: hypothyroid, diabetes.

Clinical manifestations

- Itching, irritability, soreness, burning or foreign body sensation, increased mucoid secretion, crusting, conjunctival infection.

Management

- Lubrication with wetting agents, nighttime taping or patching.

Ectropion
Etiology

- Excessive skin and/or muscle resection.
- Suture infolding of orbital septum.
- Scar fixation of lower lid to orbital floor.
- Paresis or displacement of orbicularis muscle.
- Gravitational drag of cheek on lid.
- Scar contracture of orbicularis muscle.
- Excessive removal of orbital fat.
- Postoperative hematoma.

Clinical manifestations

- Increased scleral show.

Management

- Lower lid tape splinting or forceful eye closure.
- Gentle massage.
- Corneal protection with lubricants.
- Surgical correction deferred until wound induration resolved (3-6 months).
- Skin grafts (20% larger than final desired result), horizontal lid shortening, Z-plasty.

Epiphora
Etiology

- Anesthetic injections of orbicularis.
- Injury to lacrimal punctum (eversion).
- Ectropion.
- Lagophthalmos (incomplete eye closure).
- Corneal irritation or abrasion resulting in reflex hypersecretion of tears.

Clinical manifestations

- Improper processing of tears more likely than hypersecretion.
- Complaints of foreign body sensation.

Management

- Usually temporary, resolves within several days; if persists >3 months, ophthalmologist consulted.
- Punctoplasty, horizontal eyelid shortening, over-excision, and full-thickness skin graft.

Extraocular muscle palsy
Etiology

- Overzealous fat excision in nasal pocket of upper lid, or middle fat pocket of lower lid.

Clinical manifestations

- Diplopia.

Management

- Usually resolves within 6 months; if no resolution, ophthalmologist consulted.
- Resection of inferior rectus.
- Possible resection of superior rectus.
- Exploration of superior oblique with release of scar tissue.

Skin slough
Etiology

- Wide skin undermining followed by hematoma.
- Usually 3-4 mm below ciliary margin of lateral portion of lid.

Clinical manifestations

- Ptosis.
  - Early signs: extensive ecchymosis accompanied by superficial blistering.

Management

- Conservative.

Ptosis
Etiology

- Undetected preoperative ptosis.
- Injury to levator muscle.
- Lid edema.

Management

- Usually resolves in 6-8 weeks.
- If persists > 4-6 months, surgical correction:
  - Ptosis < 2 mm: conjunctival Muller's muscle resection.
  - Ptosis > 2 mm: graded external levator resection.

Asymmetry
Etiology
- Unequal skin excision, malposition of incisions, supertarsal fixation.

Management
- Surgical correction:
  - Skin grafts, additional skin excision, tarsal fixation.

Wound separation
Etiology
- Excessive tension during wound closure.
- Skin edge inversion.

Clinical manifestations
- Often found in lateral portions of incisions.

Management
- Sterile adhesive strips.
- Resuturing.

Infection
Etiology
- Suture abscess secondary to prolonged time prior to suture removal.

Clinical manifestations
- Orbital cellulitis, blindness.

Management
- I & D, compresses, topical antibiotics.
- Minor complications:
  - Milia can form along suture lines; usually treated with pinpoint cautery; most frequent complication.
  - Subconjunctival ecchymosis.
  - Chemosis: can take up to 6 weeks to resolve.

Selected References from the Recent Literature

1. Bedrock RD, Manna LM: Postsurgical lagophthalmus treated with gold eyelid weights. *Journal of Oral & Maxillofacial Surgery* 2000;58:447-450.
2. Weber PJ, Wulc AE, Foster J: Transconjunctival upper blepharoplasty [letter]. *Plastic & Reconstructive Surgery* 2000;105:803
3. Goldberg RA: Transconjunctival orbital fat repositioning: transposition of orbital fat pedicles into a subperiosteal pocket. *Plastic & Reconstructive Surgery* 2000;105:743-748.
4. Rohrich RJ, Zbar RI: The evolution of the Hughes tarsoconjunctival flap for the lower eyelid reconstruction. *Plastic & Reconstructive Surgery* 1999;104:518-522.
5. Geroulis AJ, Kemker BJ: Transconjunctival blepharoplasty and the use of the "silent assistant." *Laryngoscope* 2000;110:174-175.
6. Hester TRJ, Codner MA, McCord CD *et al:* Evolution of technique of the direct transblepharoplasty approach for the correction of lower lid and midfacial aging: maximizing results and minimizing complications in a 5-year experience. *Plastic & Reconstructive Surgery* 2000;105:393-406.
7. Suner IJ, Meldrum ML, Johnson TE *et al:* Necrotizing fasciitis after cosmetic blepharoplasty. *American Journal of Ophthalmology* 1999;128:367-368.
8. D'Assumpcao EA: Blepharoplasty: a personal tactical approach. *Aesthetic Plastic Surgery* 1999;23:28- 31.
9. Camirand A: The surgical correction of aging eyelids [letter; comment]. *Plastic & Reconstructive Surgery* 1999;103: 1325-1326.
10. Zarem HA, Resnick JI: Expanded applications for transconjunctival lower lid blepharoplasty. *Plastic & Reconstructive Surgery* 1999;103:1041-1043.
11. Januszkiewicz JS, Nahai F: Transconjunctival upper blepharoplasty. *Plastic & Reconstructive Surgery* 1999;103: 1015-1018.
12. van der Meulen JC: Blepharoptosis repair by selective use of superiorly based muscle flaps. *Plastic & Reconstructive Surgery* 1999;103:327-328.
13. Kim JW, Lee JO: Asian blepharoplasty with a short-pulsed contact Nd-Yag laser: limited-incision resectable laser double fold with internal medial and lateral functional epicanthoplasty. *Aesthetic Plastic Surgery* 1998;22:433-438.
14. Bernardi C, Dura S, Amata PL: Treatment of orbicularis oculi muscle hypertrophy in lower lid blepharoplasty. *Aesthetic Plastic Surgery* 1998;22:349-351.
15. Botti G: Blepharoplasty: A classification of selected techniques in the treatment and prevention of lower lid margin distortions. *Aesthetic Plastic Surgery* 1998;22:341-348.
16. Farrior RT, Kassir RR: Management of malar folds in blepharoplasty. *Laryngoscope* 1998;108:1659-1663.
17. Yoon KC, Park S: Systematic approach and selective tissue removal in blepharoplasty for young Asians. *Plastic & Reconstructive Surgery* 1998;102:502-508.
18. Mahe E: Lower lid blepharoplasty—the transconjunctival approach: extended indications. *Aesthetic Plastic Surgery* 1998;22:1-8.

AGING OF THE UPPER ONE THIRD OF THE FACE

Technique

Four available techniques are effective.

Direct browplasty

1. Excise an appropriately sized ellipse of skin from above the eyebrow. Closure of the wound raises the brow and decreases the amount of excess skin. Orbicularis muscle should be suspended to the fascia of the frontalis muscle or periosteum of the frontal bone with nonabsorbable suture.
2. Prep and drape the skin.
3. Mark the elliptic area with the lower limb of the ellipse just above the upper brow margin. The ellipse should taper medially and laterally from the highest point of the brow located at the lateral limbus. The amount to be removed is determined by elevating the brow.
4. Apply local anesthetic.
5. Make an incision at the upper border of the brow (bevel the upper incision to parallel the hair follicles).
6. Excise the skin at the junction of the subcutaneous plane and the orbicularis muscle.
7. Use permanent undyed sutures to suspend the orbicularis muscle to the frontalis fascia or periosteum above to lend permanence to the correction.
8. Close the skin.
9. Slightly overcorrect the brows.
10. Perform blepharoplasty, when indicated, after the brow procedure.

Midforehead browplasty

This procedure begins with an incision in a natural transverse forehead rhytid above the level of the brow. Placing the incisions in natural lines allows for hiding of the scar.

1. Prep/drape the skin.
2. Select a natural horizontal forehead rhytid above the brow on each side. This is usually the first or second wrinkle above the brow. Often rhytids of unequal distance from the brows are selected. This is advantageous because scars at different height above the brow are less noticeable.
3. Inject local anesthetic and then incise along the previously marked line.
4. Dissect inferiorly at the level of the junction between the subcutaneous tissue and the intrinsic facial musculature. Dissection is carried down to the orbital rim. Take care not to enter the frontalis muscles, orbicularis muscles, or supraorbital nerve.
5. Suspend the orbicularis muscle to the frontalis muscle or periosteum with permanent suture.

6. Excise excess skin for the wound to close without tension.
7. Perform blepharoplasty after the brow procedure.

Midforehead rhytidectomy

This procedure begins with an incision all the way across the forehead in a natural transverse rhytid. This is an extension of the midforehead browplasty wherein the incisions above the brow are connected in a natural transverse forehead rhytid. This small increase of the incision allows the entire brow-glabella-forehead complex to be explored and treated. This is most commonly performed in men with deep transverse forehead rhytids or in older women with pronounced forehead creases. Incisions have to follow the natural forehead creases precisely, even though it is often asymmetric and slightly irregular. This scar will be hidden within the crease.

- Prep and drape the patient.
- Mark the first or second natural horizontal forehead rhytids that go all the way across the brow, and then inject local anesthetic.
- Incise and dissect between the subcutaneous tissue and intrinsic musculature of the face, down to the level of orbital ramis in the plane superficial to the musculature.
- Take care to avoid the supraorbital nerves.
- If desired, excise a section of the corrugator and procerus.
- If desired, elevate a superior flap in the subgaleal plane and incise the central portion of the frontalis muscle horizontally. Do not extend this incision lateral to pupils in order to preserve lateral frontalis function.
- If desired, excise a segment of frontalis and suture the edges, elevating the glabellar and medial brow tissues.
- Suspend the orbicularis to the frontalis muscle.
- Place a drain and the close the incision.

Forehead rhytidectomy (coronal lift, forehead lift, frontal lift)

This procedure begins with an incision behind the temporofrontal hairline (coronal approach) or in the frontal hairline (trichophytic). The preferred incision is 5 cm posterior to the hairline.

- Braid the hair anterior to incision.
- Inject local anesthetic about 2 cm above the ear, extending across to the other side.
- Bevel the incision from anterior to posterior to parallel the fair follicles.
- Dissect the flap in subgaleal plane just superficial to pericranium and deep temporalis fascia laterally.
- Carry dissection laterally over the rim and medially to the root of the nose.
- Preserve the supraorbital neurovascular bundle.

- Make horizontal relaxing incisions in the frontalis muscle to the midpupillary lines; carrying the incision laterally may result in denervation of the forehead.
- Excise corrugator muscle; improves glabellar frown lines.
- Return the flap back to original position and excise the excess skin.
- Apply galeal suture with permanent sutures to hold the flap.
- Overcorrect for brow ptosis.
- Place a drain and close the skin.
- Perform blepharoplasty after forehead lift.

Advantages and disadvantages of the different techniques

Direct browplasty
- *Advantage:* Quick, easy to perform, low morbidity, less expensive, very effective and rarely any postoperative recurrence of brow ptosis.
- *Disadvantage:* Presence of scar. This procedure is rarely used anymore.

Midforehead browplasty
- *Advantage:* Quick and easy procedure, complications rare, relatively inexpensive, and effective with minimal postoperative recurrences.
- *Disadvantage:* Scar may be noticeable and may require revision or dermabrasion.

Midforehead rhytidectomy
- *Advantage:* Direct approach problems of brow ptosis, forehead and glabellar ptosis, and rhytids.
- *Disadvantage:* Residual scar.

Forehead rhytidectomy
- *Advantage:* Scar is camouflaged behind the hairline, therefore no visible scar is present. It has long-lasting results and can be used to treat all the problems associated with forehead aging.
- *Disadvantage:* It is a more extensive operation with greater likelihood of complications. It requires longer OR time, is more expensive, and requires more experience and expertise on the part of the surgeon. The operation actually raises the frontal hairline, which may be a disadvantage in some patients.

Indications and contraindications

Direct browplasty
- Indicated in a patient with:
  - Brow ptosis.
  - Soft, non-oily skin.
  - No tendency for hypertrophic scarring.
  - No objection to using makeup to camouflage the scar.

- Sagging lateral two thirds of the brows and little or no ptosis or furrowing at the glabella (very effective).
- Contraindicated in any patient with:
  - Thick, oily Mediterranean-type skin.
  - A history of abnormal scarring.
  - No acceptance of a facial scar.
  - An unusually low temporal hairline.

Midforehead browplasty
- Indications
  - Male patients with brow ptosis.
  - Female patients (rarely) who are not candidates for a forehead rhytidectomy and have deep horizontal forehead creases.
- Contraindications
  - Patients with smooth, nonwrinkled forehead skin and in most women, except those with deep horizontal forehead creases.
  - Patients with history of abnormal scarring.
  - Patients who cannot accept facial scars.

Midforehead rhytidectomy
- Indications
  - Male patients with prominent forehead rhytids who have significant ptosis and rhytidosis of the glabellar complex and brow ptosis.
  - Older women with deep horizontal forehead rhytids.
- Contraindications
  - Patients with abnormal scarring or smooth, non-wrinkled forehead skin.
  - Patients with inability to accept a facial scar.

Forehead rhytidectomy
- Indications
  - Significant brow ptosis and deep transverse forehead creases, lateral hooding, glabellar frown lines, and crow's feet. This operation is primarily performed in females.
- Contraindications
  - High frontal hairline and thin, sparse anterior hair. This is why the procedure is performed less frequently on male patients.

Complications
- Infections are quite rare because of the forehead's excellent blood supply.
- Hematoma: risk increases progressively with midforehead browplasty, midforehead rhytidectomy, and forehead rhytidectomy, in that order.
- Visible scar present.
- Numbness or hypesthesia from supraorbital nerve stretch. In forehead rhytidectomy the plane of dissection is deep to galeal layer, whereas in the other three operations, the level of dissection is between the

subcutaneous and muscular layer. If these planes are maintained, minimal nerve damage is expected.

Botulinum A Toxin Injections

Clostridium botulinum produces a neurotoxin, botulinum A toxin, that inhibits the release of acetylcholine at the presynaptic terminal of the nerve. By blocking this release, paralysis of the innervated muscles occurs and results in an effacement of the dynamic wrinkle lines. The major dynamic lines treated are the glabellar furrows (corrugator and procerus muscles) and the orbital crow's feet lines (orbicularis muscle).

Endoscopic Brow Lift

Indications
- Brow ptosis.
- Forehead/brow rhytids.
- Weaken hyperdynamic musculature.
- More favorable:
  - Generalized asymmetric brow ptosis.
  - Horizontal and vertical forehead rhytids.
- Less favorable:
  - Thick sebaceous skin.
  - Marked brow ptosis requiring skin excision.
  - Facial paralysis.

Advantages
- Decreased alopecia.
- Decreased numbness.
- Decreased postoperative recovery.

Technique
Elevation
1. With patient upright, apply local anesthetic.
2. Make three incisions, placed 1.5 cm posterior to hairline, 1.5 cm in length; one midline, two paramedian.
3. Perform a subperiosteal forehead dissection with Cottle elevator and then endoscopic elevator to create optic cavity.
4. Use a 30-degree endoscope; visualization important in superior to brow to avoid neurovascular structures.
5. Carry out blind posterior dissection, extended 2-3 cm posterior to coronal suture line.
6. Carry out anterior dissection over orbital rim.
7. Release periosteum over the arcus marginalis to reveal retro-orbicularis oculi fat pad (ROOF).
8. Identify and divide:
   a. Corrugator muscles for glabellar rhytids (try to preserve supratrochlear nerve fascicles).
   b. Procerus for correction of horizontal rhytids.
9. Elevate temporal pockets over temporalis muscle:
   a. Anterior margin: orbital rim.
   b. Superior margin: temporal line.
   c. Inferior margin: zygomatic arch.
10. Make vertical incision 1-1.5 cm with hairline, superior and anterior to auricle.
11. Perform dissection through temporoparietal fascia (contains frontal branch of facial nerve).
12. Perform inferior dissection deep to temporoparietal fascia and superior to deep temporal fascia overlying temporalis fascia. Use 0-degree endoscope.
13. Perform complete dissection when sentinel vein is encountered at lateral canthus.
14. Join the temporal pocket with the central pocket, dissecting lateral to medial, cutting through the attachments to the temporal line (periosteum, galea, temporalis fascia).

Suspension (numerous techniques)
- Scalp plication.
- Scalp excision.
- External taping.
- Compression and suture fixation to miniscrews or plates:
  - Suture temporoparietal fascia to deep temporal fascia for maximal correction.
  - Sutures (× 3) anteriorly through periosteum, galea, frontalis.
  - Sutures secured to "T-plate" placed 6-8 cm posterior to central portal through separate incision.

Complications
- Less than traditional bicoronal flap.
- Paresthesias.
- Scalp itching.
- Temporary paresis of frontalis branch of facial nerve.

Selected References from the Recent Literature
1. Miller TA, Rudkin G, Honig M, *et al:* Lateral subcutaneous brow lift and interbrow muscle resection: clinical experience and anatomic studies. *Plastic & Reconstructive Surgery* 2000; 105:1120-1127.
2. Wolfe SA: The subcutaneous forehead lift, revisited. *Plastic & Reconstructive Surgery* 2000; 105:449-450.
3. Knize DM: Muscles that act on glabellar skin: a closer look. *Plastic & Reconstructive Surgery* 2000; 105:350-361.
4. Kennedy BD, Pogue MD: Fixation techniques for endoscopic browlift. [Review] [24 refs]. *Journal of Oral & Maxillofacial Surgery* 1999; 57:588-594.
5. Lassus C: Elevation of the lateral brow without the help of an endoscope. *Aesthetic Plastic Surgery* 1999; 23:23-27.
6. Knize DM: Reassessment of the coronal incision and subgaleal dissection for foreheadplasty [letter; comment]. *Plastic & Reconstructive Surgery* 1999; 103:1326-1327.
7. Fortune DS, Ries WR: Options in the management of the aging face. An otolaryngology-facial plastic and reconstructive surgeon's perspective. *Medical Clinics of North America* 1900; 83:283-301.

8. Knize DM: Limited incision foreheadplasty. *Plastic & Reconstructive Surgery* 1999; 103:271-284.

9. Marten TJ: Hairline lowering during foreheadplasty. *Plastic & Reconstructive Surgery* 1999; 103:224-236.

10. Macdonald MR, Spiegel JH, Raven RB, *et al:* An anatomical approach to glabellar rhytids. *Archives of Otolaryngology–Head & Neck Surgery* 1998; 124:1315-1320.

11. Nassif PS, Kokoska MS, Homan S, *et al:* Comparison of subperiosteal vs subgaleal elevation techniques used in forehead lifts. *Archives of Otolaryngology–Head & Neck Surgery* 1998; 124:1209-1215.

12. Knize DM: Reassessment of the coronal incision and subgaleal dissection for foreheadplasty [see comments]. [Review] [20 refs]. *Plastic & Reconstructive Surgery* 1998; 102:478-489.

13. Kobienia BJ, Van Beek A: Calvarial fixation during endoscopic brow lift. *Plastic & Reconstructive Surgery* 1998; 102:238-240.

14. Steinsapir KD, Shorr N, Hoenig J, *et al:* The endoscopic forehead lift. *Ophthalmic Plastic & Reconstructive Surgery* 1998; 14:107-118.

15. Friedland JA: Open approach for upper facial rejuvenation. *Plastic & Reconstructive Surgery* 1997; 100:1040-1042.

16. Michelow BJ, Guyuron B: Rejuvenation of the upper face. A logical gamut of surgical options. [Review] [20 refs]. *Clinics in Plastic Surgery* 1997; 24:199-212.

RHYTIDECTOMY (LOWER TWO THIRDS OF FACE)

Evaluation and indications

- Self-image issues: desire for appearance change is sufficient indication for surgery.
- Questions to ask patient:
  - What are the expectations of the patient?
  - Are the patient's expectations realistic and reasonable?
  - Can the expectations be met?
  - Is this patient likely to be satisfied?
  - Are there medical issues that complicate surgery (hypertension, diabetes mellitus)
- Preoperative assessment needs: patient-surgeon agreement on deformity to correct.
- Patient and surgeon need to be comfortable with each other.
- Identification of areas to correct:
  - Superficial rhytids better for peels or laser. Deeper rhytids respond better to surgical intervention.
  - Atrophy and loss of muscle tone lead to enhancement of nasolabial crease, jowls, ptotic submandibular glands, submental laxity, and platysma laxity (blunting of cervico-mental angle).
  - Inferior displacement of malar fat pads.
  - Upper eyelid laxity, hooding, fat herniation of lower lid area.
- Good candidate: moderately thick skin, minimal sun damage, good skin elasticity, strong facial bony structures, prominent cheek bones, shallow cheek-lip grooves, nonsmoker.
- Poor candidate: thin skin, obese, low hyoid (obtuse cervicomental angle) receded chin, ptotic submandibular glands, deep nasolabial grooves.

Submuscular aponeurotic system (SMAS)

- Fibromuscular layer continuous with the superficial cervical fascia.
- Variable thickness.
- Located lateral but adherent to parotid fascia, thick in this area.
- Anterior to parotid, SMAS overlies masseter and buccal fat pad and is thinner.
- Further anteriorly, it surrounds mimetic facial muscles:
  - Mimetic muscles are innervated from deep surface with exception of buccinator, levator anguli oris, and mentalis.
- Superiorly, adherent to the zygomatic arch (with the temporal branch of the facial nerve lying deep to the SMAS), then is continuous the temporoparietal fascia, and ultimately continues as the galea.
- Inferiorly envelops the platysma.

Skin incisions

- Extends from temporal region to the root of the helix:
  - Incision is parallel to hair follicles through inferior temporal hair tuft.
  - Plan incision such that hairline laterally is not lifted superior than insertion of superior helix.
  - Skin flap elevation is deep to hair follicles.
- Extends inferiorly to the tragus:
  - Posttragal in female to minimize visibility of scar.
  - Pretragal in males to prevent need for shaving on tragus,
- Beneath lobe around to postauricular area:
  - Many extend incision onto the posterior concha area because the tightly adherent fascia prevents webbing of postauricular incision.
- Extending posteriorly (6-8 cm) into the hairline over the occiput.

Approaches for facelift

- *Classic (superficial) approach* involves development of facial skin flaps only and excision of excess skin. However, undermining of the skin in a single layer puts increased tension on closure and gives only short-term improvement. It generally is not used today.
- *Contemporary: two-layer cervicofacial approach* (sub-SMAS):
  - A skin flap is developed superficial to the SMAS in the periparotid region, as is a sub-SMAS flap, which extends anteriorly to the border of the parotid gland/masseter muscle. Postero-inferiorly, the skin flap dissection proceeds in subcutaneous plane 5-7 cm to the posterior aspect of the platysma (to permit suspension). The SMAS is fused with fascia of sternocleidomastoid muscle, making dissection more difficult in this region (it is easy to injure great auricular nerve at this point). Mandibular branch of the facial nerve is avoided by staying lateral to SMAS. This branch becomes superficial 2 cm lateral to the oral commissure.
  - The short flap (4-6 cm) is used most commonly. Long flaps are cheek-neck flaps connected in the submental region. A medium-length flap is first elevated as a short flap, which is then extended to the melolabial fold and oral commissure with blunt dissection. The longer the flap, the greater the risk of hematoma formation and facial nerve damage.
  - SMAS suspension: different techniques:
    - Elevation and suspension. Flap is elevated, overlapped, and suspended. Damage to facial nerve is avoided by elevating the flap 1 cm inferior to the zygomatic arch and 1 cm superior to the ramus and not extending it anterior to the parotid gland.

- Plication (folding on itself) in the preauricular region. Indicated in patients with a mobile SMAS and cheek depression. May leave preauricular fullness.
- Imbrication. Resection of SMAS strip in preauricular and infraauricular regions, with elevation of an anterior SMAS flap (2-4 cm). Flap is pulled in posterosuperior direction and secured with nonabsorbable sutures.
- *Subperiosteal plane:* good for work in periorbital area only, poor for lower face; some have described this approach for midface with transoral access.
- *Deep (composite) plane:* developed to address midface area:
  - Increased redundancy of melolabial folds caused by inferomedial descent of cheek fat.
  - Descent of the malar crest caused by inferolateral descent of ptotic orbicularis oculi.
  - Flap is elevated as follows:
    - Neck: preplatysmal.
    - Malar region: suborbicularis.
    - Face: sub-SMAS, extending anteriorly to include malar fat pad, superficial to the zygomaticus muscle.
  - Suspension of the anatomic regions in vectors opposite to the direction of ptosis. Skin is used to position deeper elements.
  - Technique controversial because of increased risk of injury to the facial nerve innervating the orbicularis and in the zygomatic and buccal regions.
- Skin is redraped in posterosuperior direction to allow for closure without tension.

Submental region

- Excess skin only: addressed with rhytidectomy and SMAS suspension.
- Excessive fat in submental and submandibular regions:
  - Open lipectomy via submental incision.
  - Defatting of flap.
  - Liposuction.
- Platysmal bands:
  - Minimal: sectioning through lateral approach.
  - Moderate to severe: midline transection and plication through a submental incision.

Complications

- Great auricular nerve most common nerve injured.
- Danger areas of the facial nerve.
- Temporal branch (most commonly injured branch):
  - Courses deep to the SMAS but pierces the SMAS at the lower border of the zygomatic arch and lies superficial to the temporoparietal fascia.
  - Lies within 2 cm of the lateral brow.

- Enters frontalis muscle on the deep surface.
- Marginal mandibular (second commonly injured branch):
  - Courses beneath SMAS to within 2 cm of lip and runs within 2 cm of inferior border of the mandible, posterior and then superficial to facial artery.
- Hematoma: most frequent complication (8.5%):
  - Signs and symptoms: unilateral pain, swelling, buccal firmness, intraoral ecchymosis.
  - Treated with aspiration, pressure dressing, or formal drainage in the operating room (required immediately for expanding hematomas to prevent compromise to skin flap).
- Skin slough (3.6%): postauricular region caused by excessive skin tension
  - Risk factors include tobacco use (12×), hematoma formation, and longer and thinner flaps.
  - Treatment with gentle debridement and antibiotic ointment.
  - Cyanosis precedes necrosis; a few key sutures can be removed.
- Greater auricular nerve injury: most frequently injured nerve (5%), typically inured where SMAS attached to SCM fascia. Care taken to avoid cautery or suspension sutures in this region.
- Wide scar: caused by excessive skin tension
- Pixie ear: loss of lobular-facial angle. The lobule must lie tension free in apex of divided skin flap.
- Blunted tragus: associated with posttragal incision.
- Alopecia: in temporal region (0.2%-1.8%). Caused by failure of appropriate beveling of incision or tension of incision. May require hair grafts.
- Scar step-off: closure of hairline at different levels over occiput.
- Scar hypertrophy: check for history of keloids or hypertrophic scars. Treated with intralesional steroids.
- Hyperpigmentation: caused by bleeding beneath skin flap, "bone-dry closure" attempted.
- Telangiectasias of skin flap: may require steroid creams, or laser at later date.

Selected References from the Recent Literature

1. Baker SR: Triplane rhytidectomy. Combining the best of all worlds. *Archives of Otolaryngology–Head & Neck Surgery* 1997; 123:1167-1172.
2. Baylis HI, Goldberg RA, Shorr N: The deep plane facelift: a 20-year evolution of technique. *Ophthalmology* 2000; 107:490-495.
3. Calabria R: Deep plane rhytidectomy [letter; comment]. *Plastic & Reconstructive Surgery* 1999; 104:298-299.
4. Candiani P, Campiglio GL, Tremolada C: Composite rhytidectomy [letter; comment]. *Plastic & Reconstructive Surgery* 1998; 101:1411-1413.

5. Cardenas-Camarena L, Gonzalez LE: Multiple, combined plications of the SMAS-platysma complex: breaking down the face-aging vectors. *Plastic & Reconstructive Surgery* 1999; 104:1093-1100.

6. Cardoso DC: The changing role of platysma in face lifting. *Plastic & Reconstructive Surgery* 2000; 105:764-775.

7. Connell BF, Semlacher RA: Contemporary deep layer facial rejuvenation. *Plastic & Reconstructive Surgery* 1997; 100:1513-1523.

8. Evans TW: A case for deeper plane facelifts. *Journal of Oral & Maxillofacial Surgery* 1998; 56:352-358.

9. Fortune DS, Ries WR: Options in the management of the aging face. An otolaryngology-facial plastic and reconstructive surgeon's perspective. *Medical Clinics of North America* 1900; 83:283-301.

10. Ghali GE, Smith BR: A case for superficial rhytidectomy. [Review] [30 refs]. *Journal of Oral & Maxillofacial Surgery* 1998; 56:349-351.

11. Hamra ST: Frequent face lift sequelae: hollow eyes and the lateral sweep: cause and repair [see comments]. *Plastic & Reconstructive Surgery* 1998; 102:1658-1666.

12. Heinrichs HL, Kaidi AA: Subperiosteal face lift: a 200-case, 4-year review [see comments]. *Plastic & Reconstructive Surgery* 1998; 102:843-855.

13. Kamer FM, Frankel AS: SMAS rhytidectomy versus deep plane rhytidectomy: an objective comparison [see comments]. *Plastic & Reconstructive Surgery* 1998; 102:878-881.

14. Klein AW, Wexler P, Carruthers A, *et al:* Treatment of facial furrows and rhytides. [Review] [74 refs]. *Dermatologic Clinics* 1997; 15:595-607.

15. Owsley JQ: Face lifting: problems, solutions, and an outcome study. *Plastic & Reconstructive Surgery* 2000; 105: 302-313.

16. Rudkin G, Miller TA: Aging nasolabial fold and treatment by direct excision. *Plastic & Reconstructive Surgery* 1999; 104:1502-1505.

17. Tapia A, Etxeberria E, Blanch A, *et al:* A review of 685 rhytidectomies: a new method of analysis based on digitally processed photographs with computer-processed data. *Plastic & Reconstructive Surgery* 1999; 104:1800-1810.

18. Tobin HA: The subperiosteal face lift [letter; comment]. *Plastic & Reconstructive Surgery* 1999; 103:1539.

MENTOPLASTY

Indications

- Microgenia (chin eminence is diminished).
- Mild to moderate retrognathia (normal mandible size with class II occlusion).
- Mild micrognathia (hypoplastic mandible with class II occlusion).
- Ancillary procedure: often performed in conjunction with rhinoplasty or rhytidectomy. Correction of microgenia is necessary in 20% of rhinoplasties and 25% of rhytidectomy.

Contraindications

- Moderate to severe retrognathia or prognathism: will require orthognathic correction.

Preoperative measurement

- Gonzalez-Ulloa approach: line dropped from nasion perpendicular to Frankfurt line should approximate chin.
- Goode approach: perpendicular line tangential to alar crease should approach anterior to chin.
- Mentolabial sulcus should be 4 mm behind pogonion:
  - Menton: lowest contour point of chin.
  - Pogonion: anterior-most point of chin.

Technique: allograft augmentation vs sliding genioplasty

Allograft

- Implant types:
  - Silicon gel: used to be used extensively, now taken off market.
  - Silastic: preformed shapes and sizes, most commonly used.
  - Homografts.
  - Allografts.
- Actual soft tissue augmentation stabilizes in 2 years at 70%. Alloplasts are simpler, removable, and involve fewer complications than sliding genioplasty.
- Approaches:
  - Intraoral: incision located over inferior aspect of gingival mandibular sulcus with 1.5-cm vertical incision through mucosa and midline of mentalis muscle. Periosteal pocket elevated. Mental nerves avoided. Implant may be secured.

Complications

- Bothersome intraoral suture line.
- Potential contamination:
  - External: Incision made in submental crease (15-25 mm). Otherwise same as above.
- External scar.

Sliding genioplasty

- Horizontal vs vertical.
- 70%-97% tissue gain, which stabilizes after 2 years.
- Useful in:
  - Asymmetric jaws.
  - Extreme micrognathia.
  - Extreme or insufficient vertical mandibular height.
  - Failed allograft.
- Intraoral incision, periosteum reflected, osteotomy performed (>5 mm below mental foramen), fixation with titanium plates.

Complications

- Possible months of numbness in mental distribution.

Complications

- Displacement.
- Infection.
- Bony resorption.
- Mental nerve injury.
- Hypertrophic scar.

Selected References from the Recent Literature

1. Gubish W, Kotzur, A. Our experience with silicone rhino-mentoplasty. *Aesthetic Plastic Surgery* 1998;22:237-244.
2. Karras SC, Wolford LM. Augmentation genioplasty with hard tissue replacement implants. *Journal of Oral and Maxillofacial Surgery* 1998;56:549-552.
3. Frodel JL, Sykes JM. Chin augmentation/genioplasty:chin deformities in the aging patient. *Facial Plastic Surgery* 1996;12: 279-283.
4. Vuyk HD. Augmentation mentoplasty with solid silicone. *Clin Otolaryngol Rel Sci* 1996;21:106-118.
5. Guyuron B, Kadi JS. Problems following genioplasty. Diagnosis and treatment. *Clinics in Plastic Surgery* 1997;24: 507-514.
6. Ousterhout DK. Sliding genioplasty, avoiding mental nerve injuries. *Journal of Craniofacial Surgery* 1996;7:297-298.
7. Li KK, Cheney ML. The use of sliding genioplasty for treatment of failed chin implants. *Laryngoscope* 1996;106, 363-366.

SEPTOPLASTY (NASAL SEPTAL SURGERY)

- *Septoplasty:* Conservative approach to straightening the septum with preservation of cartilage.
- *Submucous resection (SMR):* excisional approach.
- *Inferior turbinectomy:* Performed on anatomically deviated, obstructing inferior turbinate or if hypertrophic mucosa continues to be obstructing in spite of medical management.

Indications
- Septal deformity causing nasal airway obstruction (subjective reports from patient).
- Persistent or recurrent epistaxis.
- Evidence of sinusitis secondary to septal obstruction.
- Symptomatic septal perforation.
- Headaches secondary to intranasal deformity.
- Preliminary step in transseptal sphenoidotomy or nasal reconstruction.
- When necessary during endoscopic sinus or cosmetic surgery.
- Harvest of cartilage for grafting purposes.

Contraindications (relative)
- Bleeding diathesis.
- Current cocaine use.
- Active granulomatous disease.
- Saddle-nose deformity.

Technique
1. Administer anesthesia:
   a. Can be performed under local or general anesthesia.
   b. Place two pledgets soaked with 4% cocaine solution into each side of nose to reach both the sphenopalatine ganglion region (posterior end of middle meatus) and the middle of the ethmoid region
   c. If required, inject circumnasal and intrainferior turbinate injections of 1% lidocaine with 1:100,000 epinephrine.
2. Make a hemitransfixion (Killian) incision (at caudal rim of septal cartilage, or 0.75-1.0 cm posterior to and parallel to the caudal septal margin).
3. Perform sharp dissection through perichondrium to cartilage (achieve an avascular plane).
4. Elevate (e.g., with Freer elevator) mucoperichondrium as an intact sheet from cartilage, proceeding posteriorly, superiorly, and inferiorly to expose perpendicular plate and vomer.
5. Incise septal cartilage just posterior to original incision, being careful to preserve mucoperichondrium on the opposite side.
6. Elevate mucoperichondrium from contralateral side in a similar fashion.
7. Resect cartilage (an example of cartilage resection is

shown). Commonly a Ballenger swivel knife is used for this purpose. Place removed cartilage in saline. Keep 0.75 and 1.0 cm of caudal septum and 1.0 cm of dorsal septum for support.
8. Remove deviated bone (if any) with rongeur.
9. Thin, strip, or crush removed cartilage and trip redundant tissue. Replace cartilage or discard (thus completing submucosal resection).
10. Approximate membranes with sutures using a small straight needle and absorbable sutures. If unstable, silastic sheets and nonabsorbable sutures can be used and the structure removed in 10-21 days. These sutures decrease morbidity, postoperative nasal congestion, and risk of intramembranous hematoma, and they increase membrane approximation
11. If caudal septum is not straight, use more complicated techniques:
    a. Excision of irregular cartilage or bone.
    b. Morselization.
    c. Checkerboard gridding: make cuts through one side of the cartilage, leaving the opposite mucoperichondrium intact, thus causing bending of the cartilage with healing.

Complications
- *Hematoma:* can interfere in cartilage revascularization, especially if infected. A saddle deformity can result. Hematomas can result from failure to obliterate dead space. Pain awareness (usually pain is minimal with septoplasty) is important. Drain through hemitransfixion incision, pack intranasally bilaterally, and start antibiotics.
- *Infection:* drain and start antibiotics.
- *Hemorrhage:* rare problem, usually from mucosal tears.
- *Nasal obstruction:* usually caused by scar formation (intranasal synechiae) or turbinate hypertrophy.
- *Septal perforation:* usually only a problem if mucosal tears are bilateral and opposing. In this case, a piece of cartilage can be placed between the membranes and sutured together, or membranes without cartilage can be reapproximated. Can also result from infection, excessive packing, hematoma formation, or tight approximation sutures.
- *Palatal and dental anesthesia* (usually transient).
- *Anosmia.*
- *Cosmetic nasal deformity* (excessive removal of cartilage during septoplasty).
- *CSF leak* has been reported.

RHINOPLASTY

Nasal-Facial Analysis
- Horizontal lines divide face into thirds:
  - Trichion to glabella.

- Glabella to nasal base.
- Nasal base to menton:
  - Lower third subdivided into thirds:
    - Upper lip (1/3).
    - Lower lip and chin (2/3).
- Vertical lines divide face into fifths:
  - Nasal base = intercanthal distance = width of each eye.
- Nose should project from face as a 3-4-5 right triangle.
- Nasofrontal angle begins at level of supratarsal crease.
- Chin and lower lip should project equally.
- Any preexisting asymmetries should be discussed preoperatively:
  - Nasal skin:
    - Thick skin does not drape well to show subtle changes.
    - Thin skin may drape too well, can show minor deformities.
    - Dorsum: thicker at nasofrontal angle, thinner at rhinion.
    - Tip: thick at bulbosity, can be thin over lower cartilages.
  - Frontal view:
    - Can evaluate symmetry.
    - Must assess curved unbroken line from medial brow to ipsilateral tip-defining point.
    - Line from midglabella to menton should bisect nasal bridge and tip.
    - Can also assess width:
      - Width of bony sidewall should be 75%-80% of width of base.
    - Two tip-defining points represent underlying dome of lower lateral cartilages; look for:
      - Asymmetry.
      - Bulbosity.
      - Excessive distance between tip-defining points.
    - Columella should hang just below alar rims:
      - Look for excess columellar or nostril show.
  - Profile view
    - Nasofrontal angle connects brow with dorsum:
      - Formed by two lines from nasion parallel to glabella and to nasal tip, typically 115-130 degrees.
    - Nasion: deepest point of nasofrontal angle.
    - Tip projection: 3-4-5 right triangle with nasion-to-tip as hypotenuse:
      - 50%-60% of tip projection from alar-facial crease should be anterior to upper lip, otherwise over- or under-projected.
    - Dorsum: should lie 1-2 mm posterior to nasion-tip line.
    - Nasolabial angle:
      - Men: 90-95 degrees.
      - Women: 95-115 degrees.

- Columella: 2-4 mm below alar margin is normal:
  - >4 mm; may be retracted alar lobule or hanging caudal septum.
  - Double break.
  - Tip of nose turns posterior, inferiorly onto infratip lobule.
  - Midcolumella, takes more horizontal course.
- Base view:
  - Isosceles triangle in thirds:
    - Lobule is anterior or top third.
    - Columella is posterior or bottom two thirds.
  - Nostrils are pear or teardrop shaped.
- Oblique view
  - Confirms previously mentions descriptors.
  - Highlights aesthetic lines and irregularities.
- Intranasal examination:
  - Adequacy of airway.
  - Position of septum.
  - Nasal valve competence.
  - Condition of mucosa and inferior turbinates.
  - Presence of septal cartilage in revision rhinoplasty must be identified.
- Nasal-chin relationship:
  - Inadequate chin projection makes nose look overprojected.
  - Line dropped from nasion perpendicular to Frankford plane should approximate chin projection or line from vermillion of lower lip.
  - Mental augmentation can be considered.
- Nasal-brow-forehead relationship:
  - Three fundamental forehead contours:
    - Protruding: diminishes appearance of nasal length.
    - Flat: can diminish appearance of nasal length.
    - Sloping: exaggerates appearance of nasal length.
- Photography:
  - High-quality photos with standard views
    - Frontal.
    - Lateral × 2.
    - Oblique × 2.
    - Basal.
  - Helps with teaching, communication, and medicolegal documentation.
- Landmarks
  - Trichion: midline, anterior hairline.
  - Glabella: most prominent point of forehead (seen best on lateral view).
  - Nasion: most posterior point of the forehead (nasofrontal suture line).
  - Radix: root of the nose.
  - Rhinion: soft tissue point above osseocartilaginous junction on nasal dorsum.
  - Sellion: osseocartilaginous junction on nasal dorsum.

- Supratip: point cephalic to the tip.
- Tip: most anterior point of nose (dome of the lower lateral cartilages).
- Subnasale: junction of columella and tip.
- Vermillion border: mucocutaneous border of upper and lower lips.
- Stomion: embrasure of the lips.
- Menton: lower border of the soft tissue contour of the chin.
- Columellar point: anterior-most soft tissue point of the nasal columella.
- Alar crease: the most posterior aspect of the nose.
- Mentolabial sulcus: depression between the lower lip and chin.
- Pogonion: anterior most projection of the chin.
- Gnathion: junction of tangential lines from the menton and pogonion.
- Tragion: point of the supratragal notch of the ear.
- Cervical point: point of intersection between line tangent to neck and line tangent to submental region.

Philosophy and Principles of Rhinoplasty

Indications
- Cosmetic modification of nasal anatomy.
- Reconstruction for nasal obstruction.
- Reconstruction subsequent to a traumatic deformity.

Contraindications
- Uncorrected bleeding disorder.
- Patient should have reasonable and specific goals and expectations.

Anesthesia
- General or local with sedation.
- Comfort without compromising oxygenation.
- 1% lidocaine with 1:100,000 epinephrine.
- Use smallest possible amount to prevent distortion of tissues.

Shaping the nasal tip
- No single technique to address:
  - Skin thickness.
  - Strength and shape of alar cartilages.
  - Domal angle anatomy.
  - Dorsal contour.
  - Length and width of nose.
  - Tip-lip angulation.
  - Tip projection and rotation.
  - Patient expectations.
- Conservative reduction of cephalic margin of lower lateral cartilage:

- Leave at least 5-7 mm.
- More aggressive techniques for more extensive deformity:
  - Interruption of lateral crural strip.
  - Resection of excess cartilage.
  - Suture reconstitution of divided edges.
- Major tip support mechanisms:
  - Size, shape, and resilience of medial and lateral crura.
  - Attachment of medial crural footplates to caudal margin of quadrangular cartilage.
  - Attachment of lower laterals to upper laterals.
- Minor tip support mechanisms:
  - Interdomal ligament.
  - Dorsal cartilaginous septum.
  - Membranous septum.
  - Sesamoid complex.
  - Skin and subcutaneous fibrofatty tissues.
  - Nasal spine.
- Procedures to repair tip deformity:
  - Prior to changing tip, must determine need for:
    - Change in projection.
    - Reduction in volume of alar cartilages.
    - Cephalic rotation with increase in columellar inclination.
    - Change in shape or orientation of alar cartilages.
  - If limited refinement is needed, can do conservative resection of cephalic margin of lateral crus.
- Surgical approaches to the tip:
  - Nondelivery approaches: less dissection and manipulation:
    - Transcartilaginous: simplest.
    - Retrograde: effective for limited tip work.
  - Delivery approaches: for more severe deformities:
    - Widely arched and bulbous alar cartilages with flared nostrils.
    - Interrupted-strip technique for more radical tip narrowing.
  - External rhinoplasty approach: best visualization, does not divide any support mechanisms:
    - Bilateral marginal incisions connected by transcolumellar incision.
    - Disadvantages:
      - Larger region of dissection with possible scar formation.
      - Prolonged tip edema.
      - Increased operating time.
    - Indications: tip is:
      - Asymmetric.
      - Markedly bulbous.
      - Severely over projected.
      - Anatomically complex (revision noses).
    - Relative indications:
      - Thick skin.

- ○ Poor tip support.
- ○ Large perforations.
- Can include:
  - ○ Columellar strut.
  - ○ Dome-binding sutures.
  - ○ Tip graft.
  - ○ Alar cartilage shaping techniques.
- ❑ Four major categories:
  - Volume reduction with residual complete strip.
  - Volume reduction with transdomal suturing.
  - Volume reduction with interrupted and resutured strip.
  - Tip refinement without volume reduction.
- ❑ Preservation of strip preferred.
- ❑ Tip projection:
  - May need to divide major tip support mechanisms.
  - Must reorient alar cartilages or add struts or grafts.
  - Avoid decreasing dorsal height.
  - Examples of techniques to enhance projection:
    - ○ Transdomal suturing.
    - ○ Lateral crural steal.
    - ○ Tip grafting.
    - ○ Columellar strut.
- ❑ Tip rotation
  - Some techniques can result in increased projection.
  - Tripod:
    - ○ Medial crura together as one leg.
    - ○ Lateral crura as other two legs.
    - ○ Can angulate infratip lobule or blunt nasolabial angle.
    - ○ Can place tip grafts.
    - ○ Generally results from planned modification of alar cartilages, can also:
      - ▼ Shorten caudal septum.
      - ▼ Shorten septum with high transfixion incision.
      - ▼ Set back medial crura on caudal septum.
      - ▼ Interrupting and overlapping residual complete strip.
    - ○ Excessive volume reduction to be avoided; causes tissue void along cephalic margin, possible valve collapse.
    - ○ Resection just lateral to domes can be considered with resuturing of cut ends to reconstitute intact strip.
    - ○ Lateral interruption of lower laterals with lateral crural overlay gives rotation with less domal deformity.
    - ○ Can do "set-back" fixation of medial crura to caudal septum.
    - ○ Can use shield-shaped tip graft.

- ❑ Profile alignment:
  - Sellion: deepest point of nasofrontal angle.
  - Dorsal line extends from sellion to tip-defining point.
  - Access dorsum through trans- or inter-cartilaginous incision or open approach.
  - Rubin osteotome to remove bony dorsum.
  - Can correct with rasps.
  - Can camouflage dorsal contour irregularities with AlloDerm.
- ❑ Narrowing bony pyramid:
  - After dorsal hump removal.
  - Medial oblique osteotomies angled laterally at 15-20 degrees.
  - Low lateral curved osteotomy started at piriform aperture at or above inferior turbinate, drive toward base of maxilla.
- ❑ Postoperative considerations:
  - Remove nasal packing as early as possible.
  - Remove columellar sutures at postoperative day 5-7.
  - Remove cast at postoperative day 5-7.
  - Can take 1 year to see final result.

Open Rhinoplasty

Scar analysis
- Columellar scar is almost negligible.
  - ❑ 1% subjective, 2% objective dissatisfied rate.
  - ❑ Skin closed with 5-0 nylon or fast-absorbing gut.
  - ❑ Closure tension decreased by extending vertical marginal incision inferiorly.

Surgical technique
- Incision and exposure
  - ❑ Transverse columellar incision with no. 11 blade.
  - ❑ Joined with vertical marginal incision above medial crura:
    - Prevents postoperative transverse columellar notching.
    - Cutting underlying crus to be avoided.
    - Elevated superolaterally over dome and lower lateral crus.
    - Dorsal skin elevated as in closed technique in subperichondrial and subperiosteal plane.
- Septoplasty:
  - ❑ Done first for functional correction and harvest of cartilage.
  - ❑ Anterior septal angle exposed down to premaxilla.
  - ❑ Helpful for columellar strut.
    - Upper lateral cartilages separated from septum. "Ouvert au ciel"—open to sky exposure—better exposure than any closed technique.
  - ❑ Must correct as needed:
    - Posterior spurs and deflections.

- Dorsal septal curvatures.
- Caudal strut deflection.
- Severe septal deformities.
- Septal perforation.
  - Related problems:
    - Synechiae: place allograft spacer.
    - Vestibular stenosis: more common after closed approach:
      - Remove bone with rongeur.
      - Postauricular skin graft.
- Nasal base
  - Done before dorsum to produce desired projection and rotation.
  - High dorsum can cause tension tip deformity, must be corrected first.
  - Medial crura.
  - Soft tissue between medial crura removed:
    - Slight columellar narrowing.
    - Wide access to premaxilla.
    - Shortened to decrease projection.
    - Incised and bunched to decrease inferior flare.
    - Scored to correct excessive crural curves.
  - Lower lateral crura:
    - Open technique allows much better exposure.
    - Can excise more symmetric amounts of cartilage.
    - Excessive excision does not further refine lobule but does weaken lateral crus.
    - A minimum of 6-8 mm of lower laterals retained.
      - More true with thick skin, needs support.
    - Accurate dissection of hinge area (junction of lower lateral and sesamoid cartilage) can give tip rotation and deprojection.
  - Lobule refinement: narrowing of lobule
    - Vertical crural division:
      - Cartilage is incised, overlapped, sutured.
      - Further scoring and 6-0 nylons maintain symmetry.
      - Double dome unit sutures draw domal units medially, narrow lobule.
    - On-lay grafts:
      - Autologous cartilage preferred.
      - Can use synthetic material (Mersilene, e-PTFE, Gore-Tex).
      - Increase projection.
      - Improve definition.
      - Camouflage asymmetries.
      - Lengthen nose.
      - Give counter-rotation.
      - Can be secured with 6-0 nylons.
  - Columella refinement
    - Premaxillary augmentation or reduction.
    - Required after iatrogenic shortening.
    - Lay graft in premaxillary pocket.

- Labial sulcus avoided.
- Gore-Tex preferred.
  - Punch holes for in-growth of tissue.
- Relative contraindications:
  - Short upper lip.
  - Dentures: should be drilled down in midline first.
  - Struts
    - Placed between medial crura, gives support.
    - Can also augment nasolabial angle or increase columellar show.
    - Placed just above premaxillary spine.
    - Secured with sutures through strut, both medial crura, and membranous septum.
    - Should not extend beyond nasal spine.
    - Help maintain tip support when cartilages are divided.
  - Battens:
    - Nonsupporting on-lay graft.
    - Can increase columellar show.
    - Can camouflage columellar asymmetries.
  - Hanging columella:
    - Caused by excessive dissection compromises blood flow to columella.
- Dorsum
  - Open approach can make anatomy more confusing.
  - Nasofrontal angle can be deepened with osteotome.
    - Can increase effect with otologic burr.
    - Can lower dorsum with diamond rasps.
    - Medial osteotomies done under direct visualization.
    - Lower lateral osteotomies performed through separate pyriform margin incisions.
    - Dorsal irregularities:
      - Trimmed under direct vision if small.
      - Sutured to close open roof deformities.
    - Spreader grafts:
      - Can open nasal valve.
      - Can widen over-resected dorsum.
      - Secured with two sutures through upper laterals and septum.
        - Sutures should not be placed over dorsum
    - Dorsal augmentation:
      - Small defect:
        - Deproject tip.
        - Dorsum elevated with transfixion sutures.
      - Larger defect:
        - Gore-Tex.
        - Puncture holes for in-growth.
    - Pollybeak:
      - 70% only require soft tissue or cartilage excision.

- ○ 30% require grafting procedures.
- ○ Tip ptosis from weakened support from medial crura with thrusting force of lower laterals.
- ○ Slow contraction of scar in supratip region allows scar to form in supratip dead space.
- ○ Can result from over-resected bone.
- ○ Cartilaginous
  - ▼ Lower cartilaginous supratip
  - ▼ Place medial crural columellar strut
- ○ Soft tissue
  - ▼ Excise supratip scar and subcutaneous tissue.
  - ▼ Score undersurface of supratip skin.
  - ▼ Transfixion suture to close deadspace.
  - ▼ Kenalog after 3 weeks repeated at 3-week intervals.
- ■ Soft tissue refinement
  - ❑ Skin management:
    - • Take care to avoid damage to dermal-subdermal vascular plexus.
    - • Can excise skin from supratip region if thick skinned.
    - • Thin skin: requires attention to fine detail of sculpting of bone and cartilage.
  - ❑ Alar advancement:
    - • Back cut along alar facial groove allows ala to be advanced as a flap.
    - • Decreases nostril size and narrows base.
  - ❑ Alar hooding
    - • Curvilinear ptosis of middle and posterior alar margin.
    - • Correct with wedge excision in caudal margin of alar rim.
  - ❑ Displaced alar cartilage:
    - • Reopen marginal incision.
    - • Make pocket for caudal margin.
    - • Z-plasty closure rotates cheek skin into sill.
- ■ Postoperative care
  - ❑ Removal of packing on postoperative day 1.
  - ❑ Columellar and alar sutures removed postoperative day 4.
  - ❑ Transverse columellar-marginal sutures and septal splints removed postoperative day 7.

Management of bony nasal vault
- ■ Basic surgical techniques
  - ❑ Hump reduction:
    - • Soft tissue envelope elevated from bony-cartilaginous framework to nasofrontal angle.
    - • Osteotome or rasp to lower dorsum.
  - ❑ Osteotomies:
    - • Aesthetic objectives:
      - ○ Close an open nasal vault.
      - ○ Straighten deviated nasal dorsum.

- ○ Narrow nasal sidewalls.
- • Should be limited to thinner aspect of nasal side wall.
- • Lateral osteotomy:
  - ○ Close an open dorsum.
  - ○ Linear (single-cut):
    - ▼ Bony cut along nasal facial groove.
    - ▼ High-low-high pathway.
    - ▼ Begins at level of attachment of inferior turbinate.
    - ▼ Small pyramid of bone at pyriform aperture left intact for suspensory ligaments.
    - ▼ Curves superior and anterior into thinner part of nasal bone at level of orbit.
    - ▼ Terminated at level of medial canthus.
    - ▼ Can use small cutaneous puncture midway between medial canthus and nasal dorsum to perform back-fracture.
  - ○ Perforating:
    - ▼ Series of transcutaneous punctures along desired fracture site.
    - ▼ Can push nasal bones out.
    - ▼ Allows maintenance of support structure in revision cases.
- • Medial osteotomy:
  - ○ Used when needed to mobilize nasal side walls.
  - ○ Angulated fashion between nasal bone and septum.
  - ○ Carried superiorly to back-fracture site.
- • Intermediate osteotomy:
  - ○ Purposes:
    - ▼ Narrow extremely wide nose with good height.
    - ▼ Correct deviated nose with one long side wall.
    - ▼ Straighten markedly convex nasal bone.
  - ○ Made parallel to lateral osteotomy.
  - ○ Via intercartilaginous incision if closed procedure.
  - ○ Must be performed before lateral osteotomy.
  - ○ Postoperative management:
    - ▼ Swelling, ecchymosis, periorbital edema are normal.
    - ▼ Elevate head of bed × 24 hours.
    - ▼ Remove splints at 1 week.
- ■ Management of middle vault
  - ❑ Internal nasal valve made up of:
    - • Caudal margin of upper lateral cartilage.
    - • Septum.
    - • Floor.
    - • Anterior head of inferior turbinate.
  - ❑ Hump reduction most common maneuver:
    - • Anatomy:

- ○ Nasal bones: small contribution to the normal hump.
- ○ Cartilaginous vault:
  - ▾ Majority of osseocartilaginous hump and dorsal hump.
  - ▾ Consists of paired triangular upper lateral cartilages and nasal septum.
- ○ Upper lateral cartilage (ULC):
  - ▾ Overlaps nasal bones up to 11 mm at cephalic part.
- ○ Male: straight/slightly convex from nasion to nasal tip.
- ○ Female: straight/slightly concave from nasion to tip.
- ○ Degree of hump removal assessed prior to septoplasty.
- ○ Tip work performed after dorsal hump removal.
- • Cartilaginous hump excised as a block with mucosa.
- • Separates upper laterals from natural connection to septum.
- • Leads to inferomedial collapse of upper laterals.
- • Problems can develop over years.
- ▢ Risk factors
  - • Inverted-V deformity:
    - ○ Posterior displacement of nasal bones and upper laterals after osteotomies with over-resection or posterior displacement of upper laterals.
  - • Short nasal bones.
  - • Long and weak upper laterals.
  - • Thin skin.
  - • Tall, narrow noses.
  - • Previous trauma or surgery.
- ▢ Prevention of middle vault problems:
  - • Preservation of middle vault mucosa.
  - • Conservative resection.
  - • Maintain soft tissue attachments between nasal bones and upper laterals.
  - • Internal splinting in early postoperative period.
- ▢ Correction of middle vault pathology:
  - • Spreader grafts:
    - ○ Rectangular cartilage grafts between upper laterals and septum.
    - ○ Lateralize upper laterals and add rigidity to nasal valve.
    - ○ Can be placed through closed or open approach.
    - ○ Best if mucoperichondrium is preserved and graft is placed in a pocket.
    - ○ Should run along dorsal septum.
    - ○ Can be layered to add bulk.
  - • Flaring sutures:
    - ○ 5-0 Nylon spans upper laterals and nasal dorsum.

- ○ Tightening suture increases valve angle.
- • Dorsal graft:
  - ○ May help with saddle nose.

Surgery of the nasal tip
- ▢ Intranasal approach:
  - • Considerations:
    - ○ Volume reduction.
    - ○ Reconstruction.
    - ○ Rotation.
    - ○ Change of projection.
  - • Nondelivery approach:
    - ○ Good for:
      - ▾ Small volume reduction of lateral crus.
      - ▾ Slight cephalic rotation of tip.
    - ○ Transcartilaginous incision.
    - ○ Best to mark resection boundaries externally for direction.
    - ○ Local injection used for hydraulic dissection.
    - ○ Currently, intercartilaginous incision with retrograde dissection, eversion of lateral crus, and resection of cephalic portion more popular.
  - • Delivery approach:
    - ○ Bipedicle chondrocutaneous flap:
      - ▾ Indications:
        - ▽ Asymmetry.
        - ▽ Bifidity.
        - ▽ Extracephalic tip rotation.
        - ▽ Alteration of tip projection.
      - ▾ Deliver cartilage with intercartilaginous incision caudal to valve around to anterior septal angle.
      - ▾ Marginal incision: stay on caudal edge of lower lateral.
      - ▾ Free cartilage from soft tissue.
      - ▾ Deliver with periosteal elevator.
    - ○ Lateral crus delivery
      - ▾ Marginal incision.
      - ▾ Free soft tissue from both sides of lateral crus with fine scissors.
      - ▾ Deliver.
  - • Pitfalls
    - ○ Nondelivery approach:
      - ▾ Asymmetric resection.
      - ▾ Over-resection.
      - ▾ Wrong incision line leading to incomplete strip.
    - ○ Delivery approach (bipedicle chondrocutaneous flap):
      - ▾ Incomplete delivery.
      - ▾ Asymmetric delivery.
      - ▾ Asymmetric resection.
      - ▾ Asymmetric inter- and transdomal suturing.
      - ▾ Overscoring and overmorselization.

▾ Compromise of tip support.
- ○ Delivery approach (lateral crus delivery):
  - ▾ Tearing of lateral crus.
  - ▾ Wrong indication.
  - ▾ Overrotation.
  - ▾ Vertical dome division (VDD).
- ❑ Rationale:
  - • Change projection.
  - • Narrow and rotate lobule.
- ❑ Goldman technique
  - • Preferred for:
    - ○ Ptotic or aging nose.
    - ○ Vertically displaced alar complex requires direct redirection.
  - • Create chondrocutaneous strut by division of alar cartilage.
  - • Deliver cartilages through marginal incisions.
  - • Must not "borrow" more than 3 mm from lateral crus:
    - ○ Avoids unnatural tent-pole appearance.
  - • Chondrocutaneous strut sutured together.
  - • Sharp edges trimmed.
  - • No suture between medial and lateral crura.
  - • Double-break accentuated.
  - • Plumping grafts used if necessary.
- ❑ Simons modification
  - • Preferred for:
    - ○ Lobule needing more subtle changes.
    - ○ Increased medial strength.
    - ○ Medial movement of lobular domes.
    - ○ Widened lobule = domal highlights >4 mm apart.
  - • Both domes delivered.
  - • Soft tissue between domes cleared out.
  - • Alar cartilages vertically incised but vestibular skin is left intact.
  - • Medial crura sutured back together:
    - ○ No deeper than inner perichondrium
  - • Medial edge should "lead" lateral edge.
- ❑ Hockey stick modification
  - • Preferred for:
    - ○ Boxy tip.
    - ○ Overprojected tip.
  - • Initial cuts medial to domal apex.
  - • Segmental sections of dome and cephalic margin resected:
    - ○ Resection shaped like a hockey stick.
  - • Can resect dorsal and caudal septum if necessary.
- ❑ Adjunctive techniques:
  - • On-lay graft of crushed septal cartilage.
  - • Columellar batten graft.

Secondary rhinoplasty
- ❑ General principles:
  - • Thorough inspection, evaluation, palpation of remaining tissue.

- • Presence of scar, contracture, lining loss, synechiae assessed.
- • Outcome less predictable because of preexisting scar, loss of blood supply.
- • Needed for previous under- or over-operation
- ❑ Guidelines:
  - • Ensure that improvement is possible.
  - • Make accurate diagnosis.
  - • Give patient realistic expectations.
  - • Time carefully; usually wait at least 1 year.
    - ○ Exceptions:
      - ▾ Inadequate, "Greenstick" osteotomies.
      - ▾ Alar base reduction.
      - ▾ Correct alar retraction.
  - • Diagnose and correct functional problems.
  - • Plan for the unexpected at time of surgery.
  - • Limit surgical dissection.
  - • Use only autologous tissue.
  - • Maximize concepts of "illusion":
    - ○ Use on-lay and supportive grafts.
  - • Avoid revision in irreparable deformities.
- ■ Complications
  - ❑ Nasal tip:
    - • Ptotic tip:
      - ○ Change in nasolabial angle.
      - ○ Loss of tip support.
    - • Overrotated tip:
      - ○ Overresection of caudal septum.
    - • Bossae: knuckling of lower lateral cartilage at tip:
      - ○ Contracting healing forces act on weakened supports.
      - ○ Increased risk with thin skin, strong cartilage.
      - ○ Seen with cartilage splitting techniques.
      - ○ Treated through small marginal incision with minimal undermining.
    - • Alar retraction
      - ○ Etiology:
        - ▾ Congenital (rare).
        - ▾ Post rhinoplasty (most common).
        - ▾ Over resection of lower lateral cartilage.
        - ▾ Resection of vestibular skin.
        - ▾ Overly long columella..
        - ▾ Traumatic/scar retraction.
      - ○ Shortened columella.
      - ○ Treated with cartilage grafts (auricular composite grafts).
    - • Alar-columellar disproportions
      - ○ Excess show:
        - ▾ Full thickness tissue resected from membranous columella.
      - ○ Retracted columella:
        - ▾ Plumping graft, columellar strut.
    - • Pollybeak
      - ○ Supratip scar excision for high cartilaginous septum or exuberant scar tissue.

- ○ Graft shielded from septal cartilage to add projection to nose.
- ○ Lateral alar graft may add support.
- ○ Dorsal cartilaginous graft can raise dorsal profile.
- ○ Abnormal tip-supratip relationship.
- ○ Excessive bone or insufficient cartilage resection.
- ○ Kenalog injection considered if due to excessive scarring.
  - • Columellar incision
- ❑ Nasal vault
  - • Saddle nose
    - ○ Loss of support of vault with subsequent collapse.
    - ○ Causes:
      - ▾ Congenital.
      - ▾ Insufficient dorsal strut.
      - ▾ Dislocation of dorsal strut at bony-cartilaginous junction.
      - ▾ Over-resection of dorsal hump.
      - ▾ Excessive resection of septum.
      - ▾ Septal hematoma.
      - ▾ Septal abscess.
      - ▾ Severe nasal trauma.
    - ○ On-lay graft to repair
    - ○ Autologous tissues have least resorption and extrusion
      - ▾ Fascia.
      - ▾ Septal/auricular cartilage.
      - ▾ Iliac or skull bone.
    - ○ Other biologic grafts tend to have high rates of absorption.
    - ○ Synthetic materials have lifelong risk of infection/extrusion.
    - ○ Dorsal onlay grafts
      - ▾ Mild to moderate cases, no loss of nasal airway.
      - ▾ Need to have adequate tip support.
    - ○ Septal strut/replacement
      - ▾ Severe saddle deformities, with nasal obstruction or loss of tip support.
      - ▾ Almost always requires secondary donor site:
        - ▽ Often cranial bone.
      - ▾ Graft formed into L-shaped strut.
      - ▾ Placed via open rhinoplasty approach and fixed to remaining dorsal bone and to nasal spine.
  - • Inverted-V deformity
    - ○ Caudal edge of nasal bones visible in relief.
    - ○ Inadequate support by upper laterals.
    - ○ Inadequate in-fracture of nasal bones.
  - • Nasal valve collapse:
    - ○ Rhinoplasty most common cause.
    - ○ Excessive narrowness or flaccidity at nasal valve.
    - ○ Normal angle 10-15 degrees in Caucasian nose.
    - ○ More obtuse angle in African-American and Asian nose.
    - ○ Cross sectional area 55-83 square mm.
    - ○ Primary incompetence: occurs secondary to intrinsic problem in strength or relationship between skeletal framework of the valve or its coverings.
    - ○ Cartilaginous deformity:
      - ▾ High septal deviation.
      - ▾ Weakening and/or deformity of ULC.
    - ○ Mucocutaneous abnormality that thickens covering of cartilages and thus decreases angle.
    - ○ Overresection of lateral crura.
    - ○ Loss of middle vault support.
    - ○ Correct with spreader grafts, batten grafts.
  - • Deviated nose
    - ○ Greenstick fractures.
    - ○ Inadequate osteotomies.
- ❑ Upper third
  - • Rocker deformity:
    - ○ Osteotomies taken too high.
    - ○ Rocks laterally.
  - • Dorsal irregularities:
    - ○ Open roof.
    - ○ Insufficient removal of resected tissue.
  - • Open-roof deformity:
    - ○ Inadequate lateral osteotomies after dorsal hump removal.
  - • Greenstick fracture:
    - ○ Memory of bone returns it to preoperative location.
- ❑ Skin-soft tissue envelope
  - • Compromise to vascular supply.

OTOPLASTY

Embryology

- Auricular development is first seen in the 5-week embryo and stems from six mesenchymal proliferations of the first and second pharyngeal arches, surrounding the first pharyngeal cleft.
- Six hillocks correspond directly with the following structures:
1. Tragus
2. Helix
3. Cymbum
4. Scapha
5. Antihelix
6. Antitragus
- Initially, the external ear arises from the lower neck and ascends to level of eyes as the mandible develops.

Anatomy

- Important topographic landmarks of external ear in the evaluation for otoplasty:
  - Helix.
  - Superior crus.
  - Inferior crus.
  - Scapha.
  - Antihelix.
  - Conchal bowl → cymba concha + cavum concha.
- Muscles of ear:
  - Intrinsic muscles: major and minor helixes, tragus, antitragus, transverse, oblique.
  - External muscles: anterior auricularis, superior auricularis, posterior auricularis.
- Vasculature:
  - Arterial supply: superficial temporal, posterior auricular, occipital.
  - Venous supply: posterior auricular, external jugular, superficial temporal, retromandibular.
  - Lymphatics: anterior to parotid lymph nodes, posterior to cervical lymph nodes.
- Nerves
  - Motor: CN VII.
  - Sensory: lesser occipital, greater auricular, auriculo-temporal, Arnold's (from CN X).

Proportions and aesthetic considerations

- "Line of balance": slope of ear should approximate the slope of the nasal dorsum (approximately 20 degrees from the vertical).
- Ear width is approximately 60% of its height.
- Average ear height and width in adult male is 63.5 and 35.5 mm, respectively.
- Average ear height and width in adult female is 59.0 and 32.5 mm, respectively.
- Superior aspect of ear is usually level with brow.
- Normal ear has angle of 20-30 degrees between the auricle and head.
- In a normal ear, the helical rim extends <20 mm from the mastoid.
- Conchal protrusion is typically 12-15 mm from head.
- Distance from lateral edge of helix to mastoid skin is approximately 20-25 mm.
- Incidence of congenital ear deformities and malformations is approximately 5%.

Preoperative evaluation

- Photographic evaluation should encompass the following views:
  - Frontal full-face view.
  - Oblique.
  - Lateral.
  - Rear.
- Evaluation of auricle:
  - Size.
  - Relationship to scalp.
  - Interrelationship among components (helix, antihelix, concha, lobule).
- Most common deformities appreciated preoperatively:
  - Lack of antihelical fold.
  - Overdeveloped concha.
- Thickness of cartilage in both ears should be evaluated.
- Analysis of preoperative symmetry between two ears is crucial.
- Darwinian tubercles and other preauricular skin tags should be noted.

Timing of surgical correction

- Ideal age of child for surgery is between 5-6 years of age:
  - Prior to grammar school age (avoidance of peer ridicule).
  - By age 6 years old, auricle is 90% of average adult size.
  - Child is old enough to participate in the postoperative care (i.e. not disturbing the wound).

Surgical techniques

Mustarde technique

- Most common technique for repair of most common indication (lack of antihelical fold).
- Postauricular skin incision.
- Markings may be made with ink-dipped fine needles.
- Several horizontal mattress sutures are placed (using permanent suture [e.g., Ti-Cron]) along the scapha to create the antihelical sulcus.
- Sutures are placed through the cartilage and anterior perichondrium but not through the anterior skin.
- It does not address protruding conchal bowl.
- Problems may arise when sutures are not placed in properly.

Converse technique

- Somewhat more complicated than Mustarde sutures, requiring more experienced surgeon.
- An "island" of cartilage is created that is placed anteriorly to the rest of the remaining cartilage.
- Allows for more permanent and gentle curve to correct antihelical deformities.

Farrior technique

- It creates an island of cartilage, similar to Converse technique.
- One incision through cartilage is made on the conchal rim only.
- However, multiple longitudinal wedges are removed at the level of the superior crus and future antihelical fold ("cartilage sculpting" technique).
- It is technically more challenging, requiring an experienced surgeon.

Pitanguy technique

- Uses smaller island flap and conchal setback suture.
- Ideal for patients with limited amount of antihelical cartilage.
- Technically more challenging, requiring an experienced surgeon.

Furnas technique

- Used for reduction of conchal bowl.
- As with Mustarde technique, it is a suture procedure.
- When used in conjunction with conchal-reducing procedure, permanent retraction of auricle can be achieved.
- Excessively anterior placement of the suture to mastoid may cause forward buckling of the bowl at the external canal os, leading to possible stenosis at external auditory canal.

Postoperative Care

- Regardless of otoplasty technique, a conforming dressing is used postoperatively.
  - Cotton soaked in mineral oil placed into creases of conchal bowl and antihelical folds, as well as behind the ear.
  - Fluff dressing with Kerlex wrap.
  - Oral antibiotic.
  - Small drain (e.g., rubber band) is recommended.
  - Dressing removed from postoperative day 1 to 5, depending on surgeon.
  - Headband should be worn around the clock for at least 1 week postoperatively.
  - Thereafter, patient is instructed to wear a headband at night for 2 months.

Complications

- Early complications:
  - Hematoma:
    - Incidence 1% in postoperative otoplasty.
    - Symptoms include unilateral postoperative pain within first 48 hours.
    - May lead to perichondritis/loss of cartilage from pressure of hematoma.
    - Treatment involves immediate evacuation of clot, debridement of necrotic tissue.
  - Infection:
    - Manifests postoperative day 3 or 4.
    - Treatment involves implementation of systemic antibiotics, including coverage for *Pseudomonas aeruginosa*.
- Late complications
  - Suture extrusion
    - May occur at anytime following Mustarde technique.
    - Results from incorrect suture placement, excessive tension, wound infection.

- Treatment involves removing offending suture and potentially performing revision surgery.
  - Aesthetic complications:
    - Involves abnormalities in relationship of auricle to scalp or distortion of auricle itself.
    - Asymmetries between left and right ear.
    - Classic deformities:
      - "Telephone ear" deformity:
        - ▼ Caused by overcorrection of the middle third of a prominent ear.
        - ▼ Overcorrection can result from excessive removal of postauricular skin or mastoid soft tissue, or from excessive tightening of conchamastoid sutures.
      - "Reverse telephone ear" deformity:
        - ▼ Results when the midauricle protrudes after overcorrection of the superior pole and lobule.
        - ▼ May result when concha is not adequately set back during surgery.
    - Unsightly postauricular scars:
      - Hypertrophic scars.
      - Keloids.
      - Bowstringing of suture: seen in suture otoplasty, excessive tension of postauricular incision results in draping of skin over sutures.

SURGICAL MANAGEMENT OF ALOPECIA

General Considerations

- Two general techniques: free graft (hair plugs) and local rotation/advancement of hair-bearing skin (scalp reduction). Local rotation/advancement used to cover temporal-parietal areas, punch grafts used to recreate a normal frontal hairline.
- Normal frontal hairline triangular, with lateral corners placed on line vertical to lateral canthus of eye. If the hairline has receded lateral to the lateral canthus, scalp reduction will be required.
- Do not transplant or use for flap areas of scalp that are at risk for further hair loss, because this may expose unsightly scars.

Procedures

Punch Grafts

- Donor site should have at least eight hairs per 4-mm diameter circle; light hair/light skin and dark hair/dark skin combinations give best results:
  - Powered instruments used to harvest adjacent 4-mm grafts in one or two rows, closed primarily. Careful attention is required to avoid transecting hair follicles and ensure consistent size/quality.

- Recipient holes are made slightly smaller, spaced evenly apart by the width of a recipient hole. Subsequent sessions will be required to fill in the interspaces with more grafts.
- Second transplant session delayed by 6 weeks, then 3-4 months before subsequent procedures. Hair requires several months to grow in new location.
- Minigrafts (four hairs) and micrografts (one hair) are used to refine the anterior areas of new hairline by creating more natural transition.

Scalp reduction
- Primary reduction
  - Multiple incisions have been described, including midline sagittal ellipse (leaving a midline scar), a Y ellipse (to advance occipital skin forward), and various crescents (intended to leave scar hidden at edge of advanced hair).
  - Incision through galea, subgaleal flaps raised, skin excised, wound closed primarily.
  - Indications can be extended through the use of tissue expanders to stretch hair-bearing skin and allow more aggressive advancement of flaps.
- Extensive reductions (bitemporal [BT] flap, bilateral occipitoparietal [BOP] flap)
  - Requires multiple-staged procedures but allows excision of up to 9 cm of bald scalp.
  - Flaps are based on superficial temporal arteries (STAs). Ligation of occipital vessels is required 6 weeks prior to flap elevation so that entire flap develops collaterals from STA, decreasing complications.
  - BOP flap consists of incision along occipitoparietal skin line, carried down to the superior portion of ear. The hair-bearing skin is extensively undermined down to and onto the trapezius muscles, then advanced and sutured, leaving a horseshoe area of scalp at the vertex of the skull. This remaining bald area is closed 2-3 months later with the BT flap, which is similar except for the removal of a wedge of occipital hair to prevent a dog-ear and to recreate a natural appearing cowlick.
  - The BOP/BT flaps do not provide any hair coverage for the anterior scalp; punch grafts are still required to restore this area.
- Juri Flap
  - Pedicled transposition flap for anterior scalp coverage. With bilateral flaps, 12 cm of anterior scalp coverage is possible.

- Based on STA. Has a 4-cm–wide flap with STA at center of base, angles superiorly into temporal flap, then postero-inferior across occiput. Also requires multiple stages.
- Posterior portion of flap is incised though galea. After 1 week the flap is elevated, then laid back down into its original location. One week after that, the flap is elevated and transposed to its new, frontal location, and the donor/recipient defects are closed. Finally, 6 weeks later, the dog-ear is revised.

Contraindications
Patients who are young and have the potential for significant further hair loss must be approached very carefully. Often the best course is to delay surgical reconstruction of alopecia until hair loss is complete. Cosmetically unacceptable outcomes occur when the natural process of hair loss exposes surgical scars that were designed to be in the hairline.

Other than progressive hair loss, few specific contraindications exist. Obviously, the patient must be able to undergo anesthesia, must have an acceptable scalp blood supply, must have no chronic wound healing problems, and must be psychologically suitable and realistic about the potential outcomes.

Complications
- Flaps: Flap necrosis, skin loss, or healing problems are rare but real possibilities. Patients who have had punch grafting in the past tend to have poorer scalp blood supply, and therefore a higher risk of serious complications. Hypertrophic scars are also difficult problems but can often be managed by performing micro hair grafts directly into the scar, offering excellent camouflage. As mentioned previously, further hair loss can cause previously hidden scars to become exposed, a difficult problem with no good solutions.
- Punch grafting complications include transient forehead edema, hypertrophic scars around graft sites, "cobblestoning" (grafts raised around surrounding scalp), and rarely, necrosis of donor site or grafts. Infections occur in less than 1% of cases. In general, serious complications occur much less often in punch grafting than in the aforementioned flap procedures.

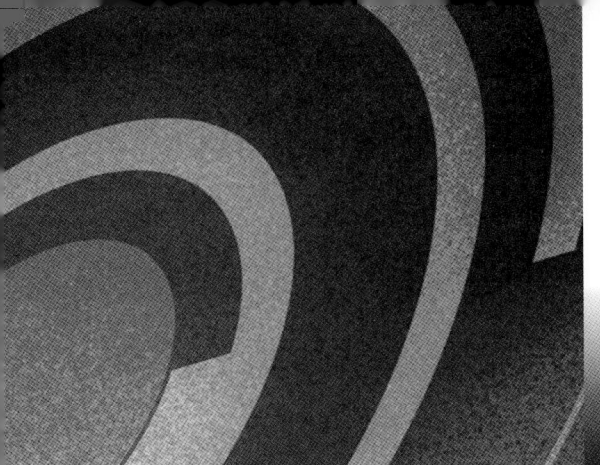

Index